AN
AMBULANCE
ON
SAFARI

MCGILL-QUEEN'S/ASSOCIATED MEDICAL SERVICES STUDIES
IN THE HISTORY OF MEDICINE, HEALTH, AND SOCIETY

Series editors: J.T.H. Connor and Erika Dyck

This series presents books in the history of medicine, health studies, and social policy, exploring interactions between the institutions, ideas, and practices of medicine and those of society as a whole. To begin to understand these complex relationships and their history is a vital step to ensuring the protection of a fundamental human right: the right to health. Volumes in this series have received financial support to assist publication from Associated Medical Services, Inc. (AMS), a Canadian charitable organization with an impressive history as a catalyst for change in Canadian healthcare. For eighty years, AMS has had a profound impact through its support of the history of medicine and the education of healthcare professionals, and by making strategic investments to address critical issues in our healthcare system. AMS has funded eight chairs in the history of medicine across Canada, is a primary sponsor of many of the country's history of medicine and nursing organizations, and offers fellowships and grants through the AMS History of Medicine and Healthcare Program (www.amshealthcare.ca).

AN AMBULANCE ON SAFARI

*The ANC and the Making
of a Health Department in Exile*

Melissa Diane Armstrong

McGill-Queen's University Press
Montreal & Kingston · London · Chicago

ISBN 978-0-2280-0329-8 (cloth)
ISBN 978-0-2280-0330-4 (paper)
ISBN 978-0-2280-0423-3 (ePDF)
ISBN 978-0-2280-0424-0 (ePUB)

Legal deposit third quarter 2020
Bibliothèque nationale du Québec

Printed in Canada on acid-free paper that is 100% ancient forest free (100% post-consumer recycled), processed chlorine free

This book has been published with the help of a grant from the Canadian Federation for the Humanities and Social Sciences, through the Awards to Scholarly Publications Program, using funds provided by the Social Sciences and Humanities Research Council of Canada.

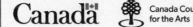

Funded by the Government of Canada   Financé par le gouvernement du Canada

Canada Council for the Arts   Conseil des arts du Canada

We acknowledge the support of the Canada Council for the Arts.
Nous remercions le Conseil des arts du Canada de son soutien.

Library and Archives Canada Cataloguing in Publication

Title: An ambulance on safari : the ANC and the making of a health department in exile / Melissa Diane Armstrong.
Names: Armstrong, Melissa Diane, 1990- author.
Series: McGill-Queen's/Associated Medical Services studies in the history of medicine, health, and society ; 53.
Description: Series statement: McGill-Queen's/Associated Medical Services studies in the history of medicine, health, and society ; 53 | Includes bibliographical references and index.
Identifiers: Canadiana (print) 20200268597 | Canadiana (ebook) 20200268856 | ISBN 9780228003298 (cloth) | ISBN 9780228003304 (paper) | ISBN 9780228004233 (ePDF) | ISBN 9780228004240 (ePUB)
Subjects: LCSH: African National Congress. Health Department—History—20th century. | LCSH: Medical care—South Africa—History—20th century.
Classification: LCC RA552.S6 A76 2020 | DDC 362.10968—dc23

Contents

Figures

Acknowledgments

The medical sector developed by the ANC in exile has been the subject of my academic attention for the past seven years. I stumbled onto the topic at the start of my master's degree in Oxford in 2012, was warned that there may not be enough material to support an entire thesis but encouraged, particularly by Colin Bundy, to pursue the project. While I expected to struggle to find relevant primary sources, I was fortunately proved entirely wrong in this expectation; with a little bit of digging, I found that the ANC's medical endeavours were well documented. Indeed, from that initial research sojourn to Alice, South Africa in 2013, it was evident that this project could not possibly be contained in a short master's thesis. Following its completion, I applied to continue the work as a PhD student under the guidance of Susanne Klausen at Carleton University in Ottawa. Subsequently, I sought to convert the dissertation into a book, adding important new sections that I had been unable to include in the dissertation. Over the seven-year process of research, writing, and revision, I was met with generosity, graciousness, and support from close friends and complete strangers; both were essential to the success of this project.

At the beginning of this research, Colin Bundy lent both his extensive expertise in the area to provide me with direction and equally his considerable patience to editing initial drafts of muddy prose. Additionally, Hugh Macmillan – whose work on the subject is both well known and inspiring – met with me on a number of occasions to discuss some of his research and connect me with others who were publishing on the subject of the ANC in exile. Both men were instrumental in getting this project off the ground.

The Department of History at Carleton University in Ottawa was also important to the continued work on this project. I was met with consistent support and encouragement from members of staff and fellow students. In particular, Will Tait went out of his way to help me navigate what being a PhD student was all about. He and his partner Jennifer Gosselin left me an open invite to their house (and their dinner table) and continue to offer me a place to stay while in Ottawa. At Carleton, I enjoyed the freedom to pursue the project without limitation and was given financial support by the University to do so. Additionally, I gratefully acknowledge the Vanier Canada Graduate Scholarship for its financial support. This scholarship gave me the opportunity to complete multiple research trips to South Africa and ample time to search the archive in a thorough manner.

The staff at the ANC archive at the University of Fort Hare were exceptional. When I first arrived, I was immediately made to feel comfortable and at home in the archive. I am especially thankful for the assistance of archivists Ike Maamoe and Vuyo Feni-Fete. Not only were they able to offer their assistance to find needed files, they were also considerate enough to text me with updates about the level of safety on campus during the university student strikes in 2015. In order to make up some of the time lost, Ike was willing to stay late so that I could continue working as needed after the archive closed.

Once, I was told that there are no great writers; instead, there are people tenacious enough to revise, revise, and then revise again. Fortunately, I have not had to undergo that revision process alone. Particularly, special thanks goes to my Auntie Sharon Westberg for the hours she spent meticulously marking this book with her sharp red pen. Each and every sentence added after her final comments suffers grammatically. Perhaps one day, I will learn the definition of a "dangling gerund" and be able to place commas appropriately on my own. In addition, the staff at MQUP have been exceptionally helpful. In particular, Kyla Madden provided points of consideration while converting the dissertation into a book and has made important comments and suggestions about how to improve the final draft. Kathleen Fraser and Elli Stylianou outlined the formatting guidelines for publication in a step-by-step fashion in order to make the process as painless as possible. Finally, Shelagh Plunkett edited the final draft; it was very reassuring to have a fresh pair of eyes comb the manuscript prior to final submission.

Outside of the university and formal channels of academic support, this book benefited from more individuals than could possibly be listed here. Among the most essential of these individuals are those that I encountered in South Africa. I am still blown away by the warmth, generosity, and hospitality of the families that I had the pleasure of meeting. When I arrived in Johannesburg in 2013 as a master's student, I was without a clear research plan and knew no one that could help me navigate living in South Africa. Tristan Gevers, a previously unknown friend of a friend, agreed to pick me up from the airport and guide me towards a hostel in the city. Tristan brought me back to his family home where I met his parents Ron and Rozanne and sisters Stephanie, Melissa, and Caitlyn. Rather than a hostel, I found myself the possessor of a key to their front door. Since then, the Gevers have become like family to me; they have included me in their family outings, painstakingly explained the finer points of cricket and rugby to me, taken me to the doctor, helped me to buy, register, and license a car, and most importantly been open, honest, and completely without pretence. They have welcomed my friends and family with equal gusto and love. Without the reassurance of their love and hospitality, I may not have had the nerve to continue the project.

I was greeted with a second outpouring of kindness in the Eastern Cape. After contacting a local church in 2013 and asking if someone in the congregation had the gift of hospitality, I was pointed, without hesitation, straight up the hill in Grahamstown to the Robertson's house. There I was greeted by Sue and Ian Robertson and their daughters Laura and Emily. I stayed with the Robertson's for many months between May 2013 and February 2017 while commuting from Grahamstown to Alice to visit the archive. Every day, I returned to their home to enjoy a hot meal, warm fire, and great conversation. Once again, I was welcomed in as family and have been treated as such ever since. I have learned so much from Sue and Ian and appreciate them more than they will ever know. Without their love and support, the months of archival research in the Eastern Cape would have been unbearably lonely.

When I applied to work with Susanne Klausen in 2013, I already knew that I would be under the supervision of an excellent scholar. What I did not know was that I would also gain a friend who continues to stay invested in this work as well as in my life away from South African history. We were hiking Table Mountain in Cape

Town, when I told her I would be shifting my future life plans from historian to a career in medicine. I am grateful that her response was characteristically gracious and encouraging; she continued to support my work as well as provide me with time off to apply for medical school. As I have attempted to juggle the formidable challenge of medical school while also writing this book, Susanne has shown continued enthusiastic interest, read and reread drafts, offered suggestions, and made this process feel do-able. Discussing South African history with Susanne over the past two years has reminded me of how much I miss being immersed in history and that I truly do still love this project. There are no words to express how grateful I am for her influence both on this work and in my life.

I have been given the most unbelievably kind, loving, and encouraging community of friends and family. In particular, Sherryl Friesen has been there over the past three years to sit with me while I struggled to balance work with wellness. We set up internet hot spots at the lake so that I could work on the book and not miss out on sitting around summer campfires, and she changed her schedule so that she would be available to road trip with me when I needed a break.

I am also so grateful for my three sisters Krista Friesen, Kerri Korol, and Andrea Gonzalez along with their families for unflinching support and unconditional love. While I was still in the initial writing phase, Krista travelled to South Africa with me so that she could better understand and appreciate what I was working on. In times of stress and anxiety, Kerri has alleviated some of the pressure with laughter, elaborate cakes, and thoughtful cards. Andrea constantly makes me feel loved with her daily messages, invitations to hang out, and reminders about the things that truly matter. I don't know what I would do without each of them in my life.

My parents Chuck and Holly Armstrong have been my invaluable coaches, teammates, and cheerleaders throughout all of my academic and nonacademic exploits. Dad, where would I be without the hours you poured in to encouraging my efforts, challenging my thought process, and providing my ideas with new perspective? Your enthusiasm in life is contagious and conviction to your beliefs is inspiring. I am grateful that you have walked beside me in all of this. Mom, thank you for patiently listening to hours of South African history; as a verbal processor, I have needed you. I am grateful for your encouragement to persevere; there are days that it is hard to have the motivation to focus and work, and you have always helped me to be productive. I hope that you fully know that your constant behind-the-scenes acts of service have made all the difference. Mom and Dad, without you both, this book would not exist; it is, therefore, to the two of you that I dedicate this work.

Abbreviations

AAM	anti-apartheid movement
ANC	African National Congress
CPSU	Communist Party of the Soviet Union
DKK	Danish krone
ECC	External Coordinating Committee
FPA	Family Planning Association (South Africa)
FRELIMO	Frente de Libertação de Moçambique (Mozambican Liberation Front)
HIV/AIDS	human immunodeficiency virus/acquired immune deficiency syndrome
ICARA	International Conference on Assistance to Refugees in Africa
ICASC	International Contraception, Abortion and Sterilisation Campaign
IDAF	International Defence and Aid Fund
IPPF	International Planned Parenthood Federation
MASA	Medical Association of South Africa
MCH	mother and child health
MHQ	military headquarters
MK	Umkhonto we Sizwe
MKA	Medisch Komitee Angola (Netherlands)
MPLA	Movimento Popular de Libertação de Angola (People's Movement for the Liberation of Angola)
NAT	National Department of Intelligence and Security
NAMDA	National Medical and Dental Association
NEC	National Executive Committee
NP	National Party
NPA	Norwegian People's Relief Association
OAU	Organisation of African Unity
PAC	Pan-Africanist Congress of Azania

PMC	Politico-Military Council
PTSD	post-traumatic stress disorder
RHT	regional health team
RENAMO	Resistência Nacional Moçambicana
SACP	South African Communist Party
SADET	South African Democracy Education Trust
SADF	South African Defense Force
SAMDC	South African Medical and Dental Council
SEK	Swedish krona
SIDA	Swedish International Development Cooperation Agency
SOMAFCO	Solomon Mahlungu Freedom College
SWAPO	South West Africa People's Organisation
TCDC	Technical Cooperation amongst the Developing Countries
TRC	Truth and Reconciliation Commission
TZS	Tanzanian shilling
UFH	University of Fort Hare
UN	United Nations
UNDP	United Nations Development Programme
UNESCO	United Nations Educational Scientific and Cultural Organization
UNHCR	United Nations High Commissioner for Refugees
UNICEF	United Nations International Children's Emergency Fund
US	United States
USD	United States dollar
USSR	Union of Soviet Socialist Republics
UTH	University Teaching Hospital (Lusaka)
WHO	World Health Organization
ZMK	Zambian kwacha

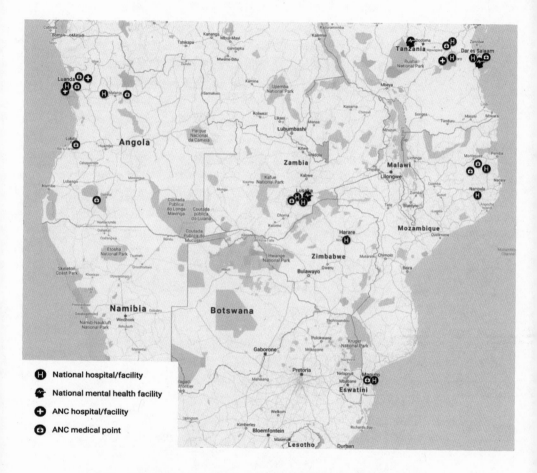

Legend:

- (H) National hospital/facility
- National mental health facility
- (+) ANC hospital/facility
- ANC medical point

0.1 Map of medical points in southern Africa. The differentiation between hospital and medical point was often blurry and changed over time. The locations marked on this map are not conclusive and are, in some cases, geographic estimates. This map is included to provide a visual approximation of where the ANC and MK were able to receive healthcare in the 1980s.

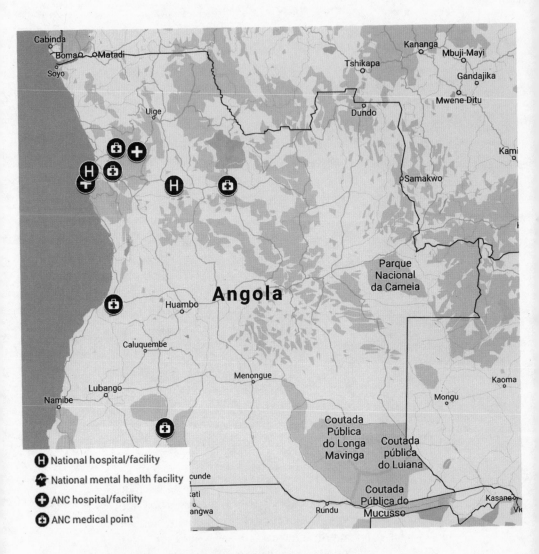

0.2 Map of medical points in Angola

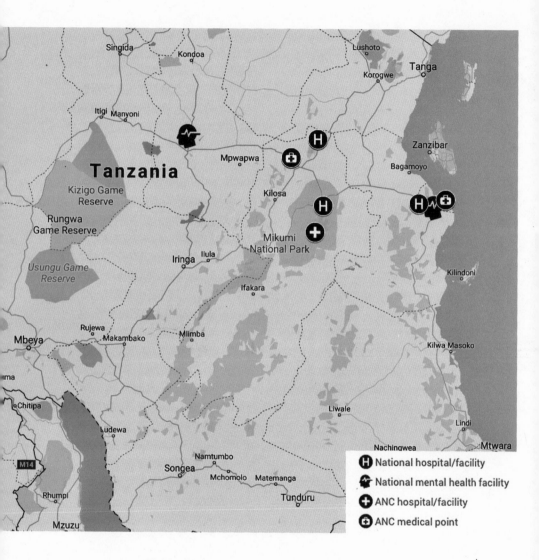

0.3 Map of medical points in Tanzania

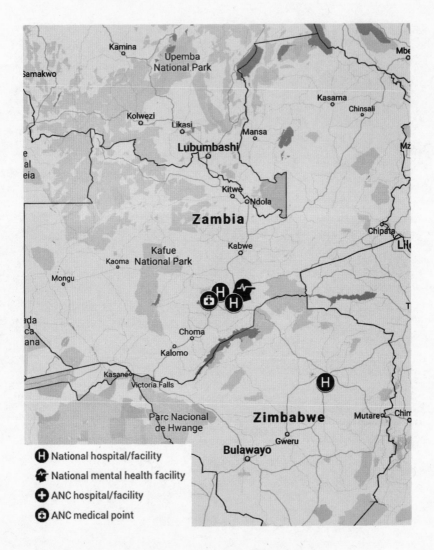

0.4 Map of medical points in Zambia and Zimbabwe

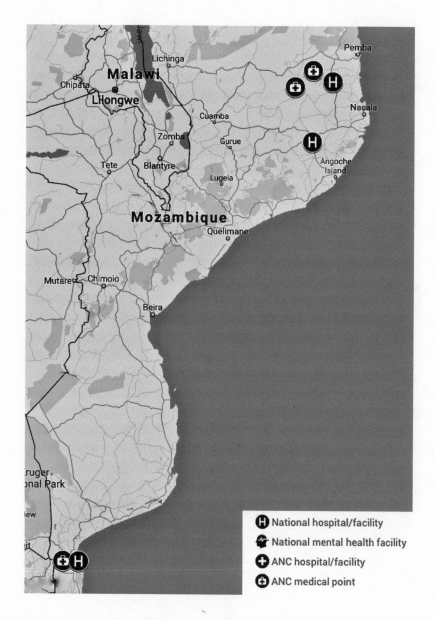

0.5 Map of medical points in Mozambique

AN
AMBULANCE
ON
SAFARI

Introduction

The provision of healthcare in South Africa has long been the subject of national and international criticism, both during and after the apartheid era (1948–94).[1] In 2009, *The Lancet* published an article that pointed to a number of systemic deficiencies in the South African public health sector, including the lack and under qualification of medical personnel, poor managerial capability, the absence of monitoring and evaluation of policies and programs, and the absence of stewardship.[2] In 2010, the World Health Organization (WHO) shone a spotlight on the uneven quality and access to healthcare by pointing out that 80 per cent of the population was without private medical insurance and therefore condemned to the over-burdened and under-equipped public service. The public sector receives less than half of South Africa's total health expenditure and is dependent on less than a third of the country's doctors and specialists.[3] All of these shortcomings have contributed to continued massive health inequalities in the post-apartheid era.

Historians have shown that South Africa's history of colonial rule in the era of segregation (1910–48) and, subsequently, apartheid are centrally to blame for some of the systemic inequalities within the healthcare system. In order to justify such slow progress towards better health for all, the authors in *The Lancet* point to the economic policies that damaged African health in the preapartheid era, and the continued exploitation of labour and entrenchment of a race-based two-tiered health system that grossly favoured whites in subsequent decades. In essence, today's ruling African National Congress (ANC) government inherited a relatively well-developed healthcare system that was steeped in institutionalised racism.[4] While the ANC government should be held accountable for subsequent poor policy decisions and pushed to provide better care for South African citizens in the future, the historical culture of inequality has plagued the national Department of Health ever since the onset of liberal democracy in 1994.[5]

Undoubtedly, one of the legacies of colonialism generally and apartheid in particular was to *entrench* race-based health inequality in South Africa. The apartheid era created the conditions for poor health and provided poor healthcare for black South Africans. However, little research has been done on the history of health and healthcare provision for the South Africans who were exiled by the National Party (NP) in 1960 and more specifically on the medical sector developed by the ANC for exiles in civilian settlements and military camps based in newly independent, sympathetic nation-states in southern Africa, with the notable exception of Carla Tsampiras's work on the history of the ANC in exile and their confrontation with HIV/AIDS in the late 1980s.[6] Exiled South Africans were affected by the legacy of colonialism, exposed to the repression of apartheid, and subject to the first efforts of the ANC's medical sector and (eventual) Health Department[7] while they were in exile. Indeed, many health professionals who filled leadership positions in the post-apartheid Department of Health were trained in exile and had been part of the medical sector in the liberation struggle during some portion of the thirty-year period that the ANC was in exile.

The medical sector developed by the ANC in exile played an important role in the liberation struggle and cannot, therefore, be ignored. On the international stage, it fuelled anti-apartheid support and helped to legitimize the ANC politically. As a medical entity, it dealt with sick and injured South Africans on a daily basis and its capacity to deliver medical services had life and death consequences for patients. For these reasons, the exiled medical sector warrants closer examination.

The ANC's Move to Exile

Four years following the 1948 election of the NP in South Africa, the ANC officially began the Defiance Campaign, a series of coordinated nonviolent strikes and protests. Throughout the mid-1950s, the ANC, initially supporting an Africanist nationalist movement, began adopting a policy of greater nonracialism and joined efforts with anti-apartheid groups such as the South African Communist Party (SACP) and the Natal Indian Congress. The policy towards nonracialism was radical at a time when pro-Africanist groups across the continent were gaining independence in the ideological spirit of a more assertive and African-centred form of emancipatory politics – later to grow into the black power and black consciousness movements. Consequently, the ANC's policy created a rift between some of its members; those against nonracialism formed the Pan-Africanist Congress (PAC) in 1958. Both of these groups fought against apartheid in exile after 1960; they often operated as jealous neighbours in exile and vied for international and South African support.

Spurred by the growing continental unrest under colonial regimes, many ANC members were impatient for a turn to military action and some members of the movement travelled abroad looking for international support for armed struggle against apartheid. Meanwhile, in 1960 the PAC arranged a massive antipass strike in Sharpeville. The police opened fire on the protesters, killing sixty-nine people. The event escalated the struggle between the NP and African political movements to new heights, and 1960 saw both the ANC and the PAC banned from South Africa. Despite ANC leader Albert Luthuli's staunch opposition to a policy of violence, in 1961 it was agreed that Umkhonto we Sizwe (MK) would be founded, as a separate wing and independent of the ANC.[8] However, by 1962 the pretence of this separation collapsed when international advocates of the ANC neglected to make a distinction between its political and armed wings.

From 1960 to 1963 elite members of MK and the SACP began military training in China, Algeria, Morocco, and Egypt.[9] In 1961 the

ANC planned its first official attack; on 16 December MK members exploded bombs near South African government buildings with the intent to cause damage without killing civilians. Between 1961 and 1964 MK engaged in 200 acts of sabotage primarily by bombing government infrastructure. The ANC's momentum was abruptly halted when in 1963 a number of ANC leaders including Nelson Mandela, Walter Sisulu, Ahmed Kathrada, Govan Mbeki, Arthur Goldreich, Denis Goldberg, and Lionel Bernstein were caught and arrested while devising new MK tactics. These men were sentenced to prison on Robben Island leaving MK crippled and lacking leadership.

Even without its key leaders, Tanzania offered the ANC space to establish its first official headquarters.[10] From their camp at Kongwa (discussed in chapter 1) they drew on their communist allies including China, the Union of Soviet Socialist Republics (USSR), Algeria, and Egypt to help equip and train their small contingent of approximately 400 to 500 military cadres. They remained headquartered in Tanzania[11] through most of the 1960s, shifting slowly to new headquarters in Lusaka, Zambia by 1969, which remained the home of the ANC's political base until the end of its tenure in exile. Over the years the number of South Africans in exile increased dramatically. While there are no absolute figures, there were at least 2,000 cadres in the mid-1980s scattered across camps in Angola and Mozambique and several thousand civilian refugees throughout southern Africa. In response to the growing health needs of the exiles, in the 1970s the ANC formed a health department to coordinate medical efforts. They gained funding from their communist allies but also from United Nations (UN) affiliated departments like the WHO and countries that considered themselves unaligned in the Cold War.

When the ANC was banned and banished from South Africa, formed its liberation army MK, and began to launch its undercover war with the NP in the early 1960s, its goal was to quickly liberate South Africa from its colonial oppressors, end apartheid, and reenter a free democratic society. The ANC gained confidence from the dozens of newly independent African nations, and the "wind of change"[12] should have blown in favour of the ANC's efforts to overthrow South Africa's racist white government. However, unlike in the former colonies to the north, the ANC continued to struggle for South African independence until the 1990s, not coincidently coinciding with the end of the Cold War. Over the course of its thirty-year tenure in exile, the ANC's economic, social, military, geographical, and political positions shifted, and its survival strategy in exile was forced to adapt accordingly. The hoped-for quick military engagement, backed by strong international anticolonial pressure, did not in fact occur, and the ANC found itself increasingly responsible for the long-term health and well being of MK cadres, ANC members, and the steady stream of South African refugees fleeing South Africa. While the organisation was still attempting to train and deploy cadres to fight against the apartheid government – indeed this was the leadership's main emphasis – it became progressively more dependent on humanitarian instead of strictly military aid. Instead of subverting the NP government through military tactics alone, it became preoccupied with its position as a "government-in-waiting."[13]

Corresponding to this gradual shift from primarily capital "P" political agendas to small "p" political efforts, the delivery of healthcare grew over time from a case-by-case, reactionary, military-focused form of care to a fully fledged Health Department complete with administration, infrastructure, and an international training and support scheme. At its height, in the 1980s the department had offices around the world and medical teams treating patients in Tanzania, Angola, Mozambique, Zambia, and Zimbabwe. It also partnered with local facilities across southern Africa under a banner reading Technical Cooperation amongst the Developing Countries (TCDC) in order to deliver better medical care to South Africans in exile. The ANC became responsible for the health and wellbeing of thousands of cadres and refugees, and for a new generation of South Africans born in exile and raised in ANC settlements.

The Internal and International Thrust of the ANC's Department of Health

Despite the low status awarded to the medical sector by the ANC's political and military administrations from the start, the medical sector in exile had a significant effect on the liberation struggle, both diplomatically as well as in the everyday lives of South African people in exile. At times, the ANC's medical sector operated to the organisation's political advantage. Not only did the ANC's medical staff make an effort to publicize the illegitimacy of the apartheid health system, it also promoted its Health Department as the rightful representative of healthcare in the future post-apartheid South Africa. The ANC bolstered its claim to be a government-in-waiting by creating a bureaucratic health department and sending delegates to international health-related conferences to establish an autonomous political identity at international events.

While its success off the continent, particularly in Europe and North America, was considerable, its actions in southern Africa were also significant. On a practical level, the healthcare provided by the ANC was critical to the lives of South Africa exiles – civilians and cadres alike. The ANC sought to provide primary healthcare to South Africans and use their allies' medical facilities to supply secondary care.[14] However, the department's inexperience and lack of clear lines of authority between its own members and members of other departments prevented the medical sector from consistently providing primary care. Further, staff negligence and poor intraregional communication within the Health Department made it difficult to effectively coordinate their patients' secondary care. As a result, the department's efforts left much to be desired. The medical sector's fluctuating capacity to treat patients and the systemic departmental problems had an immediate effect on patients and their experience of exile.

In this book, I elected to examine two important themes that were overwhelmingly dominant in the archive: the bureaucratic structure of the Health Department and patient care. First I explain how and why the Health Department in exile was formed, examine the particular shape that the department took on the ground both in southern Africa and off the African continent, and explore the relationship between the department and its international allies. This first concern makes up the bulk of the first three chapters but is also featured in chapters 4 and 5. Second, after establishing the Health Department's structure and function, I seek to demonstrate the very personal nature of health and illness in exile and examine the effect that the Health Department had on patients and staff. There were a large number of ways that I might have approached this theme, but I chose to provide a detailed discussion of the interpersonal relationships between staff members – specifically ANC staff experience within the Tanzania regional health team – and show how specific patients had the potential to be directly affected by ANC leadership and department staff decisions. I also explore the politics of reproductive health and its impact on women in exile. Finally, I dedicate an entire chapter to mental health in exile. This illness-specific case study is well placed to bring the arguments of each chapter together; it demonstrates the structure of the department in action in southern Africa and further abroad as well as the impact that the department had on the treatment of individual patients.

The first chapter provides an overview of medical provision in exile. Beginning with an examination of the 1960s and early 1970s, it argues that despite the lack of a central health administration, the ANC found ways to provide medical support for its cadres using its own medical supplies or the national infrastructure of its benevolent hosts. Furthermore, it found international support for motivated students to enrol in medicine in a number of different countries worldwide. Already the medical sector was becoming a necessary and international point of contact between the ANC and its allies. The chapter then discusses the political developments in the mid to late 1970s that enabled the ANC to develop a formal health department. While struggling to assert its authority in all ANC – and MK – occupied areas, an official health administration helped to facilitate acceptance of international donations and provided yet another means of proving its status as a government-in-waiting.

Chapter 2 demonstrates that the ANC Health Department was reliant on its southern African hosts and their ministries dealing with health matters. While the Health Department did offer its own people access to primary healthcare, it did not do so consistently. Consequently, the ANC needed its hosts to provide secondary *and* some level of primary care to South Africans. As the chapter highlights, ANC had a generally positive relationship with its hosts, attempted to collaborate on health initiatives with their hosts' health departments, and, when possible, provided primary care to thousands of local southern African patients. The effects of the bilateral relationship extended beyond patient care. Host countries provided ANC doctors and nurses with opportunities to complete their medical and nursing training and take up employment in their facilities. This was advantageous to host countries because it helped to address some of their national staff shortages, and it was essential for the ANC; without employment in southern Africa, the Health Department would not have been able to keep its doctors in the region.

This chapter then traces the history of the ANC's battle with malaria to underscore the complexity of these relationships in southern Africa. Each country had unique expectations of the ANC's healthcare priorities and delivery system, and the ANC struggled to consistently meet these varied expectations; the situation resulted in significant tension and provides another angle from which to consider the international linkages between health sectors in southern Africa. Furthermore, the malaria story also provides a bridge to the following chapter, which considers the ANC's off-continent international relationships. Taken as a whole, chapter 2 shows that the ANC developed unequal but important relationships with the national health departments of countries neighbouring South Africa. The ANC depended on these ties throughout their term in exile, but these relationships came at significant cost to the host nations.

Chapter 3 looks more closely at diplomacy between the ANC Health Department and international organizations. It demonstrates that one of the Health Department's central aims was to illuminate the gross inadequacy of the apartheid government's administration of healthcare to black people in South Africa. The ANC medical staff strategically piggybacked on the momentum of the growing international anti-apartheid movement and demand for justice in global healthcare – especially the WHO's 1977 campaign "Global Strategy for Health for All by the Year 2000" – to draw attention to medical injustice in South Africa. While emphasizing the NP's inadequacies, the ANC tried to appear as a coherent political entity and promote itself as a viable alternative representative of South African healthcare needs. It attempted to model its policies and initiatives in exile after those emphasized at global conferences in order gain approval and legitimacy from the international community as the future national Department of Health in a post-apartheid era. Despite the contradictions between their international rhetoric and the realities on the ground, this chapter argues that the Health Department was effective internationally and contributed to the strength of the anti-apartheid movement and eventual political victory of the ANC.

Chapter 4 demonstrates that the Health Department's capacity to deliver healthcare services to South Africans had an immediate, direct effect on the lives of individuals in exile. Because of the ANC's international success, the department was the recipient of considerable financial support from allied countries and sympathetic nongovernment organisations (NGOs) around the world. The funding provided the Health Department with an opportunity to practice statecraft, but its inexperience and lack of clear lines of authority between its own members and members of other departments crippled its capacity to provide consistent and quality healthcare. The chapter first examines the department's use of donor funding to establish two clinics in Tanzania where medical staff would be able to care for patients. It then assesses the staff's capacity to operate within these bureaucratic structures as a cohesive unit. Both infrastructure and staff ability left patients wanting. The case study of a South African patient, presented at the end of the chapter, demonstrates how the Health Department's deficiencies sometimes translated into serious negative outcomes.

The final chapter highlights many of the issues discussed previously by examining the ANC's treatment of mental illness in exile. It shows that the ANC was able to capitalize on the WHO's initiatives on mental health in southern African to better understand mental health and utilise the new regional plans and programs for their own patients' needs. It was also able to partner with the WHO to expose the psychological effects of apartheid. By illuminating apartheid's direct negative effect on South Africans, the ANC had yet another platform to further the global anti-apartheid movement. While the ANC gained success internationally, its treatment of mental illness among exiles was poor. Its efforts were not a significant departure from national treatment programs in the rest of sub-Saharan Africa, however, unlike the political circumstances in the nations around them, the ANC's internal security fuelled silence, secrecy, and paranoia and affected the way that patients could be treated. Negative psychosocial behaviours committed by South Africans in exile also damaged the relationship between supportive national governments and the ANC. The ANC's hosts, especially Tanzania, did not want the influence and effects of the ANC's violent activities near their major centres. For example, in Tanzania, the ANC was pushed out of the capital, Dar es Salaam, to occupy remote areas of the country.

Methodology

Most of the material deposited at the ANC archive is arranged by regional office; the archive catalogue calls these regional offices "missions," including the Lusaka Mission, Mozambique Mission, London Mission, and so on. Within these missions, documents are sorted by department or by file type (e.g., correspondence or newspaper clippings). In total, I copied more than 3,000 documents related to the ANC's medical sector in exile. These included health reports, circulars, memoranda, personal correspondence, financial reports, project proposals, patient reports, patient letters, speeches, and minutes of health meetings. I also drew from documents found in files from other sectors of the ANC, including the National Executive Council (NEC), the Politico–Military Council, the Women's Section, the Department of International Affairs, and the Department of Manpower and Development. Almost all of these documents are written in English, however English was often not the author's first spoken language. Consequently, many of the letters and reports have numerous grammatical errors and frequent spelling mistakes. In this book, I have used direct quotes from this primary source collection and transcribed the words as they were originally written but in order to avoid interrupting the flow of the statement, I do not include *sic erat scriptum* (*sic*) after every error.[15]

The heavy reliance on archival material in this book has weaknesses. Because the documents in the Fort Hare archive belong to the ANC, the party has the power to determine which documents are open for public research and which documents are to be categorized confidential. A glaring example of withholding important documents concerns the files relating to MK. From the ANC's submission to the Truth and Reconciliation Commission (TRC) (1996–98) and the testimonies of individuals who lived in exile, it is clear that the ANC has many secrets and it is likely that certain files have been deemed undesirable for public access.[16]

Another challenge presented by this archive is that documents held at Fort Hare pertain mainly to the 1980s and early 1990s. Relatively speaking, the 1960s and 1970s are not well represented in the archives. This is understandable because of the fact that the ANC established a more comprehensive bureaucratic structure in exile in later years, and therefore a greater number of reports and internal communications were generated at that time. Similarly, as will be discussed in chapter 1, the Health Department was developed in the late 1970s and so material on health and healthcare from the earlier period is relatively scarce.

While the outline archive was relatively straightforward, finding the relevant files was not. The ANC archive at Fort Hare was given the collection by the ANC in stages; the initial documents were given to the archive in the mid-1990s, and in the early 2000s another series of documents was added. As a result, the documents have been sorted and classified by at least nine people. At times folders were misplaced or else mistakenly placed in the wrong box. If an individual file was misplaced but found elsewhere, I have indicated both the catalogued and actual location.

In order to fill in some of the gaps in the ANC archive at Fort Hare, I was able to draw on existing interviews from oral history projects.[17] Specifically, the Hilda Bernstein collection at the Mayibuye Centre at the University of the Western Cape has been instrumental in creating a better understanding of what it meant to South Africans to be in exile. She conducted hundreds of interviews in the late 1980s and early 1990s. Among those interviewed were Dr Prenaiven Naicker and Dr Freddy Reddy; both doctors trained abroad and returned to work in southern Africa for the ANC in exile. Academics and researchers with the South African Democracy Education Trust (SADET), established as a result of Thabo Mbeki's assertion that there was not enough published history on the struggle for democracy in South Africa, also conducted a number of illuminating interviews for their five-volume series titled *The Road to Democracy*. Unfortunately, only the material concerning the 1960s and1970s was transcribed and published because the records of interviews in the later period were damaged before they could be transcribed. However, SADET drew on the interviews regarding the latter period in their five-volume collection and therefore provided secondhand access to these interviews.

Adding to these available oral testimonies and personal accounts, I conducted a handful of interviews with individuals who had either worked with or observed some element of the ANC's activities related to the health and well being of its members in exile. There were two periods of time in which I conducted interviews. During research for my master's degree in 2013, I was able to arrange two interviews while in Johannesburg. The first was with Sherry McLean, an Irish social worker who arrived in Mazimbu, Tanzania at the end of 1985 and continued her work with the Mazimbu and Dakawa (also in Tanzania) communities until 1987. After speaking with her, she put me in touch with Dr Ralph Mgijima, a doctor with the ANC in exile starting in 1977 who worked in Angola, Mozambique, Swaziland, Zambia, and Tanzania. He was a part of the Health Department's central administration and eventually held the leading role in the Health Department beginning in 1987. I am grateful to both Ms McLean and Dr Mgijima because they were able to give me some general insight into the nature of the medical sector and the social climate at Mazimbu and to better orient my subsequent use of the archives by providing me with key names and events. Neither interview was directly used in my master's research.

In March 2016 I was able to contact five additional people who agreed to be interviewed. During our discussions, I asked general questions about the background of the individual, their relationship to the ANC, what they knew about the Health Department, their level of interaction with the Health Department or related activities, and for any reflections on their experiences. I spoke for two hours with Dr Vuyo Mpumlwana, a South African clinical psychologist who was given a scholarship in exile to do her master's and PhD in psychology in Canada in the 1980s. Her PhD dissertation concerned the effects of torture on South African exiles, and she was able to visit the Mazimbu and Dakawa communities in the 1980s in order to conduct her research. I had a forty-five minute interview with Dr Pia Mothander, a Swedish clinical child/infant psychologist who was working in Swaziland with the Swedish Save the Children Fund in the late 1970s and early 1980s. I spoke with an American couple, Dr Felton Earls, a child psychiatrist, and his partner, Dr Mary Carlson, a neuroscientist. The two were anti-apartheid activists in the US and visited Mazimbu for three days in 1986. Finally, from March to November 2016, I corresponded by email with Dr Per Borga. Dr Borga is a psychiatrist who worked with the Swedish International Development Cooperation Agency (SIDA) in Tanzania from 1974 to 1978 and closely collaborated with Namibia's liberation movement, the South West Africa People's Organisation (SWAPO), and the ANC in the 1980s. While trying to ask open-ended and neutral questions, I recognize that these interviews were conducted within a period of critical reflection and have the potential to reflect that bias. I also run the risk of an opposite problem: I chose to interview people who were a part of the ANC or who were allied with the movement at that time. Therefore, there is the possibility that the interviewees remembered an overly romanticized version of events. In either case, the interviews are considered with these biases in mind. Given the backgrounds of these individuals, the interviews were mainly related to the topic of mental health and the use of international solidarity workers more generally. For the most part, these sources are used in chapter 5 to buttress archival material and to add personal opinions and reflections on the mental health status of South Africans in exile. However, it should be noted that my interviews were a small supplement rather than a central component of my research. Some of the interviews were not quoted in the book, though they helped to guide some of my analysis, and others are used sparingly.

The history of the ANC's medical sector in exile sheds new light on the importance of health to the international legitimacy of the ANC but also to the individuals whose lives were at risk in exile. Moreover, it begins to show that the Department of Health was also a product of apartheid in the sense that it emerged as a political response to the inequalities in South Africa and was forced to contend with exiles that had been damaged by the South African system. Attempts to understand the post-apartheid national Department of Health in South Africa must first contend with this history of health and healthcare in exile.

1

"Some Kind of Government-in-Exile": From Medical Sector to Department of Health, 1962–1990

The ANC's development of a formal health service and attempts at health provision for its comrades and South African refugees in exile had political and social significance.[1] Even at a distance, it is possible to see that medical supplies, provisions, and training had repercussions, albeit changing, for the ANC at a diplomatic level in southern Africa and further abroad. Furthermore, as an informal medical sector or a fully fledged health department, the capacity of the medical staff to provide for the needs of its patients had immediate life or death consequences for South African exiles. The bird's-eye view of the medical sector in exile, presented in this chapter, contextualizes the more specific actions and exploits of the department in the late 1970s and 1980s discussed in subsequent chapters.

The Medical Sector's Initial Services, 1962–1977

Medical provision played an early role in establishing favourable international relations between the ANC and Tanzania starting at least as early as 1962.[2] At the time, a number of white nurses who were discontented with the new independent Tanzanian government planned to leave their hospital posts, an action that would leave many hospitals and clinics sorely short-staffed.[3] The ANC leadership and the Tanzanian government cooperated to smuggle twenty South African nurses to Tanzania in order to replace those who would soon abscond.[4] This was undoubtedly an early statement of solidarity on the part of the Tanzanian government, but it was also not completely altruistic. The government gained a contingent of qualified medical staff to work in their health institutions. One of these twenty nurses, Kholeka Thunyiswa, recalled the risk of leaving for Tanzania: "The situation was tense because if there was a leak, we could have been sent to prison, like the others who ended up on Robben Island."[5] Thunyiswa spoke of her experience of going with other South African nurses to a central hospital in Tanzania in order to get acquainted with the medical system.[6] After a brief adjustment period, the women were split up and sent around the country to clinics especially in need of nurses. In Thunyiswa's case, she and one other South African nurse entered a clinic that was about to lose all eight of its qualified nurses. The two were expected to pick up the workload previously shared by eight. While many of the South African nurses later capitalized on opportunities even further abroad, some of the original twenty remained in Tanzania bolstering the local system and treating patients referred to them by the ANC.

The ANC may have provided the Tanzanian government with immediate assistance but it also had the foresight to capitalize on, and support, South Africans who were against apartheid and who had the ambition to pursue a medical education. Most notably Dr Manto Tshabalala – the longstanding second-in-command for the ANC's Department of Health in exile from 1977 to 1987 and the second post-apartheid minister of health – went into exile in 1960. She studied medicine in the USSR, graduated in 1969, and opted to further specialize in obstetrics and gynaecology at the University of Dar es Salaam in Tanzania, finishing in 1972.[7] Similarly, Dr Nomava Shangase, one of the nurses recruited for Tanzanian hospitals, went into exile in 1962. In 1963, she moved to Moscow with her husband and began a course in medicine two years later. She also graduated with a specialization in obstetrics and gynaecology and returned in the early 1970s to work at the Lusaka University Teaching Hospital (UTH) for one year.[8] She was transferred to Angola to work in MK camps on more than one occasion and was tragically killed in a car crash in Angola in October 1981.[9] She was the first medical casualty in the liberation struggle. Dr Peter Mfelang, the secretary of the ANC's Health Department, enrolled in medicine in the USSR in 1966 and graduated in 1972. He then did his internship at Muhimbili Medical Centre in Tanzania between 1973 and 1974.[10]

Several more medical personnel followed these three early USSR graduates.[11] Dr Prenaven Naicker – the head of the ANC's Mozambique Regional Health Team (RHT) starting in March 1983 – gave an interview detailing his educational trajectory in the 1970s.[12] The interview shed some light on the trials he and other medical students in exile faced:

[M]y father told me ... we don't have any money to put you into these universities. He's going to contact the ANC and see whether there are scholarships available and would you consider Socialist Countries and I did ... I then went to the Soviet Union [in] 1971 ... I did a year, I studied the language and the crash course that we were given, I must say, we had to burn the midnight oil everyday ... by six months we were able to talk freely [in Russian] and by ... in [sic] a year's time we were able to understand lectures ... The course was six years, so from 1972 to 78 I was at the First Moscow Medical State Institute.[13]

Striking a precarious balance between his Zambian and ANC medical responsibilities, Dr Naicker began work in Zambia in March 1981. By 1983 he was leading the Mozambique RHT. The common theme within the life trajectories of these doctors was that immediately after graduation, they were pulled back to serve and support the ANC community in exile and formed the core of the future Health Department.

The ANC was a central player in orchestrating these efforts to corral nurses and train doctors but there was a second, subtly different development that was later extremely relevant to the ANC. In the 1960s a number of people not yet affiliated with the ANC went into exile hoping to escape the apartheid system and get an education. In many cases, these exiles sought a *medical* education abroad. Most of these individuals had anti-apartheid sympathies but were not directly connected with the ANC. However, their departure from South Africa at this early juncture was crucial to the future successes of the Health Department in exile (and later in South Africa) and, therefore, merits discussion.

Dr Freddy Reddy was a psychiatrist who consulted for the ANC in exile in the 1980s. In the 1950s he was working as a porter at King Edward VIII Hospital in Durban where his pursuit of a wage increase made him supremely unpopular with management. He left South Africa in 1957 and proceeded on foot towards London.[14] When he reached London a year later and met anti-apartheid activists like Vella Pillay and Mac Maharaj, he joined them in their anti-apartheid activist work. Using his history as an anti-apartheid South African exile, Reddy pleaded his case to the Norwegian Student Association in the hope that he might be given an opportunity to further his education. He started medical school in Oslo in 1961 and contemplated moving to Zambia to practice in 1968. Instead, he decided to stay in Norway, build a family, and specialize in psychiatry. Dr Reddy was in contact with the ANC while working in Oslo, but it was only after 1979, when he finished specializing in psychiatry, that the ANC was able to draw on him for medical assistance.[15]

Alpheus Mangezi, the director of Mazimbu and Dakawa civilian ANC settlements in 1989, found a different way of getting an education in exile. In an interview with Hilda Bernstein, Mangezi reflected:

> I was very, very keen on education. My ambition had been to become a doctor or a lawyer but there was no money to get me to university. So I trained at the Jan Hofmeyer School of Social Work in Johannesburg and became a social worker ... I just wrote to the [British Association of Psychiatric Social Workers], and they said they would find me a placement in Glasgow if I could find money for the ticket. And so, family and friends went around, literally bowl in hand, until the fare was raised. And in May 1960 I went to Scotland to specialise in psychiatric social work.[16]

He worked as a social worker in Glasgow until 1962 when he received a scholarship to study psychiatric social work at the London School of Economics. Between 1964 and 1976, Mangezi worked in Zambia, studied in Nigeria (on a scholarship from SIDA), lived in Copenhagen, married, fathered three children, and completed his PhD. It was only in 1976 that he reported having any direct communication with the ANC; he accepted a research job at the University of Maputo and worked closely with anti-apartheid activist Ruth First at the Centre of African Studies. He worked from 1976 to 1987 at the university, all the while in contact with and playing a minor role in ANC activities. In 1988 Mangezi attended a seminar on social welfare in Lusaka and at the seminar, the ANC asked him to work for the ANC full time at Mazimbu. Undoubtedly, his training in social work was a welcome resource to the school and community. He remained in Mazimbu until the NP lifted the ban on the ANC in South Africa.[17]

The life stories of these medical personnel provide a sense of the character of the people who took leadership roles in the delivering of healthcare to South African exiles. These individuals went into exile, scraped a living through odd jobs, and attempted to complete competitive university degrees in a foreign language. As Dr Freddy Reddy reminisced on his own experience, "[there were] the pangs of pain that is involved in being in exile. To begin with the coping with new situations, coping with new conditions, coping with work conditions and inter-personal relationships ... and this continuous longing to go back to something."[18] These individuals were strongly motivated and tenacious and often somewhat traumatized by the reality of being exiled. The life trajectories of these medical staff members also demonstrate their international reach; these individuals invariably achieved a sphere of influence on their host campuses and within their cities and countries. They were generating anti-apartheid awareness among their fellow students and colleagues abroad and were creating an important international network of solidarity that could be drawn upon later. The future doctors on staff in the Health Department were well-trained and well-connected global citizens.

While these important international qualifications and relationships were being forged, the ANC was also faced with the immediate medical needs of between 400 and 500 MK cadres in Kongwa camp, Tanzania.[19] The military force was small but still large enough to

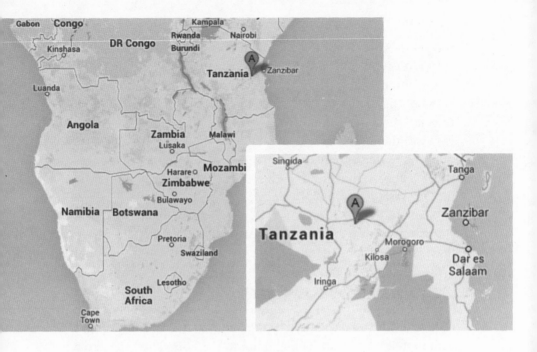

1.1 Geographical location of Kongwa camp

have medical requirements.[20] The short-term needs of MK cadres at that time did not warrant the necessity for highly qualified specialist staff; instead, the provisions were humble, geared at basic first-aid treatment for nonacute illnesses and injuries.[21] The goal of healthcare in Kongwa was to maintain military effectiveness. Evident by the medical bills paid by the ANC to host facilities, cadres frequently used the urban resources of host countries, but, to its credit, the ANC managed to establish a medical presence at Kongwa camp. At times, the care provided there was better than the local alternative – demonstrated by the many Tanzanian patrons that frequented the ANC's medical services.[22]

In August 1964 the ANC/MK joined SWAPO and the Frente de Libertação de Moçambique (FRELIMO) in a camp christened "Kongwa." Much like Ghana's pan-Africanist role in West Africa, independent Tanzania was supporting the "second wave" of liberation movements in southern Africa (this discussion will be expanded on in chapter 2). In this case, the Tanzanian support provided liberation guerrilla armies from Angola, Namibia, Mozambique, Zimbabwe, and South Africa lands to establish military camps. As a result, the ANC settled just outside of Kongwa, a village with a population of 1,000 Tanzanians, next to FRELIMO and SWAPO, and shortly became neighbours to the Movimento Popular de Libertação de Angola (MPLA) and the Zimbabwe African People's Union.[23] Not only was there solidarity among the liberation armies at Kongwa camp, all of these groups were recognized as legitimate challenges to colonial governments in southern Africa and given assistance by the Organisation for African Unity (OAU).

Accounts of the medical services in Kongwa emphasize different aspects of the service and differ on some of the details. However, there is agreement that ANC's Kongwa camp had its own medical clinic containing four, possibly five, beds (at least two for females and two for males) in the camp. The disease burden (especially foot fungus and eye diseases) in Kongwa had made medical provision a necessity; this was recognized by the OAU that occasionally assisted with supplies, but much of the time the ANC did not receive these supplies in an expedient fashion and was forced to purchase drugs from local stores.[24]

Especially because the small camp clinic was without the services of a doctor, the medical needs of the cadres could not be adequately met.[25] In order to overcome this inadequacy, the ANC fostered a positive relationship with the local medical services. Patients could travel 25 km to Kongwa's local hospital, Mpwapwa Health Centre, or they could be sent to the two facilities in Dodoma – the Dodoma Regional Hospital and Mirembe Psychiatric Hospital – located 75 km away. The three health institutions were usually sufficient for minor illnesses and injuries, but cadres needing intensive care were sent to Dar es Salaam.[26] Some of the previously mentioned South African nurses working in Tanzanian hospitals took care of ANC cadres that were not in camp or could not be sufficiently cared for at Kongwa.[27] Furthermore, international allies such as the USSR or the German Democratic Republic (GDR) saw a revolving door of ANC patients (a practice that continued into the late 1980s).[28] While ANC members used Tanzanian facilities, Tanzanians were also frequenting the ANC's medical clinic, and in some circumstances, it was reported that Tanzanians sometimes preferred the ANC's service to that provided by the local equivalent.[29] The bilateral relationship between medical sectors of host countries and the ANC, most often favouring the needs of the South African exiles, was a foundational element of the ANC's ability to offer an even remotely viable medical service throughout its time in exile.

Historical accounts begin to diverge on their recollection of who worked in the clinic. One account sang the praises of nurse Ntabenkosi Fiphaza who worked in the clinic and simultaneously trained future medical department players Salele Ratlabiane (MK name: Isaac Salele)[30], Ethel Mkhize, Simon Rantao (Tax Mosala), Rooi (Roy) Campbells, John Mathatha, Thoko Msimang-Williams (Rachael Tshounyane), Fish Mekgwe, Conny Zondy, and Davidson Themba Masuku (Haggar McBerry).[31] It reiterates that the policy in the camp was to utilize previous medical experience as well as identify those inclined to assist in healthcare in order to produce in-service trainees.

Another account neither mentions Ntabenkosi Fiphaza nor the medical trainees. Instead, it relies on an interview with Isaac Makopo, the chief logistics officer stationed in Kongwa between 1964 and 1967.[32] Makopo relates that based on experience, albeit limited, as a medical orderly at a hospital in Durban, Leslie Sondezi became the medical officer at Kongwa and Jackson Mbali (a medical orderly on the South African mines) joined him shortly thereafter. It was after Mbali joined the two-man crew that they established the small four-to-five bed clinic. While both Sondezi and Mbali had been medical orderlies in South Africa, according to Isaac Makopo Mbali was better at providing Kongwa clinic with a sense of structure and competence.[33] These two accounts of the staff are significantly different; the former suggests a relatively well-established contingent of medical support staff while the latter suggests a somewhat competent but dramatically reduced staff. However, discrepancies aside, both accounts show that the ANC wanted to semi-independently provide for the primary healthcare needs of its cadres in Kongwa and was able to do so, if on a minimal level.

Despite these accomplishments, the ANC was not without its critics. As was the case throughout the thirty-year period of exile, MK cadres were frustrated by the leadership's inability to consistently provide for their basic needs, which included healthcare.[34] However, of perhaps greater consequence to the cadres, was evidence of two-tiered treatment availability; leadership was sent abroad for top-notch treatment while most had to contend with what little was available in the camp. In 1969 ANC defector Maurice Mthombeni, broadcast a rancorous accusation against his former political overseer; his complaint was published in the socialist UK newspaper *The Black Dwarf*[35] and included a short statement about his perception of the ANC's health services:

> [M]edical facilities were very poor. There was a small camp clinic of 12 feet by 14 feet, which housed five patients of varying diseases at a time. The "Medical Officer" wasn't very well acquainted with his medical supplies which consisted largely of pain killers, mercurochrome, purgatives and suchlike. All bodily pains were treated alike, and a neurotic case was treated in the same way as a case with a simple headache. The medical supplies in the clinic were insufficient for the four hundred freedom fighters in the camp.[36]

When the ANC Youth and Students' Section in London saw the article, it sent a copy to the leadership in southern Africa and then penned a rebuttal provocatively titled "'Black Dwarf' Talks White Trash." [37] Based on the political position of Mthombeni, it would be a mistake to accept the account published in *The Black Dwarf* at its word, but it should be noted that while the Youth and Students' Section refuted most of Mthombeni's allegations, it did not comment on their accuser's account of the health facilities quoted above.

A second complaint about the ANC's capacity to provide medical care came in the same year. In the wake of the failed Wankie Campaign (a 1967 military effort to infiltrate South Africa, described below) Chris Hani drafted the "Hani Memorandum" – a list of items that pointed to poor leadership and a need for change. Item fourteen of the memorandum specifically highlighted the differences between the medical treatment provided for the leadership and the treatment available to the "rank and file." Hani emphasized that this two-tiered practice was particularly out of step with the socialist political underpinnings of the movement.[38] While Hani may have been disappointed with the two-tiered system, the growing inequality was not unexpected nor was it ever fully addressed. Due to the limited amount of medical treatment available and the low level of accountability required of the staff, access to the best care was often dictated by political and military rank.

The lack of accountability was subtly noted in some of the first Health and Welfare Department Committee meeting reports in 1969. The Fort Hare archive contains four reports compiled from these meetings held in the ANC's burgeoning political headquarters in Lusaka.[39] In one of these reports, the medical officer in charge – comrade Barney[40] – stated that a number of comrades were complaining about unequal food distribution. The care for the health and welfare of South African comrades in the 1960s may have been better than what was available to the average citizen in Tanzania, but it was not equally distributed; therefore, to many, including Chris Hani, it left much to be desired.

It was also clear from the four 1969 one-page reports that health-care was not a major priority for the ANC. The Health and Welfare Department was not as concerned with illness and disease as it was with the diets of comrades and the availability of sweaters for its charges in cold weather. "Health and welfare" consisted of first aid courses as well as the opportunity for the comrades to see films, play a variety of sports, enjoy dance lessons, and have access to indoor games like chess or checkers.[41]

The overall lack of interest in explicitly medically focused care is better understood when the ANC is analyzed through an economic lens and by considering the political position of the ANC at that time. As has been previously alluded to, the earliest support to the ANC and MK came from newly liberated African countries and the Soviet Union. Members of the ANC and MK received military support and training in the USSR, Morocco, Algeria, Ethiopia, and Egypt (which extended to medical training in the cases of the aforementioned four ANC doctors).[42] Southern Africa and, initially, Tanzania provided the ANC with land, and it was the desire of newly independent African countries to see the ANC launch a successful armed struggle against the apartheid government rather than establish social services like healthcare aimed at the long-term needs of South Africans. The initial turn to exile was an optimistic and idealistic time for the ANC; the organisation did not envision a prolonged thirty-year conflict and its decolonized African supporters were liberation-focused.

The fight against the NP had also become a Cold War struggle and the communist military allies were essential to the survival of the ANC and MK.[43] Ideologically, the ANC's leftist political platform bore semblance to communist ideals, and the USSR and China had already been heavily invested in liberation movements worldwide. Consequently, the ANC was the recipient of considerable military support from the USSR. On top of its trade embargo of South Africa in 1962, the Soviet Union's communist party channelled money to the ANC and MK.[44] In 1963 they sent their first instalment of US$300,000 and funding continued for several years.[45] Not only did communist political parties and national governments from nations like the USSR, Romania, Yugoslavia, and the GDR provide financial assistance, conventional military supplies, and training, but the ANC's Cold War allies also helped to provide for the immediate medical needs of cadres as well as to train cadres to become "medicos" – individuals with some basic medical knowledge who could be used to strategic military ends.[46] Even with this modest medical support, the emphasis on military action left the medical sector understandably neglected and underfunded.

It was undoubtedly disappointing to the ANC and its financial supporters that the first decade of military struggle showed MK to be ineffective at infiltrating South Africa and engaging the South African Defense Force (SADF). South Africa was surrounded by a "buffer zone" of colonial states: the Portuguese occupied Mozambique and Angola, and white Rhodesian settlers occupied Southern Rhodesia (now Zimbabwe). MK cadres, therefore, had to cross hostile colonial territory before entering South Africa. For example, in 1967 the ANC sent a contingent of MK cadres across the southern Zambian border into Rhodesia.[47] The Rhodesian state army, assisted by the SADF tracked, captured, and killed MK cadres rendering the campaign a historic failure.[48] In 1968, the ANC attempted another military venture – the Sipolilo Campaign – to send MK cadres south to infiltrate South Africa. This effort, too, failed while also corresponding with leadership infighting and political unrest and, consequently, ANC leadership grew increasingly hesitant to send cadres south.

In 1969 Tanzanian officials told the ANC and MK that it had fourteen days to vacate Kongwa camp and the country altogether. Kongwa camp, intended as a transit camp for MK cadres, had become a stagnant, permanent camp for MK. Not only was this torpidity a security threat, bored cadres were increasingly accused of mischief and criminal activity. The indiscipline of ANC and MK comrades was a problem that plagued the Tanzanian government until the end of the exile period. In his book, Stephen Ellis quoted correspondence from the Tanzanian officials to the ANC:

> The protracted stay of the same cadres in the one place has over the years led to exposure of secrets and generally to a breakdown of security to the serious detriment of Tanzania and the freedom struggle … in particular, the enemy has been able to collect, and in all probability continues to receive, detailed intelligence information about Kongwa. In this sense the camp is a lucrative hunting ground for enemy agents. This is inevitable where the morale of the cadres has been severely weakened by years of inactivity and frustration.[49]

This was just one of the reasons that the ANC was asked to leave; the second, and perhaps more important reason, was that the ANC was suspected to be involved in a coup attempt against the Tanzanian president.[50] MK cadres were sent temporarily to the USSR before they were conditionally accepted back to Tanzania. Ultimately, by the mid-1970s the ANC headquarters officially shifted to Lusaka, Zambia, and the ANC's military activity in Tanzania was on course to be greatly diminished.[51]

The ANC's military inaction in the early 1970s did not inspire much more confidence in the organisation than it did in the late 1960s.[52] Historians have considered the early 1970s as the low point of the ANC's tenure in exile.[53] The ANC leadership's focus had turned from its revolutionary goals and was progressively targeting its internal concerns. Trapped in exile for a decade without a great deal of military engagement, members of the ANC and MK were showing clear signs of battle fatigue.[54]

Cold War contacts were vital to the survival of the ANC and MK, but the ANC was growing increasingly aware that it was not going to win victory in the near future and needed to begin to reenvision its role in exile. Therefore, the ANC needed to look for additional, nonmilitary support – a central shift to the development of an official health sector. This alternative support was not immediately forthcoming. In the late 1960s leadership of the ANC travelled to Sweden on two separate occasions asking for financial assistance; they were unsuccessful. Sweden was a logical place to begin asking for support because, since the early 1960s, Sweden had taken a positive stance towards helping African liberation movements and was the first industrialized Western national government to send these movements humanitarian aid.[55] By the time the ANC approached Sweden, the Scandinavian country was already supporting FRELIMO and the MPLA.[56]

In 1971, after being rejected twice by the Swedish government Oliver Tambo, president of the ANC, in desperation for support, travelled to Sweden himself. Yet despite his international respectability, even Tambo came home empty handed. Until then Sweden had a number of reasons to withhold support from the ANC; not only did Sweden have significant financial interests in South Africa at the time but the country's government was aware of the ANC leadership conflicts, corruption, and lack of military efficacy (not to mention Sweden's already considerable financial support for FRELIMO and the MPLA).[57] In fact, Sweden's correspondence with Tanzania was not altogether encouraging. Historian Tor Sellström wrote:

> When in mid 1972 the Swedish embassy in Dar es Salaam raised the issue of possible humanitarian support with the Prime Minister's Office, the responsible Tanzanian official disparagingly characterised the ANC as a "victim of age … which ha[s] abandoned its warrior operations"… he [the Tanzanian official] was of the opinion that "luxurious" food grants, work permits and land allocations would only lead the ANC members to "lose their sense of blood."[58]

While the Swedish government was not yet enchanted by the ANC, the country's anti-apartheid movement was growing.[59] The influence of the apartheid government extended past its own borders. In the mid-late 1960s the UN General Assembly declared its distain for the South African government's illegitimate grip on Namibia (formerly South West Africa) and Sweden was among the first to endorse financial aid to SWAPO's anti-apartheid cause.[60] While SWAPO and the

ANC were fighting for power in two distinct geographic territories, the two liberation movements shared striking similarities; they operated in camps that were in relatively close proximity to each other and had a common enemy in the South African regime. Swedish, and more broadly Scandinavian, anti-apartheid support was therefore channelled into the two movements. At times, it made practical sense to coordinate funding to develop joint ANC/SWAPO initiatives. Many future medical projects funded by the Nordic countries, especially those concerning medical education, strategically tied the two organisations together.

The Swedish government first granted SWAPO small sums of money in 1970 and 1971. However, in 1972 Swedish representatives in southern Africa called into question SWAPO's ability to handle additional funding. Consequently, there were no funds transferred to SWAPO in the 1972–73 fiscal year – a one-year hiatus in thirty years of financial assistance.[61] During that year, the ANC, rather than SWAPO, became the recipient of SEK150,000 (approximately US$34,000) in Swedish solidarity aid.[62] But the meagre sum, explicitly short-term financial aid, demonstrated Sweden's hesitancy to support the organisation. In retrospect, this 1973 donation was a tipping point for the ANC and the start of a series of increasingly lucrative aid transactions. By the 1993–94 fiscal year, the ANC had received approximately US$16.3 million from Sweden; between 1973 and 1994, SIDA had gifted the ANC approximately SEK 600,000,000 (US$101 million).[63]

Swedish and, eventually, pan-Nordic aid clearly became crucial to the ANC's ability to provide for the social needs of South African exiles. The increase in financial assistance can begin to explain why, despite the military stagnation in the early 1970s, the ANC's bureaucratic apparatus spread further across the region; this growth had an impact on health infrastructure and will be described in detail later in this chapter. While new healthcare services started to arise in this period, the unofficial medical sector remained regionally divided without a centralized authority and lacked a systematic approach to patient care.

The scant medical records found for this period also indicate that the ANC was finding new ways to use medicine to deepen their southern African alliances. In 1972, three years before Mozambican independence, FRELIMO sent requests to the ANC for medicine and food.[64] Despite the ANC's own precarious situation and reliance on international aid for supplies, they sent two truckloads of medicine, bandages, soup, and salt.[65] After delivery, the ANC secretary for administration Mendi Msimang wrote to ANC Treasurer General Thomas Nkobi stating, "we [the ANC] could have released more quantities than some of these [amounts listed above] but for lack of packing space."[66]

The increase in southern African solidarity as well as the beginnings of the financial partnership between the ANC and Sweden corresponded with a number of major events that dramatically changed the political and military position of the ANC. In 1975 Mozambique and Angola gained independence from Portugal. This had four major implications for the ANC. First, Sweden slowed its financial assistance to FRELIMO and the MPLA and the Swedish Krona was now free to be sent in a much more substantial way to the anti-apartheid struggle. Second, the SADF lost territory from its buffer zone leaving South Africa more vulnerable to MK attack. Third, the governments led by the MPLA and FRELIMO granted the ANC permission to create military camps in Angola and Mozambique, permission that provided new military possibilities.[67] Fourth, the success of these two liberation movements was inspiring to South Africans, especially young students, and many were emboldened to take greater anti-apartheid action.[68]

In the first week of June 1976, the Swedish second secretary at the Ministry of Foreign Affairs, Ann Wilkins, was commissioned to go to South Africa to interview representatives from the various anti-apartheid groups in order to compile a report that made recommendations regarding which organisations should be the recipient of considerable Swedish funding. The ANC's political absence in South Africa made Sweden anxious to look within the country for effective anti-apartheid movements. Yet Wilkins' report concluded the opposite; Tor Sellström quotes her report:

[T]hat the assistance to ANC should be seen as support to one of several organizations fighting against apartheid. The movement cannot … be considered as some kind of government-in-exile. [Nevertheless], since we are cooperating with ANC we should not support organizations which are antagonistic towards [the movement]. That would probably be the situation if Swedish support was granted to ... [the] PAC.[69]

Needless to say, Oliver Tambo was encouraged by the fact that the Swedish government would consult him regarding their future funding endeavours.

A week after Ann Wilkins had conducted her interviews in South Africa, a series of student uprisings occurred in South African townships that sent students into exile, eager to enlist in MK and fight the apartheid government. The boost in Swedish funds helped the ANC to be the main exile group able to accommodate the young refugees entering into exile after 1976. It was significant that the students joined the ANC and MK in exile. This was definitely not the inevitable fate of the students. The student ideology, which was closely aligned with Steve Biko and the Black Consciousness Movement, directed the events of 16 June 1976 and was more consistent with PAC ideology. Splitting from the ANC over its acceptance of nonracialism, the PAC was a more radical Africanist anti-apartheid movement. The PAC would have been the natural political organisation for students to join. However, the PAC had not been given the same military opportunities as the ANC in Angola and Mozambique, and the leadership was in disarray.[70] Based on the political upheaval within the PAC from 1978–81, Sweden was disenchanted with the organisation; in addition to already recognizing the ANC as more important than the PAC, Sweden dramatically limited their financial assistance to the latter organisation. Therefore, the PAC was less structurally equipped than the ANC to deal with the sudden influx of students. While not overly resource rich or adequately prepared, the ANC had more to offer new young recruits; therefore, it managed to claim the vast majority of student enlisters. The wave of new students into exile brought revival to the ANC and helped establish the organisation as the principal anti-apartheid political group.[71] Once received by the ANC, students were given the option to either enlist in MK[72] or continue their education in the ANC's settlement in Mazimbu, Tanzania (this will be discussed further in chapter 2).[73]

Due to events in 1975 and 1976, the medical sector's responsibilities changed. Rather than attempting to deal with health crises on a case-by-case basis, the neglected and poorly developed medical sector was required to be responsible across southern Africa for the long-term maintenance and health of a growing intergenerational community affiliated with the ANC. They also needed to be able to communicate with the growing MK force across a much larger territory in exile.

By 1976 the ANC headquartered at Lusaka had a major civilian camp in Mazimbu, Tanzania; operated military camps in Angola and Mozambique; had cadres moving through Swaziland, Lesotho, and Botswana; and managed to get a handful of cadres to infiltrate South Africa. Additionally, the ANC had a presence beyond the continent. The ANC had offices in London and Stockholm that sought to generate international anti-apartheid support. It had cadres in training and students on scholarship across Soviet-allied nations, and some students were also studying in Nordic countries. All in all, the network of the ANC was growing rapidly.

One of the first signs of movement towards a centralized health structure emerged in 1976. Albert Nzo the secretary general of the ANC in exile circulated a memorandum to all offices outlining a new policy to deal with individual and organisation-wide offers for health care and rest abroad. Until that point, ANC members had been approached independently by sympathetic individuals and organisations and offered opportunities to go abroad. The ANC was not in the habit of interfering with the freedom of its members to take advantage of these offers. However, in February of 1976, Nzo announced a policy change. He stated,

> [T]hat practice [of allowing individuals to go abroad] is no longer being encouraged and any such offers should immediately be reported to Headquarters for use as it deems advisable. This applies equally to general offers in your area. Comrades will appreciate the fact that the Organisation has a large membership ... At best, the Organisation has endeavoured to introduce a cycle system based on the element of urgency in so far as medical treatment is concerned and on pure rotational principle in regard to rest.[74]

His change in policy was a reflection of the growing South African population in exile and the increase in international health-related support, as well as recognition of the need to gain more centralized control over its health-related concerns. This final need for a more organized bureaucratic structure was not just for better quality patient care but also because the ANC needed to display itself internationally as the political entity that would be able to challenge the NP for political power in a post-apartheid state. Establishing an official department of health was a step towards establishing greater political legitimacy.

Inauguration of the Health Department: Bureaucratic Growth and Change, 1977–86

Backed in part by Swedish aid, in 1977 the ANC was able to inaugurate its official Department of Health. In fact, contrary to Ann Wilkins' assertion that the ANC could not be considered a "government-in-waiting" Sweden's funding was specifically geared at the long-term establishment of bureaucracy and future governing capacity. According to Tor Sellström, a consistent chronicler of humanitarian aid between Sweden and southern Africa, "Towards the end of the 1970s, the assistance to ANC assumed a much more distinct political character than the support extended to any other Southern African liberation movement. Apart from strictly humanitarian aid, it focused on institution and capacity-building, information activities and on the extension of ANC's infrastructure inside the apartheid republic."[75] Sweden's initially reluctant move to support bureaucratic development and the ANC's political dominance, was mirrored by other Nordic countries: "The political attitude of the governments in the Scandinavian countries towards the ANC is far from favourable; however, there are presently trends within these governments towards recognising that the ANC is the only rightful representative of the people in South Africa."[76] With the opening of an official health department, aid from other humanitarian sponsors could be channelled into more established long-term medical efforts rather than be aimed at immediate relief.

On 2 July 1977, Drs Peter Mfelang, Manto Tshabalala, and Fiki Radebe-Reed attended a meeting in Dar es Salaam that formally discussed the potential need for an ANC health sector. The idea had been percolating at ANC headquarters and the Dar es Salaam meeting was the first opportunity to discuss its merits and potentially operationalize a medical sector. The proposal was apparently met with a positive response: 27 August 1977 is considered the inauguration date of the ANC Health Department.[77] The ANC Medical Committee was established and the ANC Health Department gradually grew from this official starting point.[78] But this event, while historically significant, was relatively anticlimactic and not well documented. Six doctors and four additional members of the ANC were invited to a consultative meeting of the ANC Medical Committee in which Alfred Nzo restated that the ANC should centralize its medical personnel in southern Africa. The meeting was recorded in an abbreviated two-page report and was then subsequently referenced in ANC health reports that briefly discuss the origins of the medical department.[79]

The ANC leadership's primary motivation for a department of health was overtly political. The Medical Committee was to be used as part of the ANC's claim to political legitimacy; the committee was envisioned as the "the nucleus of the future South African Medical Association."[80] To further underscore this point, Alfred Nzo went on to explain the importance of the committee by stating that, "internationally, the ANC is being seen as the Alternative government of South Africa. This position has further been accentuated by the granting of Observer Status to the ANC in the United Nations and all its agencies including the World Health Organization."[81] Already, the committee was charged with the task of "map[ping] out the future programme of the nascent Medical Association of free South Africa."[82] These bold statements further highlight the important departure from the healthcare-related efforts of the ANC up to that point, efforts that had been focused on southern African alliances and immediate comrade health provision and maintenance.[83]

However, the 1977 meeting did not focus on international possibilities to the exclusion of the situation on the ground. The Medical Committee was also charged with the directive to assess healthcare efforts in each region. It was suggested that they create a registry of South African medical personnel in southern Africa and abroad, create a list of health-related requirements in each of the regions, start to coordinate health centres and educational programs in ANC and MK populated areas, and recruit students to the medical field for training.[84] The Medical Committee and its extensive ambitions were then officially established with Dr Peter Mfelang at the helm as chair. Dr Manto Tshabalala was named secretary and Drs Randeree, Radebe-Reed, and Nokwe were committee members. After August 1977 the Medical Committee was recognized by the ANC as part of the administrative machinery and was expected to report to the secretary general's office – the office that oversaw the Women's Section, Youth Section, Department of Manpower Development, the Department of Arts and Culture, and the Department of Education.[85]

The next eighteen months might be considered an audition; the ANC was still not completely convinced that a health department would be able to play an effective role in coordinating regional medical initiatives. Meetings to coordinate efforts during this inaugural year were sparse; the first, already described, occurred in August, the second was held in October, and the third meeting was not held until July 1978.[86] Luckily, the paucity of these meetings did not render the committee's efforts wasted. Most likely the strength and tenacity of Dr Manto Tshabalala drove the agenda forward. (Her foundational role in the form and character of the Health Department will be delineated below.) In an attempt to invite all South African health personnel to join the Medical Committee, the committee wrote "letters of appeal" to individual South African medical affiliates and published a broader version of the appeal within its internal ANC publication *Sechaba*. Dr Freddy Reddy reported receiving a copy: "Then in 1979 there was a notice in *Sechaba*, where the Medical health section of the ANC was inviting doctors to come over and help them in the crisis situation. But they couldn't afford to pay the tickets for the doctors to come. I thought they had grandiose ideas that all ANC South African doctors were going to just storm down there to this …"[87] While he did not respond to the call immediately, the publication was clearly a success in creating awareness of a Medical Committee among the South African community in exile.

The committee compiled an initial report on the healthcare developments in Tanzania, Zambia, Angola, and Mozambique, with the most progress seen in Tanzania.[88] Furthermore, it reported that the ANC's educational officer (Department of Education) was putting together a list of students involved in medical training and was conducting seminars on public health and hygiene at the Training Medical Centre in Morogoro. The committee drafted a "First Aid and Nutrition" syllabus and disseminated it to members of the Educational Committee in Tanzania for consideration. It was also able to report on international, mostly Scandinavian, support for the proposed plans of a health centre at the future ANC school outside the Morogoro town limits, as well as the OAU's donation of an ambulance. Significantly, committee members attended two international conferences: the WHO Regional Committee for Africa in Brazzaville in September 1977 and the World Assembly in Geneva in May 1978.[89] Their presence at these two conferences reinforced the image of the ANC as not just a parochial anti-apartheid movement but a governmental player on an international stage – a theme that will be expanded upon in chapter 3.

The report did not neglect to mention the committee's early shortcomings. First, the committee's initiatives were not met with overwhelming enthusiasm. Dr Tshabalala wrote,

> Very little effort has been made in running our health pro-
> grammes in an efficient and organized manner. The under-
> lying reason would appear to be firstly the uninspired work
> being done by way of mobilization [no response to the ap-
> peal sent by the committee mentioned above] and second-
> ly the problem of getting people to sufficiently respond to
> change. The third reason may be the lack of co-ordination
> and fluid contact between the members of this Committee
> and between Medical teams. By these is meant that for a
> long time Medical services in the Organisation were con-
> ducted on ad hoc basis and this in time became the pattern
> of doing things.[90]

The battle for authority between the previously independent regional medical teams and the Medical Committee was ongoing throughout the exile period. The committee sent out guidelines only to find out later that regional teams did not even bother to read them; the regional teams preferred to work within their own independent parameters.[91] Furthermore, Dr Tshabalala had to make a direct request to the leadership to help establish the new committee's centralized authority. Understandably, the committee wanted to be consulted on all matters related to medicine, such as the program of sending students for medical training. The conclusion of the July 1978 report made suggestions regarding how the committee could proceed more effectively. Predictably, the committee saw that it needed to develop a better internal structure, have detailed job descriptions for each member, and substantially increase its staff size to better address broad, regional concerns. Tshabalala ended the report by stating, "It is clear from this report that much still remains to be done … the bulk of the responsibilities has been left in too few hands … This does not excuse members of this Committee from failing to discharge this important task set to them … and that is 'to create a Medical association.'"[92] In retrospect, Tshabalala's conclusion would have been an appropriate ending to almost any of the subsequent health reports written by the Health Department in exile.

Part of the problem for the committee was a major disparity in political will for the department's success. The alternative approaches sometimes caused seriously detrimental personality clashes within the department. The difference in approach between Chairperson Dr Peter Mfelang and Secretary Dr Manto Tshabalala clearly accentuates this point. Tshabalala's assertive character in the ANC is first made apparent in her correspondence with the Tanzanian Morogoro project team manager in August 1977. At the time, she was employed in Morogoro in a teaching position mostly unrelated to her work as a member of the ANC.[93] As an ambitious young doctor newly involved with the ANC in southern Africa, she was anxious to attend organisational meetings, medical seminars, and workshops. On at least two occasions in 1977, she applied for leave to Lusaka: the first was to attend the August inauguration meeting and the second was to attend the aforementioned October Medical Working Committee meeting. While Project Manager Dr J.P. Kasiga begrudgingly allowed her leave for the August meeting, his response to the second request was less favourable: "It will be difficult if not impossible for me to permit my staff to commit themselves in other activities, however urging [sic] they may be, leaving the classes semi-parallised [sic]. I therefore wish to advise you to seriously concentrate more on the Programme … and less about extra curriculum work outside our Institution. It is your obligation."[94] Tshabalala's response was characteristically brusque: "My serious conviction is that I can not be accused at anytime of not concentrating on the Project. If anything I have exerted more time for the smooth running of the Project …

Extra-curriculum activities outside the institution are well in order. These broaden out one's outlook and I think should be encouraged for as long as they do not semi-paralyze [*sic*] the Project work."[95] She closed the letter with what was to become a staple line in many of her more confrontational letters: "I hope this will be taken in the good spirit it is meant."

Tshabalala became a powerful representative of the Health Department in part because of the somewhat negligent role assumed by Dr Peter Mfelang. The archived documents do not specify why he was given the lead position but it was clear that Mfelang's ambitions did not solely lie within southern Africa. In 1975 prior to the creation of the Medical Committee, he applied for a scholarship to do postgraduate studies in medicine.[96] The report on his application stated, "He is willing to study anywhere where a good school is available."[97] His desire to continue his studies did not cease with the creation of the department. In 1980 Mfelang was accepted into the Master's in Public Health certificate program in international health at Baltimore's Johns Hopkins University – a course that he extended for an extra six months in order to gain focused training in program design for primary health care and maternal and child health.[98] Tshabalala's reaction to the extension was not positive:

> I have to express great disappointment, at the fact that you have unilaterally decided to extend your tour without referring to the "Department". You have not forgotten that you are in effect the "Head" of this department and therefore should not depart from our decisions and agreements, at least without consultations. To be frank, I think the basics we get in the MPH [Master's in Public Health] course ... is enough for us to consolidate and cement them operationally. The amount of work is enormous and we need to do the work amongst our own people first. The communities are increasing and our physical presence is an absolute necessity. Single handed I can not manage. This is a fact.[99]

This was not the first letter Tshabalala sent regarding the issue of staff shortage.[100] In response Mfelang reprimanded Tshabalala's communication style: "[T]he information in the letter, though useful, does not answer any of the important questions I had put to you over the months, since my arrival here. And they are not sensitive."[101] Rather than finishing the Master's in Public Health course and returning to southern Africa as Tshabalala proposed, Mfelang wrote to Alfred Nzo appealing for support for the department so that he could remain in Baltimore for all of 1981.

Predictably, uneven commitment to the cause of the Health Department was found at all levels of the medical sector and sadly for the ANC this issue also meant that the Health Department was chronically understaffed. But that does not mean that the issue was completely neglected. In 1980 the Health Department was clearly still trying to identify the number of ANC students studying abroad. In January they had identified twenty-two in medicine, three in pharmacy, one in dentistry, one in radiography, one in biochemistry, one in childcare, one in physiotherapy, and two training to be medical assistants.[102] Six doctors were doing postgraduate courses abroad (including Dr Mfelang).[103] They also identified eight trained medical auxiliaries, six of whom attended the OAU school in Morogoro; three became laboratory technicians and three became medical assistants. An additional five students (alongside a number of SWAPO counterparts) were sponsored by the Norwegian People's Association (NPA) to complete a first aid course in Norway. The summary report concluded its section on education by stating, "This is about all our Department can boast about so far."[104] The statement was somewhat misleading because not all of these students were under the direct control of the ANC; the department was newly aware of these students' educational endeavours but, based on the notion that they were previously unknown to the organisation, it is safe to say that the ANC had very little say in these students' ultimate career choices. The exception to this was the students sent to the OAU School and the First Aid course in Norway. The OAU was explicitly looking to sponsor students of liberation movements who would contribute to the struggle in practical ways. Norway was also selecting ANC members who wanted to return and work for the ANC; this was evident by their choice of loyal ANC students including Lillian Booi and Sidwell Langa from Angola, Roy Campbells from Tanzania, Magdalene Gatsewe from Mozambique, and Tim Maharaj from London.[105] The five returned to educate other members of the ANC on rudimentary first aid.

In early 1979 the Medical Committee became the more authoritative and wide-reaching Health Department.[106] Interestingly, this title still did not signify confidence that a centralized health sector would be able to make much headway on the ground. The department comprised Chairperson Peter Mfelang and Secretary Manto Tshabalala, as well as elected medical representatives from each region with an established ANC presence. Angola, Tanzania, and Zambia had "health teams" because of the already existing medical structures in these regions, and these teams were, at least initially, headed by doctors; a team in Zimbabwe was added in 1984. The Mozambique Health Team did not initially seem to merit the same status due to the absence of a medical doctor. However, in January 1979 nurse Florence Maleka was posted to Mozambique and, regarding this appointment, Dr Tshabalala wrote, "you [Ms Maleka] have been posted to Maputo, to mend our medical affairs, we have no doubt that our Comrades medical and health needs will be attended to satisfactorily now."[107] The inclusion of Maleka helped to legitimize the Mozambique Health Team within the Health Department.

In addition to the health teams stationed in southern Africa, the ANC also had health teams in the United Kingdom, Canada, US, and Scandinavia.[108] These off-continent teams played a supplementary role by raising awareness and funding for the ANC's health endeavours as well as supporting the training of future medical students. While a number of medical personnel were affiliated with the ANC Department of Health, as seen in the number of students counted as a part of the ANC, the department only claimed three doctors (two of who were on leave for studies), two nurses, and ten to fifteen medical auxiliaries as part of a committed staff.[109] The department, therefore, was still an understaffed fledgling group attempting to centralize medical authority.

The internal departmental structure was a rigid, clearly defined apparatus on paper but much more complicated and mercurial in practice. In theory ANC medical clinics and dispensaries were supposed to report to the RHTs. The RHT leadership comprised a chairperson, a secretary, and two to five additional members.[110] They were responsible for coordinating health activities in the regions as well as submitting quarterly reports to the health chairperson in Lusaka.[111] In practice, RHT leadership (especially outside Tanzania) was often made up of undesignated individuals and they struggled to meet regularly or at all.[112] For instance, in Angola medical staff was expected to cover several MK camps spread out across a civil war zone without adequate transport or supplies; therefore, the added expectation of regular meetings and detailed regional reports was not reasonable. The Angolan RHT held its first official leadership meeting in 1981.

Perhaps even more prohibitive were personality clashes between members of the central administration and members of the RHTs. This friction between individuals often stemmed from the RHTs' desire for independence and the battle for authority over health provision. (The vertical tension is delineated in chapter 4.) This uncooperative attitude depleted much of the political will to report to the department, and in some cases regional teams, especially in Tanzania, addressed their reports or concerns to the secretary general or the region's ANC chief representative instead.[113] The lack of medical personnel in each region made it difficult to create a structure that would be accountable to a centralized authority; the bulk of the early communication between the regions and the department was limited to urgent medical requisitions and requests to transfer patients in need of acute care. Venting her frustration at the lack of communication, Secretary Manto Tshabalala wrote to the ANC secretary for professional bodies, Sindiso Mfenyana, explaining that the regions were not engaged with the Health Department's concerns: "We thought the centres would have the report after the NEC meeting. We have enough copies for each centre. If only they could function and communicate. They are all dead."[114]

Throughout its time in exile, the Health Department constantly sought ways to improve communication and clarify job descriptions in order to maximize departmental productivity. Another central concern of the Health Department was its lack of power to provide incentives to qualified health personnel. As a result, it was not able to offer medical professionals any sort of competitive monetary compensation for working in ANC facilities.[115] Doctors and nurses trained with ANC support far preferred working in their hosts' national facilities or in international facilities farther abroad than operating in poor, under-equipped, and understaffed ANC settlements. Furthermore, some staff believed that the ANC would not be able to keep them busy enough to warrant full-time work in their various specialties.[116] By the end of 1982, the Health Department complained that it "had not grown in strength. It had not improved the quality of health care rendered to [its] communities."[117] However, the situation of having well-trained ANC members working in local hospitals must have been one of the reasons that the Health Department was able to claim good relations with local health facilities throughout its time in exile. The downside of this situation was that the Health Department itself was more inept than it otherwise would have been.

In 1983 a new body, the health secretariat, was constituted and by October of that year, it operated out of offices at ANC headquarters in Lusaka.[118] This was put in place with the hope of establishing clearer roles and responsibilities for each member of the Health Department. Headquartered in Lusaka, the secretariat was also, seemingly, another attempt to convince the RHTs and other ANC departments of the authority of the Department of Health. It was hoped that the clear job descriptions provided each member with more extensive oversight and coordinating ability.[119]

Even so, things did not improve. At the July and August 1986 Health Council Meeting, one of the major concerns stated was that, "There has been a negligible improvement in the vertical relationship intradepartmentally ... However, there is need to re-emphasize the importance of stren-gthening [*sic*] this relationship."[120] As the Health Department was still found wanting, an additional five portfolios were added.[121] The minutes of that 1986 Health Council Meeting show that the secretariat, while growing in size, had only two full-time functionaries and that it was believed that this significantly hampered the workings of the department and centralization of authority.[122]

Another bureaucratic attempt at strengthening the Health Department was the establishment of the Health Council; the council was made up of members from the central leadership as well as members from the regions and it met once every three years to discuss possible improvements to ANC health policy.[123] While the council had ultimate power to influence health decisions, it was an advisory board rather than an actual mobilized force for the department. Members of the secretariat overlapped as members of the council, rendering

4. In January this year, the formation of a Secretariat was suggested but this has not materialised.

PRESENT STRUCTURE OF HEALTH DEPARTMENT

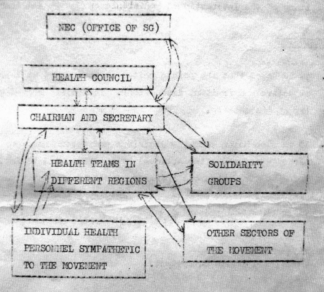

1.2 Present structure of Health Department authority. The complicated lines of authority between structures in the Health Department are indicated in this organigram. The text is unclear, but the importance of the illustration lies in the arrows between the boxes containing the names of authoritative bodies. There are sixteen arrows attempting to delineate the flow of command.

the body somewhat redundant. The creation of these multiple levels of authority caused some level of confusion (see figure 1.2).

This is not to say that the situation on the ground was not showing signs of improvement: by 1986 a total of thirty-five doctors and an untold number of associated medical personnel had completed their training and a general system for treating cadres or referring them to local facilities was in working operation.[124] The ANC had received funding from a number of international organisations, most notably in Scandinavia, and had embarked on massive health infrastructure-building projects and received a host of solidarity workers in all sectors of medical care from an array of countries worldwide.[125] The regional teams managed to collaborate in meaningful ways with local health facilities and personnel, and the ANC collaborated well with host governments on treatment, supplies, health education, and medical training.[126]

The ANC's early attempts to deal with health-related issues in exile included medical training abroad, the development of some semiformal care, and the eventual institutionalization of the medical sector in 1977. Consistent throughout this entire period was the ANC's strategic diplomatic use of healthcare; the medical sector had anti-apartheid-inclined medical students all over the world, it supplemented local health institutions with international medical personnel, and it at least partially represented South Africa at major international conferences relating to health. The ANC's strategic bureaucratization of the medical sector after the student uprisings in 1976 increased international support for the ANC's bid to be considered a government-in-waiting. Unfortunately, at the same time throughout the period of exile there was constant criticism of healthcare delivery to South African cadres and refugees. Early complaints pointed out the two-tiered nature of medical provision, and as the medical sector grew into a department it struggled to secure staff commitment to the project and centralize its authority among the regions.

2

"We Shall Continue to Treat ANC Patients at All Our Hospitals": Cooperation between the Health Department and Its Southern African Hosts

Bilateral cooperation between the ANC and its host countries was a prerequisite for the ANC Health Department's ability to deliver healthcare services. At significant national cost, the governments of Tanzania, Zambia, Zimbabwe, Angola, and Mozambique provided South African refugees with an opportunity to settle within their borders.[1] The ANC relied on this hospitality, and without it the Health Department would not have been able to build health infrastructure projects in southern Africa, train students, or register its doctors to practice medicine; in short, it would not have had an operational health department in exile. Independent nations in southern Africa already recognized the legitimacy of the ANC's anticolonial effort on a political and military level, and therefore, unlike the international realm farther abroad, the Health Department did not need to try to establish the illegitimacy of the NP and its own political viability. These southern nations had a major impact on the ANC's delivery of healthcare to its patients, and therefore the ANC's Health Department cannot be looked at in isolation from its allied neighbours.

The goal of the ANC's Health Department was to provide primary care to South Africans in exile. Primary care included curative and preventative approaches; it was necessary to be able to treat routine illnesses and injuries, provide health education to cadres and refugees, and to be proactive in preventing future illness through initiatives like providing mosquito nets. In many ways this was an ambitious goal because the department had a small medical staff, a large and diverse geographical region to cover, and was reliant on the benevolence of international donors to provide essential medical supplies. The Health Department had a fluctuating level of success in meeting its primary health goals, and, in so doing, it managed to intermittently supplement the host countries' primary healthcare needs. However, at times the dysfunctional organisation of the department warranted its hosts' support in providing even basic care. Additionally, the ANC's Health Department did not have the capacity to provide secondary, specialized care to its patients and, therefore, relied on its hosts' facilities and expertise to fill this gap in health coverage.

The provision of primary and secondary care was shaped by geographical location. Therefore, South African exiles' experience of medical care was also determined by region. The Tanzanian and Zambian Ministries of Health had a longer relationship with the ANC, and after 1977 dealt directly with Health Department leadership. ANC medical staff often worked in their hosts' medical facilities, and there was some level of mutual benefit gained by the partnership. However, the relationship in Zambia was primarily urban, and Tanzanian cooperation included both urban and rural components. Zimbabwe's Ministry of Health only formed a formal alliance with the ANC's medical sector in the 1980s. The arrangement was straightforward: when necessary, the ANC paid considerable sums of money for patients to travel to Harare and receive high quality, specialized care. The Angolan and Mozambican Ministries of Health, themselves sorely under-resourced and short-staffed, faced a mainly military South African population with scant, fluctuating medical support. These two countries supported the ANC but had less to offer in terms of medical provisions and reinforcement because they were bogged down by civil war with little chance to build up their own infrastructure and treatment capacity. However, the relationship between the ANC Health Department and its host ministries of health was different because the South African population in each area was different. Angola hosted thousands of South Africans – internationally labelled "refugees" – who were often fixed in specific locations for long periods of time. Additionally, the Namibian exiles far outnumbered the South Africans in the area and SWAPO – backed by Nordic funding – had already established some social infrastructure in the area. Consequently, there was a concerted effort to cooperate with SWAPO and access some of SWAPO's international support, while operating under such bleak conditions. Unlike the situation in Angola, Mozambique was host to less than 200 South African exiles who were typically very mobile.

The ANC's approach to malaria highlights the way that the ANC Health Department's multiregional operation placed additional strain on local ministries of health. The ANC's Health Department had varying success at dealing with malaria in each location and was, most often, unable to contend with the constant threat of malaria. Responsible for a mobile, guerrilla army as well as a large rurally based population in tight quarters, the ANC was not able to consistently deliver and monitor their population's use of the prophylactic malaria drug, cloroquine. As new resistance to chloroquine developed, the health of Tanzanian, Angolan, and Mozambican citizens was compromised and southern African health authorities insisted on keeping the ANC accountable for its negligence. Feeling the pressure from their hosts, the ANC attempted to maintain its independence from local governments and appealed to the WHO to support their attempt to care for their South African "citizens" in exile. Despite WHO involvement, the choices made by the ANC leadership impacted the epidemiology of malaria in southern Africa – much to the displeasure of their southern African hosts. Similarly, the response to HIV in exile is a product of the ANC Health Department's experience with cloroquine-resistant malaria. While HIV effected a smaller number of South African exiles and was more heavily stigmatized, the ANC leadership was quick to establish screening procedures and use HIV/AIDS conferences hosted in southern Africa to assert its solidarity with the region as well as its ability to deal with the epidemic in the future.

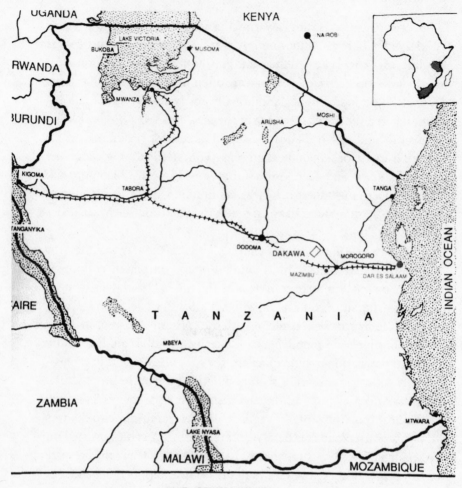

MAP OF TANZANIA

DISTANCES :
DAR ES SALAAM – MOROGORO   200 KM
MOROGORO – DAKAWA   60 KM
                    TOTAL   260 KM

2.1 The ANC in Tanzania. The geographical precision of this map
may be called into question. However, it demonstrates the
relationship between the three locations of the ANC and its
donors. "Map of Tanzania," no date.

Tanzania

Tanzania became the site of the ANC Health Department's most concerted efforts to provide medical services because, starting in the late 1970s and early 1980s, ANC involvement in Tanzania took on a distinctly civilian demeanour. Dar es Salaam became a transit hub for sick and injured MK cadres and for students coming and going from international studies, as well as a home to a number of ANC administrative facilities that were not assembled in Lusaka. A larger contingent of students, children, pregnant women, sick or disabled comrades, and professionals lived 180 kilometres west of Dar es Salaam near Morogoro in one of two ANC settlements: Mazimbu and Dakawa. The ANC's most developed RHT, the East Africa Health Team,[2] sought to provide for the primary health needs of South Africans in Tanzania while also trying to act as a triage centre for those in need of secondary healthcare. In this safer zone, patients comprised a diverse population and many of the health-related needs concerned maternal health, long-term disability, and mental health. By the mid-1980s, the ANC hospital at Mazimbu became the main referral centre for ANC patients in southern Africa. In short, Tanzania was home to a greater proportion of the ANC membership needing medical attention than the other regions in southern Africa.

Dar es Salaam's major state hospitals, under the authority of the Tanzanian government, were relatively well equipped and, therefore, ideal for comrades being flown in from frontline states needing urgent medical attention.[3] The main hospital used by the ANC was Muhimbili Medical Centre,[4] which provided specialist medical treatment and employed a handful of doctors affiliated with the ANC.[5] Consequently, a number of residences popped up in different Dar es Salaam districts operating as transit houses for the sick and injured as well as for students, cadres, and other ANC comrades. These patients also came from Morogoro and needed temporary lodging in Dar es Salaam.[6] The most important Dar es Salaam residence for the sick was the sickbay located in the Kurasini district though its medical performance left something to be desired by patients and staff alike. (The internal politics at Kurasini will be discussed in detail in chapter 4.) Rather than operating purely as a transit holding zone, Kurasini was also designed to house between fifteen and thirty patients on a longer-term basis.[7] Patients were ferried between the sickbay and the hospital; they received treatment at Muhimbili and then were supervised at Kurasini by medical support staff between appointments. Kurasini operated in some medical capacity for the ANC from 1974 to 1984 but only had any operational capacity as a sickbay due to its partnership with Muhimbili.

The ANC members were not easy guests in Tanzania's capital. The South Africans were idle and spread out in both Dar es Salaam and Morogoro town, and it was reported that, "The [Tanzanian] government is becoming concerned, they feel that Tanzania is becoming a dumping ground for the elements not needed by the organisation."[8] As had been the case in the past, many indolent South Africans in exile had problems with both alcohol and violence and both gave cause for international strain between the ANC and the Tanzanian government.[9] South African patients needing specialized attention not available elsewhere in the country were still able to use Muhimbili Medical Centre, but long-term care in Dar es Salaam was coming to an end. It was neither the government's nor the ANC's intention for Dar es Salaam to become a permanent home to South Africans. In order to move the masses of ANC and MK personnel out of the capital, the organisation was given land near Morogoro to create a more permanent "refugee" settlement.[10] In giving the ANC land to establish Mazimbu and later Dakawa, the Tanzanian government was looking to contain the growing problem by establishing exclusive ANC localities.[11]

The first South Africans arrived at Mazimbu, Morogoro in 1977.[12] In 1978 the ANC started the construction of the Solomon Mahlangu Freedom College (SOMAFCO), an institution initially envisioned as a secondary school in Mazimbu (see figure 2.1) and later expanded to include primary school students as well.[13] Due to population growth in the region, the ANC also sought to provide primary healthcare in the community by building its own health clinic with the knowledge that the Tanzanian hospitals in Morogoro and Dar es Salaam could still be called upon in cases of emergency. The Health Department staff leaned heavily on the resources of the Morogoro Regional Hospital which had the capacity to perform minor surgeries and treat most illnesses and injuries. Without a doctor in Mazimbu until 1984, even any mildly acute illness had to be referred to Morogoro and all pregnant women were sent there when it came time for them to give birth.

An ANC hospital in Mazimbu was proposed in 1978 shortly after the department's inauguration, when the Medisch Komitee Angola (MKA), a Netherlands-based donor, agreed to fund a new hospital with an eighteen-bed capacity for the ANC refugee and student community.[14] The hospital was to be called the ANC–Holland Solidarity Hospital, and it was intended to be tightly connected to the secondary school in Mazimbu while offering classes in first aid and health science to students and residents in the settlement.[15] The ANC hoped that the hospital would eventually have twenty beds for adult patients and eight for children. Much to the annoyance of the ANC leadership, when the hospital was finally opened in 1984 it, too, was unable to operate completely autonomously and relied on Tanzanian support.[16] At a secretariat meeting in Lusaka, it was estimated that the hospital would need twenty-two people to adequately run the facility.[17] On this subject the secretariat stated, "In terms of staffing, the ANC must encourage that its own resources be exhausted first. If the ANC expertise is not available, than [sic] ... local expertise should be identified. In the same spirit [of cooperation,] assistance from friendly countries will be sought, whenever necessary."[18] The Health Department was accustomed to the constant support shown by their Tanzanian hosts and fully expected to be able to draw from this important resource in order to staff their new facility.

Confidence in Tanzanian medical support was founded not only on the ANC's experience of solidarity up until that point; the Tanzanian government specifically stated that it was prepared to be of service. At the ceremonial opening of the ANC's hospital in May 1984, the regional secretary of Chama Cha Mapanduzi (ruling political party in Tanzania), Ndugu Manduka, gave a particularly strong statement of solidarity:

[T]he Tanzanian Government is behind you. We truly support the ANC and shall continue to give every support for the ANC to win the war in South Africa. We know the position you are in now ... Speakers here have said how much support Tanzania has given. This is not true – we have given nothing. We shall give more ... The Chairman had said that you get much help from the Morogoro hospital. By building your own hospital, does not mean an end to this help. On the contrary, it is only the beginning. We shall continue to treat ANC patients at all our hospitals whenever it may be necessary.[19]

The Tanzanian Ministry of Health derived some benefit from the ANC's presence in the region; the ANC's hospital did not turn Tanzanian patients away from its facility, and as a result ANC medical staff saw significantly more Tanzanians than it did South Africans. In 1985 the ANC–Solidarity Hospital staff saw 16,758 patients at the polyclinic; there were 7,081 from the ANC community and 9,677 Tanzanians.[20] The ANC medical staff fielded some of the primary healthcare needs and sent all acute cases to Morogoro. Mazimbu staff then did rounds at the Morogoro Regional Hospital in order to keep proper tabs on their patients.[21] All-in-all, the relationship between the Mazimbu and Morogoro health staff was often mutually beneficial.

In 1981 while the Health Department was still waiting on the construction of the MKA-sponsored ANC–Holland Solidarity Hospital, the Tanzanian government gave the ANC another 7,500 acres near Morogoro to accommodate the growing number of South African refugees and students. The residential centre in this land allotment, developed by the ANC starting in late 1981, was named Dakawa and was located approximately sixty kilometres north of Morogoro.[22] While not stated explicitly, the settlement was also intended to contain some of the most problematic members of the ANC: namely those who were violent, rule breaking, unskilled, or mentally ill.[23] The land was off the beaten track and located near a Tanzanian prison.

The ANC's original plan for Dakawa was that it be used as a "reception for all students both secondary and post-secondary level"; in essence, this site was meant to allow leadership to screen students, provide them with a political education, and introduce various opportunities for secondary education or work in exile.[24] The ANC also hoped that the community would be able to be self-sustaining. It sought to establish a vocational training centre, a childcare centre, and an agricultural project.[25] Coinciding with these ANC aspirations, at the end of 1981 the Health Department was already considering its future in Dakawa; Manto Tshabalala proposed to reallocate DKK235,875 (US$33,000), earmarked for the Mazimbu hospital, towards the establishment of a health centre in Dakawa.[26]

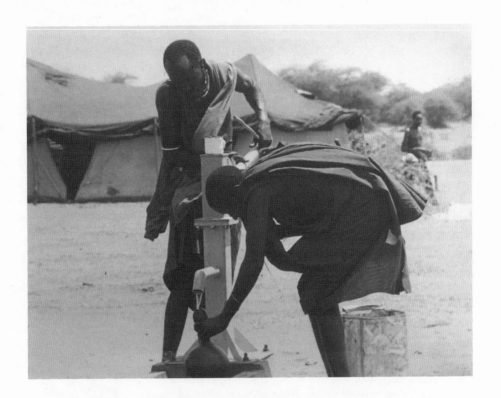

2.2 Maasai in Dakawa. This is an image of two Maasai people getting water from a pump in Dakawa. Photograph, no date.

Early in 1982 the amount of actual construction progress and infrastructure development was minimal, but the Health Department sought to provide some level of primary healthcare for the approximately one hundred South Africans currently staying in Dakawa. Regina Nzo, then regional chair of the East Africa Health Team, went to see what immediate measures could be put in place and whether it would be possible to establish a relationship with the nearby Tanzanian prison hospital.[27] While the boundaries of the relationship were not yet worked out, she found that the prison's meagre medical facilities were already serving the needs of ANC personnel.[28] Not wanting to completely rely on the Tanzanian prison, the department sought also to contribute to healthcare provision in the region.[29] By mid-year the East Africa Health Team had established a small health post and was reportedly receiving approximately 1,000 patients per month.[30]

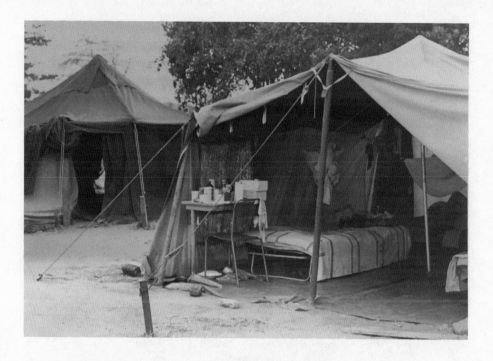

2.3 Dakawa's first health post. The image depicts a small tent with
three beds and a small desk. There is a collection of
medical supplies on the desk. Photograph, 1983.

This estimation is almost certainly an exaggeration; the number was
probably closer to 400 patients per month. Regardless, the inflated
number hints at the desperate lack of healthcare resources in the
area. The benevolence of Tanzanian regional efforts was returned at
the new health post where, undoubtedly, the majority of the patients
seen were Tanzanian.[31]

The facilities and staff available were still not enough to accommodate patient needs. Dakawa's population steadily grew and it had
a reputation of being a "dumping ground" for undesirable South
African exiles. Medical staff did not want to be assigned to posts in
Dakawa and viewed being sent there as a punishment.[32] Therefore,
posts were often filled by a rotation of staff; doctors working with
the ANC in Morogoro visited Dakawa once or twice a week to do
rounds and treat patients who were not able to travel to Mazimbu
for treatment due to a lack of transport.[33] While the health team

in Mazimbu tried to assert that being sent to Dakawa was not a punishment, the conditions in the settlement did not support their argument. Dakawa was a place to send students who were expelled from SOMAFCO for a variety of reasons including dagga (cannabis) or alcohol abuse, violence, thievery, and in at least one case having been charged with rape.[34] Fathering a child or procuring an abortion were also grounds for expulsion and banishment to Dakawa. Sick comrades were sent to the settlement despite the lack of medical resources,[35] and it was also, at least by the end of 1982, the ultimate destination for mentally ill comrades who were to receive rehabilitation through practical work-related activities.[36] At the request of Dr Manto Tshabalala, Tanzanian doctor Dr J.G. Hauli visited the site to evaluate the impact of the poor conditions in Dakawa on the mental health of the residents. He found that "people thought that they were in solitary confinement or prison camp. Some were so angry that an explosion seemed eminent."[37] In an extreme case one young woman stated that she would commit suicide if forced to return to Dakawa.[38]

One 1985 report provided a short but, nevertheless, informative snapshot of healthcare in Dakawa. There were eight distinct zones in Dakawa: plot eighteen (Ruth First), plot seventeen, plot sixteen (Lillian Ngoyi), plot twenty-two (Elias Motswaledi), plot twenty-one (Raymond Mhlaba), the Paul Peterson Residence, the Vocational Training Centre, and a location simply called "Site."[39] Among these zones, two had functioning medical points: one was at Ruth First run by two medical officers and an ANC doctor (Dr Abel Maminze) and the other was at Elias Motswaledi run by one medical officer and one ANC doctor (Dr Sandile Mfenyana).[40] Both doctors were in Dakawa because they had just completed their training and were eagerly awaiting reassignment. The two posts were one kilometer apart and the report claimed that, together, they saw between 1,500 and 2,000 patients per month.

One of the biggest problems for the ANC Health Department's operation in Dakawa was its distance to Morogoro. Sixty kilometres was a prohibitive distance for patients to travel without reliable transportation.[41] One report indicated that the team saw an average of ten patients per day who needed care that could not be afforded in Dakawa, but the lack of transportation prevented timely transfers to

Morogoro. In order to provide for these patients in an acceptable way, the anonymous author of the report estimated that Dakawa would need a car, a ten or fifteen passenger vehicle, two scooters, and four bicycles.[42] Considering the supplies in the region, it was unrealistic to ask for this level of mobility. However, the transport that *was* made available was handled in a corrupt and undisciplined manner that sometimes had deadly consequences for comrades in need of urgent care in Morogoro. The vehicles were either monopolized by administration or mishandled, leading the author of the report to state, "transport is carelessly looked after no one is called to book for damaging transport and even killing of locals. No measures are taken to correct those at fault."[43]

The two health posts in Dakawa were only able to provide intermittent treatment for nonsevere cases of malaria, provide basic first aid to minor injuries, and act as a triage centre for patients who desperately needed services in Morogoro or Mazimbu. However, the preventative and educational aspects of primary care were almost nonexistent, and the ability to give patients access to timely secondary care was dismal. The relative isolation and general punitive feel of Dakawa made working in the settlement especially undesirable, and it was a constant struggle for the East Africa Health Team to force qualified members of the medical staff to work there. ANC doctors preferred collaborating with Tanzanian medical professionals, working in equipped facilities, and serving the needs of ANC patients within those facilities. This was the relationship established in Dar es Salaam and Mazimbu, but the lack of a major Tanzanian facility close to Dakawa made a similar arrangement impossible. Without the ability to collaborate closely with the Morogoro hospital, even primary health provisions in Dakawa left much to be desired.

Zambia

Like Tanzania, in Zambia, as one of the ANC's earliest homes in exile, comrades had a long relationship with local facilities and had been drawing on Zambia's healthcare system since at least the early 1970s. However, the ANC's position in Zambia was unique: it was neither a civilian zone like Tanzania nor a military zone like Angola or Mozambique. Instead, Lusaka was the political headquarters and relatively sparsely populated in the late 1970s and early 1980s. Additionally, it was roughly the centre point between all other ANC settlements in southern Africa making it a good transit point and meeting hub. Lusaka's South African population grew, and its demographic changed throughout the 1980s. In 1982 and 1983 it was estimated that between 300 and 400 ANC comrades were in Lusaka and between 200 and 300 were at Chongella farm – the ANC's agricultural project forty to fifty kilometers from the city.[44] In 1985 the number of comrades in Lusaka had risen to more than 700 and over the next five years, the population grew exponentially. By 1989 Lusaka had an ANC population of about 2,000, reflecting the exodus of ANC and MK from Angola. The population doubled by the end of the following year.[45] The top-notch healthcare provided to the leadership in Lusaka in the early 1980s was not able to accommodate the rapid growth, and consequently healthcare available to South Africans in Lusaka became two-tiered.

In the late 1970s and early 1980s members of the ANC leadership in Lusaka were typically the most fortunate recipients of healthcare in exile because the population was small and based in Lusaka. Healthcare at the primary and secondary level in Lusaka was easily available due to Zambia's relatively well-established health system and infrastructure. In addition the Zambian Ministry of Health readily integrated ANC doctors and doctors-in-training into its healthcare system.[46] Starting in the late 1970s UTH hosted medical internships for doctors. Doctors who had completed their medical training abroad could apply to the Zambian Ministry of Health to do their "housemanships"[47] in Lusaka in order to serve the ANC while fully qualifying in their field. Others also applied for work at the hospital in order to gain experience and have the opportunity to work in a fully equipped facility. In 1978 the Medical Committee, in establishing the number of South African medical personnel available to it, reported five doctors and "a good number of qualified nurses" in Lusaka.[48] The fact that there were five doctors in the region meant that Zambia was home to the most qualified South African medical staff in exile – a consistent reality throughout the ANC's stay in southern Africa. The ANC also saw their doctors' placement in Lusaka as an opportunity to improve their relationship with their hosts. In the housemanship placement application letters written on behalf of

Dr Haggar McBerry and Dr Prenaven Naicker, the ANC reminded the Zambian ministry that the placements were "also in line with our policy to render any possible assistance to our Zambian comrades."[49] Of course, having its own ANC personnel on hand was beneficial as well to ANC patients in the city.

Hospitals were able to capitalize on this skilled ANC labour force while the ANC leadership was able to gain access to Zambian medical facilities at minor expense. The two major health centres frequented by ANC members in Lusaka were UTH and Chainama Hills Psychiatric facility. Both were well-equipped and received South African patients referred from the frontline states and Tanzania.[50] UTH was host to both ANC patients and many ANC health personnel. Chainama Hills was specifically designed for psychiatric patients, and many ANC patients were accepted for treatment throughout the 1970s and 1980s; however, unlike UTH, there was no ANC medical staff at Chainama Hills because of the paucity of qualified ANC medical professionals in the mental health field. The consequence of this close relationship between the ANC and local facilities was that the ANC made poor use of their own resources in Lusaka. Relative to other regions at that time, there was a high level of privilege and sense of entitlement to specialized healthcare.

At least as early as 1978, the ANC's Zambia RHT had a small dispensary that was supposed to act as a minor treatment and triage centre while also a repository for medical supplies, equipment, and drugs. In particular, some drugs were kept at the dispensary and provided to patients in order to save money on purchasing drugs from local pharmacies.[51] The utilization of the dispensary in the late 1970s and early 1980s served to characterize a unique problem for the Zambia RHT: the inability to persuade patients to seek healthcare at ANC facilities before attending local hospitals. In 1979 the Medical Committee was still in the process of centralizing authority, and the newly formed RHTs were attempting to formalize their role with ANC patients. The new dispensary staff felt bypassed and recommended,

Consultations should and must be run only in the dispensary, except for genuinely critical patients ... Our people must be prepared to follow the normal routine in all the Medical Centres without expecting obviously unnecessary special arrangements to be made for them at the expense of the local population.[52]

One year later, the problem had not been resolved. Rather than receiving medical attention at the dispensary, the staff used the ambulance to ferry comrades to hospitals and pharmacies; those who did intend to receive medical attention at the dispensary were let down by an absence of staff. In 1982 the underutilization of available resources and expertise was further commented on: "The ambulance was used mostly for getting prescriptions at various pharmacies around Lusaka … The Medical Assistant's time and even that of the MCH [Mother and Child Health] Aid was spent mostly in locating a drug in town."[53] It was concluded that the team was uncoordinated, needed firmer job descriptions, and clear authoritative command.

Part of the problem was the long-established pattern of seeing doctors in Lusaka hospitals. At the time of the 1982 report, there were four qualified ANC doctors at UTH and patients preferred and felt entitled to medical rather than paramedical attention. Tanzanian psychiatrist J.G. Hauli, mentioned previously, also evaluated the situation in Zambia and aptly summed it up:

> Inspite [*sic*] of the presence of a number of doctors at the UCTH [UTH] as well as Nurses, the Health Activities were in disarray and the dispensary staff morale was very low. They complained that they only work as messengers as everybody only wants to see a doctor. Obviously they will feel useless and some indicated a request to move from the health team.[54]

The doctors and other medical staff at UTH were divided on how to deal with the situation. Dr Prenaven Naicker described a rigorous schedule of attending to ANC patients during work breaks, throughout the evening, and sometimes in the middle of the night. He felt that it was his duty as a member of the ANC to provide the best and most immediate treatment to ANC comrades in Lusaka.[55]

In addition to the underutilisation of ANC health facilities, Naicker also faced opposition against his prioritization of ANC members. He noted that the opposition was "[b]ecause some felt that our people wanted to be … well they were getting spoiled by this form of individual attention that I was giving then [sic] and they thought this was unfair on our community, that I'm not really setting the example, of people actually using the facilities of this Zambian hospital and that I was actually drawing people away from a set pattern."[56] The ideal "set pattern" was for the ANC members to queue to see a doctor rather than have special access to immediate healthcare. Naicker's opposition was merely calling for the ANC to use the proper channels, on par with what was available to Zambians. However, without a clear policy or ability to police doctors' behaviour, it was Naicker's prerogative to treat patients as he saw fit.

The RHT was not a coordinated or cohesive unit accountable to the health secretariat. The team meetings showed poor attendance and the urgency so evident in other regions was absent in Lusaka. At the end of 1982 it was reported that the team did not record the names of patients that came through the dispensary, they did not submit financial statements, they stopped submitting strategic bulk orders for essential medicine, and the staff's efforts were disorganized.[57] In 1984 ANC Administrative Secretary Edna Miya penned her long-suffering frustration at Lusaka's negligence toward its duties as an RHT: "It is unpleasant for us to write you a letter completely different from those written to other health teams … other health teams, with less qualified personnel than your team, have compiled their reports in accordance with the guidelines … it is glaring that your team's activities are not reflected [in our yearly department report]."[58] While the Zambia RHT was not operating in a cooperative manner, their Zambian host's health support shielded South African patients from the ANC's inability to provide optimal care.

Unlike other regions where problems included inadequate care, staff shortages, and, consequently, suffering patients, the problem in this region in the early 1980s was underutilization of the available resources and overuse of the Zambian state facilities. Indeed, one 1984 letter reported that one Lusaka health team member's negligence in duties could be chalked up to the fact that the region was "overstaffed."[59] Another discussion paper stated, "statistically we have in exile one of the highest ratios of doctors/population probably in the world" and relative to the other ANC-occupied regions in exile, the evidence of this beneficial ratio was most clear in Lusaka.[60]

Even though the dispensary in Lusaka was not used adequately in the early 1980s, the ANC decided to produce a fully fledged clinic to serve ANC medical needs.[61] The clinic opened in the Emmasdale district of Lusaka in 1984 and "comprise[d] a reception room, file store, consultation room, dressing room for staff members who are on night duty, a drug store, kitchen, two toilets and one bathroom."[62] Unlike the Mazimbu hospital, Emmasdale clinic did not have inpatient services, but it, too, was focused on primary healthcare delivery.

Just as Emmasdale was opening it was evident that the healthcare provided to the expanding number of ANC/MK residents in the city was two-tiered. In January 1985, Dr Sipho Mthembu and one other clinic staff member, Nomna Jobodwana, visited the ANC residences in Mtendere district in Lusaka and discovered that the living conditions were subpar and that the comrades were in urgent need of access to consistent health services.[63] This district was home to a number of MK cadres. Mthembu reported, "The faces of all comrades were expressionless and there was no happiness at all."[64] The residences were unsanitary and residents were living in squalor. Within the next year, an ANC health post was set up in the district, and Dr Naicker was made the officer in charge of the post. Between March and October 1986, Naicker saw 332 patients. Typically, the patients complained of fever/flu, "coughings," gonorrhoea, and fungal infections.[65]

Emmasdale clinic was not initially within the reach of those in Mtendere. The clinic was a unique project; despite the up-to-then reliance on Zambian health facilities, it was the only clinic that was not immediately set to serve the needs of locals as well as ANC members. In June 1985 ANC leadership considered a system in which locals would have to pay for services rendered. This may have been a reflection of the locally prevailing system in Zambia; the bigger public hospitals were less equipped but free while the smaller private clinics provided excellent if expensive care.[66] For its size the Emmasdale clinic was well staffed and had the *potential* to offer better healthcare than in the public hospitals. In addition to one ANC doctor consulting from UTH, there were six medical officers working at the clinic, and the team collectively saw 360 patients per month. However, the fee-for-service principle attempted at Emmasdale was not easily maintained. The last quarterly report for 1986 noted that one of the problems of the clinic was that ANC comrades brought Zambian friends for treatment, and it was nearly impossible to turn these residents away.[67] The ANC medical sector in Zambia was too intertwined with Zambia's Ministry of Health to be able to execute a policy of exclusion against Lusaka dwellers. Moreover, in order to legitimately be able to charge for service, the clinic would have to qualify for registration by the Zambian Ministry of Health. To accomplish this it needed to improve its overall treatment capacity. The clinic would need a permanent doctor on staff, provision for inpatient treatment, and a general upgrade of the available services.[68] In addition, the behaviour of the staff would have to be brought up to professional standards. One report mentioned that patient confidentially was not kept, causing ANC members to be reluctant to use the clinic. This was particularly a problem in the face of the HIV/AIDS epidemic where stigma against HIV+ patients was dangerously high.[69] Furthermore, junior staff members, without seeking the advice of senior and more qualified personnel, sometimes made poor judgement calls.[70]

With the growing MK population in Lusaka, Emmasdale, like the Mtendere health post, slowly began to address the needs of the military. In 1986 the clinic added to its facility a twenty-patient rehabilitation centre called "the annex." This was an attempt at community-centred treatment for mentally ill patients transferred from the military frontline.[71] Patients were given an initial assessment and treatment at UTH or Chainama Hills and subsequently accommodated at the annex. Those who caused problems in Lusaka at the annex were sent to Dakawa, home of the main rehabilitation facility. The efficacy of both rehabilitation facilities will be discussed in chapter 5, but it should be mentioned here that the annex was left somewhat neglected and governed by untrained staff. A report on the health provisions in Zambia in late 1987 stated, "Life at the centre [the annex] is a bit monotonous. You find comrades resorting to their rooms and sleeping. For better results to be achieved in this centre, something had to be done urgently in a way of rehabilitating these cdes [comrades]."[72] By 1988 the medical staff at Emmasdale allocated the supervision of the annex to junior medical staff on a rotational basis. Unfortunately, this was not an effective care model. A March 1988 report stated that the person in charge did not take his responsibility seriously, was not often found at the clinic, and only occasionally checked on the evidently bored "inmates."[73]

The situation in Lusaka clearly illuminates the interconnected-ness between the ANC's medical efforts and the Zambian Ministry of Health. The system of medical provision in Zambia changed throughout the 1980s as the population increased. When the population was small and urban, the ANC leadership drew heavily on its host's resources and underutilized its own healthcare provision. As the population grew, the level of care became more evidently two-tiered. The previous system of immediate care in Zambian facilities could not accommodate the hundreds of South African newcomers in Lusaka, and consequently, they were left to use the ANC's underdeveloped primary healthcare structures. However, relative to other regions, if an ANC member needed medical attention, it was probably most advantageous for that member to be sick or injured in Zambia. The clinic staff had struggles amongst itself, but, based on local availability, the care in Zambia had the capacity to be nearly immediate and specialized.

Zimbabwe

In the late 1980s, Zimbabwe was a destination that rivalled Zambia for care. A report commissioned by the Norwegian Trade Union Research Centre in 1987 claimed that "very complicated and serious cases" were sent from Zambia (or elsewhere) to Harare.[74] The short distance between Lusaka and Harare further facilitated this custom. Manto Tshabalala weighed in on the practice of transferring patients between Zambia and Zimbabwe:

> [We] are equally concerned about the medical ethics, and the political impression our Organisation potrays [sic] both to the doctors attending our people and the health services of Zambia as a whole, by transferring our patients back-wards and forward from equally competent health services. This is, in fact, silently declaring that we have no confidence in the services offered in our countries of refugee [sic]. We need to re-examine this exercise.[75]

Significantly, Tshabalala pointed out that the ANC health service's only job in this process was to be the facilitator of patient transfers.

The ANC only established an RHT in Zimbabwe in 1984, and the extent to which it settled into the region was minimal relative to the longer relationships developed in Tanzania and Zambia. However, Zimbabwe had a lot to offer the ANC in terms of healthcare. The new government of postcolonial Zimbabwe was the beneficiary of a relatively well-developed medical infrastructure, the best of which had been previously established for the settler population. The facilities, expertise, and medical schools in Harare were used by the ANC in Zimbabwe's postindependence period.

Some of the earliest connections made between the medical departments in Zimbabwe and the ANC were to do with their efforts to deal with mental health. Both the ANC and Zimbabwe joined the African Mental Health Action Group in 1982 and were a part of discussions about how to establish programs and facilities for mentally ill patients. In 1983 Roy Campbells was the first student accepted for a scholarship to study social work and rehabilitation in Harare.[76] That same year discussions commenced between Tshabalala and the deputy minister of health in Zimbabwe regarding the provision of positions for ANC students to study medicine and nursing at the Zimbabwe medical school.[77]

In January 1984 two students were accepted for placement in the medical school in Harare.[78] There were also ANC patients being treated in facilities in Harare as well as a slow trickle of medical professionals attempting to get accreditation and work in Zimbabwe.[79] In keeping with the Health Department developments elsewhere in southern Africa, the department sought to operationalize its own RHT in Harare. In April 1984, led by social work student Roy Campbells, a "health team nucleus" of five members came together and by October of that year, the group officially became the new Zimbabwe RHT.[80] However, from 1984 to 1990 the team did little more than find Zimbabwean physicians and other medical care providers in the region who would be willing and able to treat incoming ANC patients.[81] Medical services in Zimbabwe were based entirely on Zimbabwean rather than ANC resources.

Throughout 1985 Zimbabwe accepted additional medical staff to work in its hospitals and new students to study at its medical school. Consequently, the ANC was building a considerable medical community in the area.[82] By 1987 the team rivalled Zambia for being the most medically qualified team; there were six doctors, two medical students, two pharmacists, a nurse, and a physiotherapist.[83] In late 1987 the team also acquired a residence-cum-sickbay and an ambulance to transport patients to and from the hospitals. The sickbay was a way to house patients who were visiting Zimbabwean facilities and needing extra care between treatments, but the focus of the team at the sickbay was not to provide treatment but to move the patients from the sickbay to proper care in the city.[84]

The practice of treating patients in Harare was of considerable expense to the movement. Based on healthcare spending in 1986, the health team put together an approximately US$25,000 yearly budget for hospital fees, doctor fees, and prescriptions in addition to their own vehicle upkeep and the daily needs of patients.[85] This budget, however, was seriously expanded in the 1989 to 1990 project proposal to Finnida (a Finland-based donor). The team reported that it would need nearly US$210,000 in order to pay for local care, equip its own sickbay, and cover the costs of secondary medical caregivers for the residence.[86] Until the unbanning of the ANC in 1990, the comparatively low number of patients seeking treatment in the area meant that healthcare was characterised by expensive, Zimbabwean-provided, high-quality care.[87]

Military Zones

The political and military situation in Angola and Mozambique presented unique challenges to the ANC Health Department. In the late 1970s and 1980s, both countries were newly liberated, host to thousands of South African and Namibian "refugees," and still in the middle of civil war. Consequently, the ANC's host governments' health infrastructures were grossly underdeveloped, leaving the cadres in regions with minimal options for local ongoing medical support. Cadres were transient and often unable to benefit from any level of healthcare consistency. In addition to their cooperation with local governments, the ANC Health Department sought to partner with the medical sector serving the Namibian refugee population. As early as 1979 the ANC's medical leadership reported, "The general feeling is that it is time we explored possibilities of having closer working relations with the Medial Department of the Patriotic Front and

SWAPO. This will help us to exchange views and experiences and possibly come to one another's assistance whenever the situation demands."[88] But, the ANC did not have much to offer in the partnership; many ANC health professionals found the conditions in military zones undesirable, and without proper equipment and supplies in the camps, trained personnel thought they would not be properly utilized, the environmental conditions left much to be desired, and enemy attack was a constant threat. Therefore, the leadership put pressure on the Health Department, which then tried to persuade medical professionals to work in military regions, and the professionals often pushed back against what could be interpreted punishment. As a result the military zones suffered from a serious and chronic lack of qualified staff and medical attention.

For many of these reasons the ANC was often unable to provide even basic primary healthcare in military zones. Without medical attention, minor health issues escalated into major, acute health problems, and the department typically sought to transport the comrades from the military front lines to Dar es Salaam or Lusaka to receive specialized treatment. As a result and because the quality of medical provision on the part of all three parties was low, the relationship between these two Ministries of Health and the ANC Health Department was thin. However, this did not mean that the separate medical sectors were not interconnected. Within the realm of available healthcare , it is clear that the ANC worked cooperatively with SWAPO and the Angolan and Mozambican Ministries of Health in order to achieve better health outcomes.

Angola

Between 1977 and 1979 there were two main MK camps in Angola situated south of Luanda: Bengula and its successor, Novo Catengue.[89] Novo Catengue was the political and ideological training ground for new MK recruits. It was estimated by Gwendolyn Sello, a member of the Angola Health Team, that between the two camps and Luanda, there were about 500 cadres, twenty-five of whom were female.[90] At this early stage, the ANC relied on Cuban support and leadership in the camp and, consequently, were also the beneficiaries of Cuban medical services.[91] The ANC provided medical staff to the camps and actively sought support for drugs and first aid supplies. From May 1977 to August 1978 Novo Catengue received medical equipment and supplies from their hosts in Angola as well as the Red Cross, the MKA, Romania, the GDR, and Secours Populaire francais.[92] Furthermore, the camps had relatively steady access to two ANC doctors (Dr Peter Mfelang and Dr Novama Shangase) and two nurses (Gwendolyn Sello and "nurse Alice").[93] Healthcare was nothing to boast about in the two camps at that time, but it was significant that some level of primary care was made available.

Medical attention slowly began to decline after Novo Catengue was destroyed in the March 1979 attack and as the level of internal security and militarization within the zone increased. There were two reasons for this decline. First, cadres were spread out even further between newly created camps so that a future airstrike would not be disastrous. Regarding the social effects of this spread, MK cadre Thula Bopela wrote, "with camps located in different regions and different countries the feeling of togetherness that had been experienced at Novo Katenga was lost. The camps established in Angola were Quatro, Camp 13, Pango[,] Quibaxe, Viana Transit Camp and Caculama."[94] In addition to ebbing morale, the increased number of camps meant that the medical support available was stretched thinner than before. Some reports claimed that, due to the poor road conditions, the camps were three to five days' drive from Luanda. The great distances between camps coupled with a lack of transport made the availability of medical expertise, equipment, and supplies unreliable. The overall quality of care was low in the camps. There was a lack of experienced personnel – often the camp "medical staff" included one in-service medical trainee – and a shortage of medical equipment and supplies.[95]

Thus far there are no figures available to indicate exactly how many cadres were in Angola from 1979 to 1990. Additionally, it is not possible to determine exactly how many South Africans living in Angola at this time were directly involved in MK and how many were refugees or the families of cadres. Certainly, the labels "refugee" and "cadre" had international political significance with respect to their donors' financial contribution. Some international donors, wishing to appear neutral to military positions, were able to politically justify assistance to South African "refugees" rather than military "cadres."

This politicization of the South African population in Angola must certainly contribute to the discrepancy between historical accounts.[96]

In 1979 the United Nations High Commissioner for Refugees (UNHCR) had deemed there to be 1,000 South African refugees in Angola; in October 1981 the UNHCR estimated the number had risen to 5,000.[97] These numbers are much higher than the estimates given by the ANC, which alleged there were approximately 500 cadres in Angola between 1977 and 1979.[98] It is likely that the ANC's estimates did not include the children of MK men and Angolan women or people escaping the apartheid government but not explicitly a part of MK. Supporting this notion is the fact that of the 1981 UNHCR estimate of 5,000 "refugees" nearly 40 per cent were thought to be female. It is improbable that MK had recruited that many women into their ranks.[99]

In any case, the ANC Health Department had to care for a combination of MK cadres and South African refugees and, while seeking to cooperate with the Angola Ministry of Health, it also deepened its relationship with SWAPO. SWAPO was operating in camps in Angola and receiving funds for social infrastructure projects from primarily Sweden and Norway.[100] The Swedish government and a number of Swedish humanitarian agencies partnered with SWAPO to serve thousands[101] of Namibian exiles at their Kwanza Sul camp (located within Kwanza Sul province).[102] The medical projects at the camp provided Namibian refugees with better healthcare than their Angolan counterparts in the area.[103] As was the case in Tanzania and Zambia, the ANC sought collaboration with the major state hospital in the capital, Luanda. Manto Tshabalala visited Angola for over two weeks in July and August 1980 to meet with the Angolan Ministry of Health. The health minister agreed to formally register ANC doctors working both in and outside of Luanda.[104] As with other regions, this action was vital for the ANC to entice South African doctors to the region. If the doctors worked in local hospitals they would be paid for their work and able to serve the needs of MK from within the hospital. Without registration, the doctors would be isolated in the camps.[105] The collaboration between the ANC and MPLA medical services also opened up opportunities for further education. In 1982 the University of Angola agreed to take ten medical students from the ANC, sponsored by the WHO, to study medicine.[106]

While Dr Tshabalala was in western Angola, she also assessed one hundred patients, ensured that MK cadres got treatment at Angolan facilities, and referred several acutely ill or injured patients out of the country. Even her visits to local hospitals were done with the intent of entrenching solidarity; she explicitly stated that she wanted to visit patients but also to "strengthen working relations with the Health Personnel [in Angola]."[107] Optimistically, with the new ability for doctors to be registered in Angola, the ANC hoped to send two doctors to work in Luanda by the end of the year. The placement would be good for its bilateral relationship with Angolan medical services.

In early 1984 a health centre and clinic were planned for Viana, a small town about twenty kilometers from Luanda (the camp at Viana was used as a transit camp for MK).[108] Having the ANC health facilities close to Luanda made it more realistic for doctors to be stationed there. Those doctors would have the ability to see more patients and the option of also seeking employment with the Angolan Ministry of Health, and the centre and clinic would be accessible for doctors who were only in Angola for brief periods of time. Furthermore, the clinic was strategically positioned close to SWAPO's camp at Kwanza-Sul. With the two liberation movements in close geographic proximity, it was easier to coordinate and maximize Nordic support. For instance, a coalition of Nordic organisations was able to provide first aid instructor training to both ANC and SWAPO students at Kwanza Sul.[109]

The ANC's Viana clinic was, at least initially, designed to provide primary healthcare for 250 to 300 people including members of the ANC community in Luanda and Viana as well as Angolan citizens. The clinic also acted as the main referral centre for those in the camps who were sick but could not be treated in the abysmal camp facilities. However, due to the clinic's limited capacity to treat seriously ill or injured patients, it was mainly a triage centre to refer cadres to Angolan facilities or, when possible, another host country's facilities. The ANC and its international donors hoped that Viana would become a self-reliant centre with the capacity to make the South Africans in Angola somewhat self-sufficient. Furthermore, the future vision for Viana was to include an ANC health education centre that would act as a training school for ANC and SWAPO students interested in the medical field. The project was designed to build ANC autonomy and reduce its draw on its host's paltry social resource supply.

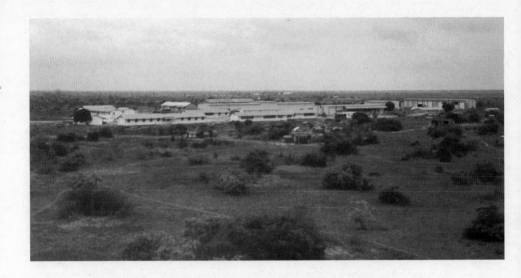

2.4 Viana health project. The archive's description of this
     photograph stated, "The project included the buildings
     for the Vocational Training and Health Care Centre in Viana.
     Phase I the building types were classroom and library
     blocks, dining hall/kitchen, dormitory and ablution blocks,
     semi-detached houses, mechanics' and tailors' workshops,
     administration and storage blocks and truck parking."
     "Makrotalo oy: Vocational Training and Health Care
     Centre, Viana, Angola," no date.

In 1987 a report commissioned by the Norwegian Trade Union
Research Centre found that the health education centre had been built
and was enrolling ten ANC and ten SWAPO students into one-year
medical training courses.[110] While this was a step towards generating
some level of autonomy, the conditions at the school were poor. The
ANC leadership struggled to find qualified teachers, and the students
were left without transport, adequate diet, or appropriate housing.
The report described the clinic, then designed to treat 500 to 600
patients per month, as serving only 200 to 300 patients per month
with more than half being Angolans.[111] Several factors contributed
to this underachievement: there was very little medical equipment
available, the mother and child health facilities were inadequate, the
clinic had only a single six-bed ward, and the workforce operating
the clinic was inadequate. In essence, the clinic was not even able
to provide basic primary healthcare services. This lack of healthcare

capacity was in keeping with the general quality of care available to the ANC and MK in Angola. While the ANC and the Angolan Ministry of Health had a collaborative relationship, the healthcare available in the country was such that, typically, the ANC sought supplementary secondary healthcare outside of Angola.

Mozambique

The health collaboration in Mozambique was much the same as in Angola except that in the case of Mozambique, the relationship was dramatically downsized after the Nkomati Accord was signed in March 1984, and MK was pushed out of the country. Until then ANC-affiliated civilians and cadres in Mozambique were split between two regions: Maputo in the south and Nampula/Cabo Delgado provinces in the north. The south carried the larger percentage of the population. Similar to the situation in Dar es Salaam, the ANC had residences in and around Maputo, which were used as transit or semipermanent housing, and it was within these residences that the health team was able to see patients. The northern regions had several small MK camps and one refugee camp, reminiscent of the camps in Angola, all with equally sparse medical provision. The South Africans in the northern regions relied heavily on the taxed Mozambican medical facilities available, which were often several hours' drive away. Reports from Mozambique seldom provided demographic breakdowns of the ANC population in the country because the MK force was very mobile in this region. However, the 1981 UNHCR report estimated that there were about one hundred South African refugees in Mozambique.[112]

As mentioned in chapter 1, in October 1978 registered nurse Florence Maleka was posted to Maputo and, as the most qualified ANC medical person in the region, was made head of the RHT.[113] By 1979 the team was made up of three women: Maleka and two medical auxiliaries with limited practical experience. The three operated out of a small clinic at a Maputo residence that mostly housed trained MK cadres. They were able to treat minor ailments and injuries, but more importantly, due to the ANC's convenient location in the capital, they were able to draw on local clinics or the Maputo Central Hospital. Without an ANC presence in the main Maputo health facility, as was the case in Zambia and Tanzania, specialist services offered by doctors in Maputo treated ANC patients as they did local patients. They only accepted people with appointments and charged money for consults. It cost the treasury between US$120 and US$150[114] per month just to purchase extra medication that had not been supplied from donors.[115]

In essence, the small medical residence and staff operated as a triage unit. While it was able to treat very minor health problems, cadres were generally screened by the women and then sent to Mozambican facilities or away from the front line to Tanzania. However, the staff was limited in its ability to complete even this task. One of the major complaints of the medical staff in Maputo was the lack of transport. The healthcare residence was too far from the Maputo Central Hospital to travel on foot; a makeshift ambulance and driver was very necessary but often not available. Furthermore, the ANC's health residence building was unsanitary and in complete disrepair.[116] The ANC staff was not able to effectively treat its own comrades and therefore had no hope of providing primary care to Mozambicans as was customary in the other regions.

Tshabalala recognized that the team in Mozambique was in desperate need of a doctor. The doctor would work in Maputo Central Hospital to provide an ANC presence, albeit minuscule, to the region's major medical facility. The Health Department in Lusaka began its attempts to get Dr Naicker released from his position at UTH in order to be posted to Maputo.[117] Based on an agreement between the department and the Mozambican ministry, a position for an ANC doctor in a Maputo Medical facility was made available to the ANC in the early 1980s.[118]

Midway into the preparations to send Dr Naicker to Mozambique, he got cold feet and decided that he wanted to stay in Lusaka.[119] Dr Naicker recounted some of his fears about going to Mozambique:

[I]t made me think, what am I going to expect ... Speaking to people who'd been in Mozambique, I got a bit frightened because in 1981, I had to deal with our people here in a meeting, learning for the first time how the Boers had hit at Matola, and then subsequent to that was Maseru, etc. etc. So we are dealing with a war situation at that time. And my fear was ... was that I was not trained at all and will I be able to cope in that sort of situation, a war situation.[120]

The environment described was contributing to poor healthcare provisions in the country. Dr Naicker's sudden change of heart was bad for the ANC's Health Department diplomacy and the department worried about the long-term implications of his reneging on their agreement. The relationship between medical sectors was already quite limited and, therefore, this early agreement was important in the ANC's efforts to establish better lines of communication. Fortunately, in May 1982 they were able to make new arrangements with Mozambique and at the start of 1983, Dr Naicker was persuaded to take up the post in Maputo.[121]

In March 1983, Dr Naicker arrived to find ANC health provisions as expected: the small clinic was nearly inutile, there was limited transport, and the staff residence was poor.[122] He began a preliminary, noncomprehensive, health screening of cadres in the region.[123] Many of the MK cadres that had been shuttled through Mozambique into South Africa were falling sick and therefore rendered ineffective as military agents. In his two-week study of fifty-one cadres, there were a number of medical complaints but nothing to warrant serious Health Department concern. However, one month later, the situation in Mozambique began to change. An MK cadre travelling from Angola was discovered in Maputo with a threatening strain of malaria. Dr Naicker wrote to Edith Pemba in Zambia:

> Although accommodation for our clinic still remains a problem the local authorities are begining [sic] to see some light in our work and are offering slow, but reassuring [?] assistance. We study disease patterns and in this task our medical assistants are gaining knowledge e.g. we have highlighted a chloroquine resistant malaria case history imported from Angola. This has proved invaluable not only to our future work in this particular region but also to the local Ministry of Health where this frightening disease is being studied. So, we are working jointly and building a foundation.[124]

New interest from local authorities was clearly linked to the new and potentially dangerous imposition of malaria (discussed below).

The mid-1983 report written by Manto Tshabalala after her visit to the Mozambican region provided the first glimpse of the solidarity shown by the Mozambican facilities and medical staff in northern Mozambique. Two Mozambican facilities helped to serve the South Africans: the military hospital in Nampula and NAMAPA.[125] Nampula's military hospital, was the largest of the available facilities in the region and important to the health and well-being of the South Africans there. If cadres could not be treated at the hospital, they were sent to Maputo or abroad. Although perhaps the best in the region, it was not a well-staffed and equipped hospital relative to what was available in Maputo, Dar es Salaam, or Lusaka.

NAMAPA was a smaller clinic located about three kilometers from the Lurio River and the border between the Nampula and Cabo Delgado provinces. The clinic helped to supply the ANC with necessary medicine, but the clinic had a number of shortcomings. On a visit to northern Mozambique in 1983, Manto Tshabalala provided the Health Department with a bleak report:

> The NAMAPA centre is a health hazard ... Immediately in-front [sic] and behind the residential area are two swamps, indeed fertile ground for mosquito breeding. It can be expected therefore, that the prvalence [sic] and incidence rates of malaria are high, especially during the rainy season ... We were made to understand that the place is usually inudated [sic] by crocodiles once the river is full. Communication also becomes practically im possible ... There are lots of venomous snakes, from report. For these health considerations, it is recommended that the comrades be moved from the area.[126]

In her report, Tshabalala insisted that, in the spirit of solidarity, the military hospital and NAMAPA be reinforced with ANC staff because both facilities saw many South Africans and neither facility was functioning well.

Trying to provide some level of its own primary health coverage in the north, the ANC Health Department had a small health post at its agricultural project.[127] One solitary health worker with minimal knowledge and experience staffed the small clinic at the agricultural centre and greeted one hundred to 150 patients on a daily basis. Almost certainly, the vast majority of those patients were

Mozambican mothers and their children. While not an ideal situation, the popularity of this small health post is testament to the lack of medical facilities available in the northern part of the country. Recognizing this, Tshabalala noted, "he [the health worker] does a valuable job, providing primary health care for which the population is appreciative."[128] The alternative to this health post was a facility approximately ninety kilometers away.

Unlike Tanzania, Zambia, and Angola, Mozambique never developed its own medical clinic in Maputo. A centre had been proposed, but the project never had a chance to get off the ground because of political developments at the beginning of 1984. In March the governments of Mozambique and South Africa signed the Nkomati Accord, which, among other things, pushed MK out of the region and minimized the priority placed on South African health care in Mozambique. Starting in April, Tanzania began making preparations in Dakawa for the arrival of seventy to one hundred South Africans from Mozambique and Swaziland.[129]

In this transition period Dr Naicker remained behind at the Maputo Central Hospital for another fourteen months; his relationship with the staff there was reasonably positive and he awaited a transfer to the USSR to continue further medical study. In 1989, in order to keep the relationship with the Ministry of Health alive, the ANC sent another ANC doctor – Dr Gaba Magaqa – to the region to work in Mozambican facilities. While the bilateral relationship that existed between the ANC Health Department and the Mozambican Ministry of Health was on a small scale, health services provided by the Mozambican Ministry of Health were crucial to all of the ANC's healthcare efforts in the region.

Malaria[130]

This chapter has thus far illuminated the Health Department's bilateral relationships in a region-by-region fashion, but these individual snapshots do not fully capture the interconnectedness of the ANC's population across southern Africa and the difficulties faced by local governments in dealing with a health department that was subordinate to the ANC's wide political and military interests. The ANC's relationships with host nations was pivotal to any success in providing care, but the ANC Health Department also had to accommodate the secrecy of its military operations and serve the ANC's ultimate goal of liberation. The ANC's treatment of malaria across its population in exile represents just one example of this tension.

Malaria was a relentless and often deadly threat to the ANC. Without previous exposure to the disease, South Africans, unlike their African neighbours to the north, had no level of acquired immunity and consequently the ANC Health Department was inundated with malaria patients. The Health Department had to find ways to treat infected refugees, local nationals, and MK cadres as well as prevent others from becoming infected within environments particularly well suited to mosquito breeding. There was always a balance to be struck between preventative and primary care approaches to malaria; the Health Department wanted to practice the former but was often in situations where they were stuck with using the latter. In essence, drugs were sent while mosquito nets were put on hold.

The ANC and MK's exile situation in southern Africa inadvertently created ideal conditions under which drug-resistant malaria strains could spread across the region.[131] Antimalarial drugs were, for the most part, limited to quinine prior to WWI. The transfer of Western troops (nonimmune soldiers) into high malarial zones during the war spurred interest in developing new drugs that would be cheaper and have few side effects. Chloroquine was developed in 1934 as an effective alternative to quinine, and by the end of WWII it was made available at a relatively low cost. With chloroquine, the WHO was optimistic about the global eradication of malaria. The WHO, bolstered by its success with the eradication of smallpox and the promising discovery of chloroquine, embarked on a global eradication campaign in 1955.[132] Optimism ebbed when, in 1960, chloroquine-resistant *Plasmodium falciparum* (CRPF) was recognized in Venezuela, and in 1962 found in Southeast Asia along the Thai–Cambodia border. Both locations were epicentres for the spread of CRPF. Resistance moved south from Venezuela across Brazil to northern Paraguay. From Thailand and Cambodia CRPF spread southeast to Papua New Guinea and the Philippines, and northwest towards India. Miraculously, during the 1960s and 1970s, sub-Saharan Africa's malaria parasites escaped this trend and were still effectively controlled with chloroquine. However, based on the emergence of CRPF, the WHO eradication project was deemed unattainable and abandoned in 1969.[133]

Even with chloroquine's efficacy intact in southern Africa, malaria had had a devastating effect on South Africans throughout their time in exile and was the most common illness treated at the various health centres;[134] however, it was the spread of chloroquine resistance in the early 1980s that grabbed the attention of the WHO and, more importantly, southern African ministries of health. Consequently, the ANC had to confront the newly politicized health issue directly. Starting in mid-1983, malaria became an important item of discussion within nearly every ANC Health Department report.

Concern from host countries was certainly justified. Despite the fact that malaria is not infectious, its presence within larger populations of a region does have some impact. The more infected a population is, the more chance that mosquitos will ingest infected blood and possibly then infect new persons. It is therefore critical to aggressively treat and take preventative measures to decrease the prevalence rate of malaria in order to protect a region. However, the ANC was not able to consistently accomplish this. South Africans were pooled in stagnant groups, prophylactic drugs were not provided or enforced, and mosquito nets were a rarity. Not only did malaria outbreaks occur in ANC-occupied regions, local populations living in areas immediately surrounding the ANC were at higher risk of being infected. Furthermore, the ANC's method of treating malaria – occasional subtherapeutic doses of chloroquine – made the spread of CRPF highly likely. The reality of CRPF meant that future medical treatment of malaria would rely on alternative, expensive, and potentially less effective drugs.

In some ways, the cards were stacked against the ANC's ability to prevent malaria. For instance, the rapid spread of malaria depends on there being relatively good conditions for Anopheles mosquitos to breed.[135] Typically, low-lying areas with standing water are preferable environments; this preference is most apparent when malaria prevalence rises during the rainy season in tropical Africa. The ANC's settlements usually fit the mosquito's requirements. The ANC military camps were set in rural and often undesirable areas of Angola or northern Mozambique where malaria was most common. Moreover, despite best intentions, the Health Department's lack of consistent physical presence in the frontline states made effective monitoring and treatment nearly impossible. Compounding the issue was that South Africans were particularly susceptible to malaria infection.

There are two types of defenses that humans have against malaria. The first is genetic. The sickle-cell gene – a protective genetic mutation against malaria parasites – is found predominantly in tropical Africa (10–45% of the population) and has a much lower rate in South Africa where malaria is significantly less prevalent.[136] The second defense is acquired. When an individual is constantly exposed to malaria parasites, that person gains a small level of immunity to infection. Therefore, environment and immunity considered, the ANC's over-crowded communities created the perfect breeding ground for the new strain of malaria – CRPF.

The spread of CRPF and the ANC's relative mobility are closely interconnected. Fred Nuwaha, associate professor at the Centre for Disease Control and Prevention at Makerere University, reported that there were no confirmed cases of CRPF in sub-Saharan Africa until a single sentinel case was discovered in Kenya in 1977, followed by another isolated case in Tanzania one year later. Subsequent incidences of CRPF were confirmed in Madagascar in 1980 and Tanzania in 1981. Nuwaha then stated that CRPF "spread explosively" in the mid-late 1980s, forcing a decline in the use of chloroquine in twenty-four sub-Saharan countries by 1985 and almost all of Africa by 1989. While delayed by fifteen years, the spread of CRPF was much faster and more complete than was the case in either South America or Southeast Asia.[137] While the cause of this is not confirmed, it is likely that the presence of the ANC and MK (as well as other mobile liberation struggle groups in southern Africa) contributed to the accelerated diffusion of CRPF.

The first mention of chloroquine-resistance among South African refugees or MK cadres came on 20 May 1983 in a letter written by Dr Naicker – then located in Mozambique – to Edith Pemba, a member of the medical staff in Zambia. He pointed out the discovery of CRPF in an MK cadre that had travelled to Maputo from Angola.[138] In a relatively optimistic interview, Dr Naicker reflected on his excitement at discovering the case of CRPF:

> I present to him [a local Mozambican malariologist] with
> a suspected diagnosis of chloquin-resistant [sic] malaria
> and then ... he then provide it on the one case and it ex-
> cited him greatly because its never ever been reported in

Mozambique at that time, and this is 1983 … So he got tremendously excited because there's a breakthrough for him and wasn't it a breakthrough for me, because I had now realised that we are on the right track and he's actually somebody else who's proved this. And he did it beautifully because it was all scientifically done, with all the precautions … it was just tremendous. I mean I have all my time to this, all the coughs and colds, I ignored it, it was all my time given to this. We embarked on a seven month, tremendous, marvellous, exciting project of studying this.[139]

Clearly, both Naicker and his colleague were eager to be at the centre of a scientific discovery that had global implications. However, the repercussions of such a finding for the general population were ominous.

The Mozambican Ministry of Health's awareness of the growing number of CRPF cases in Madagascar in 1980 and Tanzania in 1981 would have, no doubt, been the cause of alarm due to Mozambique's proximity to both countries. Furthermore, Mozambique did not have the local health infrastructure and treatment capacity to adequately deal with malaria sensitive to chloroquine, never mind the new CRPF. In order to keep chloroquine as a viable treatment option in southern Africa, the Mozambican ministry sought better communication and coordination with the ANC to treat malaria.

In June 1983, comrades and refugees in Tanzania were also experiencing a disquieting decline in the usefulness of chloroquine.[140] Students at SOMAFCO experienced chronic outbreaks of malaria. Students became sick every two to three weeks resulting in anaemia and abnormal spleen enlargement. This development was not surprising. First, Tanzania was host to the second instance of CRPF in sub-Saharan Africa and by 1983 CRPF was confidently recorded more widely in the country. Second, in April 1983 the Health Department had commented on the lack of drug compliance in Tanzania: "As regards anti-maleria [sic] tablets, it was noted that, while some students take them other [sic] do not."[141] The lack of staff in Tanzania made health surveillance difficult and treatment was not proactive.

The resistance found in Tanzania in 1983 was not complete and therefore chloroquine was still somewhat effective, but the East Africa health team was concerned with the need to increase the dose of chloroquine in order for the drug to take effect.[142] Students at SOMAFCO, were especially vulnerable because they lived in cramped dormitories in a malaria-endemic region. Local Tanzanian doctor Dr. Ebba Mokoena indicated worry that without intense diligence a child could overdose on the amount of chloroquine now needed for effective treatment of the parasite. He suggested an increase in preventative efforts including an attempt to confront the mosquito-friendly environment by draining standing water, cutting long grass, and spraying the area. While acknowledging the high price of mosquito nets in Tanzania and the complications of administering antimalaria prophylaxis, he emphasized their necessity for those who seemed most prone to the disease.

On 13 June 1983, Dr Naicker – stationed in Mozambique – provided an extensive and official report to the Health Department detailing the case histories of two cadres who had both come from Calucuma and Caxito camps in Angola and were strongly suspected of carrying CRPF.[143] The individual mentioned in the first case had spent September and October of 1982 in Caxito camp and had been repeatedly treated for malaria to some positive effect at that time. She was later transferred to Mozambique and experienced successive relapses of malaria in January, March, and April 1983. In May she was admitted to hospital, and despite aggressive treatment, the reprieve was worryingly brief. The second case had also shown symptoms of malaria while stationed in Caxito in September and October of 1982. She, too, was given chloroquine, which apparently had some efficacy. When she transferred to Mozambique, she again presented with malaria in March and April, and treatment, again, provided some level of reprieve. However, hers was clearly also a chronic case; she was readmitted to hospital on 13 May 1983, and the administration of chloroquine provided progressively shorter periods of remission. Chloroquine was subsequently stopped and both were given Fansidar – an alternative antimalarial drug – with the hope that the new drug would produce long-lasting results.

Reacting to Dr Naicker's report, the Health Department sought medical staff reinforcements to help address Mozambique's malaria problem and attempted to conduct an extensive malaria screening campaign.[144] It was important to be proactive not only for their own comrades' health but for their relationship with the government in

Mozambique. Dr Manto Tshabalala arrived in Maputo in July 1983 to begin a region-wide investigation and report.[145] It is evident from the report that there was little data available; the areas that she visited were unable to provide her with comprehensive regional updates and were sorely equipped to help map the malaria burden amongst ANC and MK personnel in Mozambique. However, her initial medical examination provided cause for serious concern. In her report, Tshabalala stated, "Ninety blood slides of our people in Mozambique have been examined for malarial parasites. Six out of 13 positives are chloroquine resistant. Of these six, two are also resistant to FANSIDAR. It would appear their enzymes neutralise the FANSIDAR. They have responded well on Quinine so far."[146] While the numbers of infected comrades at this time were low, the ANC found it disquieting that nearly half of the cases were chloroquine resistant.[147]

The report also illuminated a number of major medical concerns to the Health Department and to the ANC more broadly. First, Tshabalala claimed that the WHO had not confirmed prior incidence of CRPF in Mozambique before the ANC study. She admitted that there may have been "an error in administering the chloroquine treatment, and in some cases, FANSIDAR as well" and that it seemed that the CRPF had spread from Tanzania – where there were known cases of CRPF previously – to the neglected and poorly supplied Calucuma and Caxito camps in Angola and from there to Mozambique. Tshabalala was indicating that she believed the ANC to be responsible for the transfer of CRPF from Tanzania to Mozambique. Due to the lack of local information, it was impossible to confirm whether or not the ANC cadres were indeed the earliest cases in the region, but the ANC Health Department was feeling semi – if not fully – responsible for an incredibly unwelcomed imposition of drug resistance into the region.

The ANC's role in the spread of CRPF was a diplomatic problem with a number of consequences.[148] First, local health authorities in Mozambique wanted greater oversight and preventative measures put in place to limit the spread: they wanted comprehensive testing of all ANC personnel in Maputo and Nampula, screening for all cadres coming from Angola into the region, a coat of antimalaria chemicals sprayed liberally over the ANC residences, and further entomological assessments of ANC occupied areas. However, any attempts by the Mozambican government to inspect whether these measures were acted on was seen by the ANC as a security threat; it was believed that the Mozambican authorities would acquire too much additional information about the underground movement, know the location of every ANC and MK residence, and get a good indication of how many cadres were in the region.[149] Tshabalala, acting under the constraints imposed by the ANC military, persuaded the Mozambican government to trust that the ANC's Department of Health would implement the insisted upon measures without surveillance, but it was clear that CRPF prevention was of the utmost importance in order to maintain their bilateral relationship.[150]

As per the agreement reached with the Mozambican Ministry of Health in 1983, Dr Tshabalala and medical assistant Solomon Molefe left for the Nampula region in Mozambique to help train local and ANC technical medical staff to properly test, treat, and prevent CRPF incidence.[151] Unfortunately, the military hospital used by the ANC in the Nampula region did not have the capacity for malaria testing, and the ANC did not have adequate staff in the area to complete the assigned tasks. Instead, Tshabalala and Molefe themselves provided Fansidar to comrades in their small settlements and took blood samples for testing once back in Maputo. It was observed that malaria was a major problem in the region as was quoted earlier in this chapter: "The NAMAPA centre [in the Nampula region] is a health hazard. The place is right on the bank of the river. Immediately infront [sic] and behind the residential area are two swamps, indeed fertile ground for mosquito breeding. It can be expected therefore, that the prvalence [sic] and incidence rates of malaria are high especially during the rainy season." While it was suggested that a new location be found to replace Namapa, in the interim ANC personnel were trained in mosquito-vector control. In addition, Solomon Molefe was left in the region to assist in the antimalaria campaign.

Unfortunately, the Department of Health efforts in Mozambique were not enough to satisfy the Mozambican Ministry of Health.[152] The ANC's Health Department had been unable to screen all of the South Africans in Maputo, and the Mozambican ministry was concerned with the lack of communication and collaboration between the ANC and its own national department of health. But this was not entirely the ANC Health Department's fault. Issues of security were at the centre of ANC concern, and the screening procedures were time-consuming and believed to have negative implications on ANC military security. Quite understandably, one set of minutes of the ANC's East Africa RHT meeting in 1983 worryingly stated, "the Mozambicans feel that our people transported this resistant strain."[153] In any case, the situation was creating tension in the previously amicable relationship between the two health departments, and the ANC Health Department was entering into bilateral health negotiations and discussions with the Mozambican health ministry without complete authority (guarded by the military) to uphold its promises.[154]

It should be stated that the Mozambican ministry's desire to be involved in the ANC Health Department's affairs was not completely without benefits for the ANC's Department of Health. While the tension complicated the lives of the military and political leadership, the Department of Health was suddenly placed in the spotlight, receiving an increased fraction of authority within the ANC and given more opportunity to be active in the frontline states, including Angola. Suddenly, health issues had the potential to damage important diplomatic political relationships.[155] The situation in Mozambique in 1983 worked to expose the poor health conditions within the yet untested Angolan camps. These camps were especially conducive to the transmission of malaria due to their location within environments particularly well suited to mosquito breeding, the lack of preventative measures against mosquito bites, and the generally inadequate medicine and transport supply. In particular, Caxito was clearly shown to be a major site of mosquito breeding, malaria transmittance, and especially good for the proliferation of CRPF.[156]

Communication with the Mozambican Ministry of Health pushed the ANC's Health Department toward further collaboration with the Angolan ministry and the WHO as it planned its response to malaria in Angola: "A plan of Action worked out by the [Angolan?] Ministry upon receipt of the report from the Ministry of Health, Mozambique include:- Inviting the A.N.C. Health Department through the M.P.L.A. Workers Party to participate in the malria [sic] programme. Working in close collaboration with the Provincial Health Office."[157] The health ministry in Angola was to provide a laboratory and screen ANC members as well as Angolans living in close proximity to ANC camps for malaria. In addition, a WHO official would be able to oversee and advise the process of malaria testing and prevention. Even before leaving to examine malaria in Angola in September 1983, Tshabalala further recommended that everyone should be tested, treated, and declared malaria-free before exiting the region. She also recommended that new arrivals be barred from Caxito and that the camp be closed down while at the same time chloroquine be phased out as the drug of choice in the region.[158]

Dr. Tshabalala arrived in Angola in mid-August 1983 to assess what was promising to be an abysmal malaria situation.[159] This proved to be the case. Not only were the health conditions in camps poor, the inexperienced and under-qualified staff was administering anti-malarial drugs irregularly and, specifically in the case of chloroquine, improperly. Most infected cadres were receiving less than half of the needed 1500mg chloroquine dose. She also found that the team was using chloroquine prophylactically, providing cadres with subcurative doses (300mg) every week.[160] As a result, each area had four to five patients treated for malaria everyday, cadres were suffering from headaches, dizziness, and blurred vision, there were reported cases of cerebral malaria, relapses were common, and, justifiably, cadres were afraid of the illness. As per the discussions with the ministry in Mozambique in July 1983, the ANC coordinated efforts with the WHO and the Angolan Ministry of Health in order to keep the lines of communication open, actions transparent, and increase effectiveness in halting the spread of CRPF.[161]

Formal testing for CRPF in Caxito and Viana began in earnest in September 1983, after Tshabalala travelled to Brazzaville with members of the Angola Health Team to become better equipped for such a process.[162] Sixty-eight cadres from Caxito and 205 from Viana were screened for malaria. Of those screened in Caxito, seventeen had malaria parasites and thirteen were chloroquine-resistant. Of those screened in Viana, eight had malaria parasites and five were chloroquine-resistant.[163] As predicted, CRPF accounted for more than half of all cases of malaria. While this was a good initial start to testing in Angola, the comprehensive testing for all camps was not completed by the end of 1983 because of the lack of reliable transport in the region.[164] Once again, it was recommended that preventative measures be taken seriously; two ANC members were being trained in "spraying methodology" and Tshabalala recommended an entomological survey be done in all of the settlements.[165]

The developing problem of CRPF was not just a military, frontline issue. The East Africa RHT's third quarterly report in 1983 started off by stating that malaria was "still a major problem with some of the patients relapsing and resistant to the drug of choice."[166] Beginning the report with a statement about malaria demonstrated the notoriety achieved by malaria in previous months. Tshabalala, however, did not appreciate the vagueness of the report nor the unsubstantiated claim that malaria in that region was chloroquine resistant: "[I]t is not enough to say malaria is a major problem. Please indicate the number of cases, the rate of relapse. It has not been proved yet whether, in fact Morogoro is an area of Chloroquine resistance ... As this stands, it may cause problems of demand from the community, based on unproven statements. We must try and avoid this."[167] Tshabalala's annoyance toward the RHT's report ran counter to her own statements in the Mozambican report in which she postulated that CRPF spread from Tanzania. Unfortunately for the Department of Health, the then unconfirmed insinuations were proven true the following year.[168]

However, the deputy secretary was evidently now well aware of the political implications of CRPF in ANC communities and was anxious to avoid rumours or speculation. Indeed, in August 1984, Dr Pren Naicker wrote to Tshabalala advising her that the Mozambican Ministry of Health was planning to publish an article that would point the finger at the ANC for the spread of CRPF. Naicker was busy looking for evidence to counter the accusation and was tentatively hopeful after reading a study on malaria done in 1982 in Cabo Delgado Province.[169] The study reported a case of CRPF in Mozambique that did not involve the ANC at all. At the 1985 Technical Cooperation amongst the Developing Countries (TCDC) meeting in Mauritius, Tshabalala thanked those who were helping control the ANC's malaria crisis but "strongly refuted the allegation that the ANC cadres were the only identified carriers of malaria to Mozambique from Angola and Tanzania."[170] Evidently, the ANC did not fancy the idea of being considered vectors of CRPF.

Between April 1983 and December 1983, the issue of malaria had gone from being treated with near nonchalance to causing the Health Department extreme anxiety. It was shown in a departmental yearly report for 1983 that in Angola and Tanzania numbers of malaria patients had risen and that the symptoms associated with malaria fever – diarrhoea, vomiting, and malnutrition – were taking a toll on medical resources.[171] It was also reported that there were at least five deaths caused by malaria in Tanzania and Angola; two were MK cadres and three were babies (belonging to comrades or South African refugees) in Tanzania. While the reports seem to indicate an increase in the number of infected South Africans, it is hard to determine the level of intensification of malaria prevalence due to the ANC Department of Health's lack of malaria awareness before the onset of CRPF. Incidence of the CPRF strain did not necessarily mean that there were more malaria cases, only that the cases now needed to be treated with different drugs. As a result of the regional emphasis on CRPF, the 1983 regional reports from ANC occupied regions put a spotlight on the ANC's involvement in the CRPF drama by reporting on malaria. I suspect that the 1983 malaria burden was similar to years past and that it was the precursor for a massive increase in actual prevalence rates over the next few years.

Malaria assessment was a priority for the ANC Health Department across all of its southern Africa locations in 1984. The department aimed to finish screening cadres in Angola and to start testing for CRPF in Dakawa and Mazimbu in Tanzania.[172] Riding the wave of interest in malaria, the ANC Health Department made a proposal to the WHO regarding malaria screening and treatment on behalf of approximately 9,000 South African refugees. This request was described as a joint venture between the ANC's Health Department and the Angolan Ministry of Health. In August 1984, Tshabalala wrote to the WHO regional director for Africa Dr Quenum to ask for just less than one million antimalarial pills (none of the varieties requested included chloroquine) and mosquito coils for the South African refugees in Angola, with the assumption that each of those refugees would get malaria five times per year and that the malaria strain would be CRPF.[173] In October 1984, for reasons unknown, Tshabalala reported that their proposed budget for an antimalaria campaign in Angola and its requisition for specific drugs and screening equipment would be cut from US$56,000 to US$4,000 quarterly.[174] However, in spite of the lowered amount, efforts in the region were producing overall positive results. The Politico-Military Council commented, "Malaria had become a real terror in our camps and valuable lives of cadres

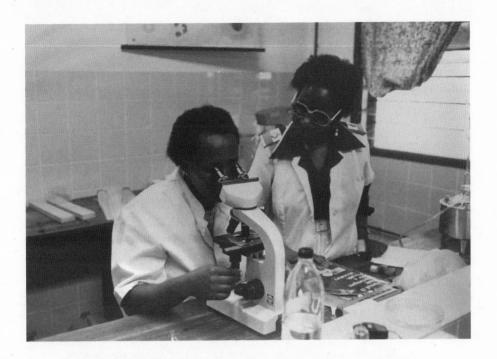

2.5 Medical microscope. The image depicts two women using a microscope in the hospital. They are most likely looking for malaria parasites on a blood smear. Photograph, no date.

had been lost. Since the crusade by the health team fatalities caused by malaria have been reduced to the very minimum."[175] Another 1984 year-end report written by the RHT in Angola commented on health improvements due to the increased number of medical staff and the provision of mosquito nets, coils, and sprays.[176]

Along with its MK cadres, the Department of Health also recognized that students attending SOMAFCO and other residents of Mazimbu and Dakawa needed attention and care. From the beginning of 1984, the Health Department was aware that CRPF was likely to have permeated the settlements in much the same way as it had in Mozambique and Angola, but the extent to which this was true was still unknown. The ANC's prioritization of the frontline states had put South Africans in Tanzania on the back burner, but the issue of malaria infection in Tanzania could not be put off longer. A February 1984 report from the health team in Mazimbu stated that malaria numbers were high and the clinic had seen 350 cases that month.[177]

The ANC proposed a US$6,000 study of their communities in the Morogoro region,[178] and with assurance of WHO support, the ANC released the money to the National Institute for Medical Research in Tanzania in order to begin as soon as possible.[179] The East Africa RHT relied on the assistance and expertise from the Ministry of Health in Tanzania for its screening investigations in the Mazimbu and Dakawa communities. Investigations began in March.[180] It was found that 22.8 per cent of those in Mazimbu and 33.3 per cent of the residents in Dakawa had malaria; of those cases 9.3 per cent and 20 per cent in Mazimbu and Dakawa respectively did not respond to chloroquine treatment, confirming the presence of CRPF in the area.[181]

In August 1984 Regional Secretary Victor Maome announced his frustration over the fact that no provisions for CRPF were made by the Health Department in the wake of confirming its presence within the ANC settlements in Tanzania: "What is puzzling is that there is no follow up on such a finding. No drugs are sent to the region so that we can combat such cases. This becomes even more serious when one considers that Tanzania has none of the drugs to be used in resistant cases."[182] Compounding the issue in East Africa was the sudden influx of South Africans from Mozambique, after the aforementioned 1984 Nkomati Accord was signed, who were possibly carrying CRPF back to Tanzania and who now would need mosquito nets or other antimalaria prevention provisions.[183]

In 1985 the Health Department continued to face challenges when attempting to improve the malaria situation at Plot 18 in Dakawa. Not only did Dakawa receive less than adequate medical attention, Plot 18 was an especially good breeding ground for mosquitos and was consequently host to a high percentage of those sick with malaria.[184] The Morogoro health inspector and, subsequently, the ANC's East Africa RHT recommended that the plot be closed and relocated in order to escape the problem.[185] Regrettably, the Dakawa political administration did not place the same priority on malaria control and did "not seem to realize how dangerous the present situation is nor the consequences of having that plot in such a highly mosquito infected area." [186] Instead, oil was poured into the standing water to reduce the number of breeding habitats. Therefore clinic reports that presented high numbers of malaria patients can be attributed in part to the poor health decision-making of leadership rather than simply in the inability of the Health Department to supply mosquito nets or adequate antimalarial drugs.[187]

The RHT in Angola also continued to attempt to combat malaria in its camps in 1985. Following an outbreak in Caculama, the medical team in Angola also went to their settlement in Malange Province and undertook a small antimalaria campaign. Earlier that year, the RHT received nearly 450 mosquito nets from the Central Committee of the Communist Party of China.[188] They distributed mosquito nets, treated infected cadres with chloroquine, Fansidar and primaquine, and tested their blood at four intervals to make sure that the "radical treatment" took full effect.[189] Cooperation between the local hospital in Viana and the ANC's health team enabled the ANC to use Angolan supplies for their laboratory test work.

After 1985, the department's reporting on malaria changed, indicating that the initial panic and sensational quality of CRPF had subsided. Mozambique was completely off the malaria radar; Naicker was able to write to Tshabalala and report that there were no longer any cases of malaria among the very few South Africans left in Mozambique.[190] In Tanzania, malaria was still the most common disease seen at the ANC facilities, especially during the rainy season, but the crisis of discovering CRPF had passed.[191] The discussions continued their trend toward prevention rather than the reaction-based curative measures that had been so necessary during the previous two-and-a-half years.[192] The antimalaria strategies emphasized were the same as before: they called for a community-oriented attack on mosquito habitats by cutting the long grass and clearing the standing water,[193] but they were now the suffix of a long, intense, and now dwindling discussion of CRPF. At the Third Health Council Meeting in 1986 local doctor Mmipe Saasa gave an educational paper specifically on malaria and the issue of CRPF was barely considered. The report listed the multitude of drugs that may be used for treatment instead of focusing specifically on the ones that were losing efficacy.[194]

Typical reporting in Tanzania also mentioned malaria more briefly or in conjunction with other health-related issues that required similar solutions: "Illnesses [sic] Malaria is still high; 2 children have had measles and an outbreak of flu is under control."[195] In at least one report in 1986, malaria was listed in the hospital disease breakdown charts but not deemed worth mentioning in the overall analysis.[196] In November the Mazimbu/Dakawa health report stated that the ANC health team was able to handle all malaria cases "including complicated ones," using a combination of chloroquine and quinine and that referrals to Morogoro hospital were no longer necessary.[197] This was a significant accomplishment in that the RHT saw 12,961 malaria patients between January 1986 and March 1987.[198]

In this way, malaria highlighted the success of the ANC's infrastructure in Tanzania in 1986 and 1987. Even in relatively damning reports about the limited efficacy of health posts or the unfulfilled potential of the ANC-Holland Solidarity Hospital, these facilities were able to treat malaria patients: "The capacity of these establishments [health post and dispensary in Dakawa] is limited to out-patient treatment of malaria and acute infections, first-aid."[199] Curative services were considered less ideal than preventative ones, and it was envisioned that these facilities would be able to do more but it is important to acknowledge the role that the ANC played in providing medical points that were able to help patients suffering from malaria, Tanzanians and South Africans alike.

The ANC was not solely responsible for the spread of CRPF from Tanzania to Angola and Mozambique. However, the lack of organization within and authority of the Health Department coupled with the reality that the ANC community was highly concentrated, non-immune and mobile contributed significantly to the rapid spread of CRPF – an established global phenomenon starting in the 1960s – in southern Africa in the early 1980s. Despite what Dr Tshabalala said in Mauritius at the TCDC, the ANC's Health Department was aware that it was contributing to the spread of chloroquine resistance and worried about the ANC's perpetuation of the "high transmission rate of a super-infection" and what that would do to their relationships in southern Africa.[200]

HIV/AIDS

In the late 1980s, the Health Department's attention slowly shifted from malaria to HIV/AIDS. The history of HIV/AIDS in exile has been covered in detail elsewhere; particularly with regard to the ANC's attempt to design education materials concerning HIV.[201] However, it is evident that the concerns with HIV share a striking resemblance to the Health Department's issues with chloroquine resistance. Once again, South African exiles were potential vectors of a deadly disease that had their hosts' attention. However, different from malaria HIV was less well understood, highly stigmatized, and the Health Department – perhaps considering the accusations that were levelled against it concerning the spread of chloroquine resistance – was worried about transmitting the disease back to South Africa.

Despite the ANC Health Department's desire to be seen as a government institution with interest in global health concerns, it was unconcerned about the rapidly spreading HIV global epidemic until 1986 and did not show earnest concern until 1988.[202] In a 1990 seminar report, the ANC Health Department tried to explain this delay:

> Because of the fact that there was a relative unclarity about the desease [sic] in the ANC the beginning, as it was the case with the rest of the world and because it related to sexuality of people – an area viewed as taboo, the Department of Health (DOH) of the ANC stated [sic] late in looking for responses to it. It was only in 1988 that the Department of health began to ponder upon this situation with the assistance of the Swedish International Development Authority (SIDA). This delayed response has caused the movement to pay a high price. The Department of Health also benefitted from the experiences of our host countries.[203]

In fact, the southern African countries were hosting, in concert with the WHO, a number of HIV/AIDS conferences, which pushed the ANC to consider the gravity of the new pandemic and then gave the ANC a platform to critique South Africa's approach to HIV.

In 1990, barely seven years after attempting to defend itself against the accusations of spreading chloroquine resistance, the ANC presented a paper on HIV/AIDS at the conference in Maputo implying its innocence in the development of the region's epidemic: "The African National Congress cannot escape the epidemic since its exile communities are in the countries with established epidemics."[204] However, the same paper declared its solidarity with and reliance on its hosts, acknowledging that the ANC benefitted from local efforts.

The paper also stated the ANC must play its part to limit the continued spread of the disease.[205] Furthermore, learning from its recent
complications regarding chloroquine resistance, the ANC's Health
Department was quick to consider the political consequences of
unchecked mobility. In 1987, the Zambia RHT reported, "The question of AIDS came up, and this time were the political implications
of such a thing as sending comrades with HIV+ inside [South
Africa]. The main reasons for this were that it would do enormous
harm to us should the enemy find it out."[206] Consequently, a decision was made by the NEC: HIV positive patients would not be able
to go home "until further notice."[207] The carelessness of some South
African exiles helped to solidify this position. In one instance, the
Zambia RHT reported that an HIV positive MK cadre transferred
from the frontline was educated about the modes of HIV transmission but proceeded to "sleep around" despite his promise not to.[208]
In the meantime, the Health Department was attempting to screen
all cadres heading for military zones as well as students and patients
travelling outside of Africa.[209]

However, as was the case with malaria, the Health Department
had little control over the actions taken by the military command and
the movement of MK cadres. The NEC charged the Health Department
to notify the military headquarters (MHQ) about the decision to
keep infected South Africans from going home. MHQ's response left
much to be desired. MHQ asked the Zambia RHT to screen the cadres
earmarked to go to South Africa but when given the results of the
tests, the military command did not inform the cadres of their test
results. This silence may have been partly due to the harsh stigma
that accompanied a confirmed positive test:[210] "The general feeling of
cdes in the army is that [HIV positive cadres] should be given suicide-
missions. Further discussions pointed out that the feasibility of such
a person being able to carry out a mission in the first place is open to
question. This is an urgent need for a serious meeting with the MHQ
because we are sitting on a time-bomb, and they must be made aware
of this."[211] Despite attempts at education in Angola, the harshness of
the stigma remained; in late 1989, it was reported that some cadres
still felt that HIV positive people should be isolated from the community or sent on suicide missions.[212] HIV status notification and
the movement of cadres remained an unresolved issue throughout

the repatriation period; the opinion of the host nations' ministries of health is not recorded in the archive.[213]

Compared to the incidence and prevalence of malaria in the region, HIV/AIDS was hardly mentioned in actual patient reports or doctor notes. Furthermore, unlike the case of malaria, the practical measures that could be taken to treat HIV positive patients were minimal. However, like malaria, HIV was of political significance to the ANC based on the diplomatic power and potential that this new epidemic carried. In addition, the ANC saw the future implications of HIV/AIDS at home. Therefore, the ANC leadership – both in and out of the Health Department – sought to show its neighbours that it was taking the threat of HIV seriously and that in the future, it would be able to design a policy to limit the damage of the epidemic in South Africa. Conferences were used to simultaneously express solidarity and independence. A paper delivered at the Maputo conference in 1990 stated, "Some people could argue that it is not necessary for the ANC to spend resources on an AIDS campaign because the host countries have national intervention programmes from which we should benefit. However ... the ANC communities are unique in a number of ways. There are language and cultural differences between ANC people and host countries which limit the benefit from local education and intervention strategies."[214] As the threat of HIV in southern Africa grew, so did the knowledge that the ANC would soon have to tackle this major health concern outside of the general surveillance of its southern African hosts.

The ANC's hosts' medical services were foundational to the Health Department's attempts to treat its patients in each region. While the ANC attempted to provide primary care in Mazimbu and Dakawa, Tanzanian facilities in Dar es Salaam and Morogoro provided access to much-needed secondary healthcare. The ANC was not able to provide seamless care to patients; however, it treated South Africans and Tanzanians whenever possible. As a result the ANC and Tanzanian medical staff had a good working relationship. Unlike those in Tanzania, medical efforts in Zambia were mainly concentrated in an urban space. In the late 1970s and early 1980s, the small cast of ANC leadership neglected its own ANC healthcare provision and drew on the resources of the local facilities. There was a high concentration

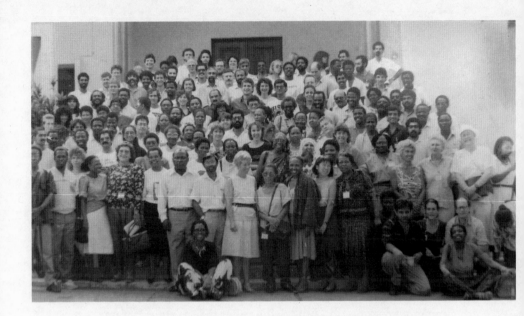

2.6 Maputo conference delegates. This is a group photograph taken of ANC Health Department staff and international solidarity workers at the HIV/AIDS conference in Maputo. "Maputo Conference," no date [April 1990].

of ANC medical personnel working in Zambian facilities, and the relationship between national and ANC medical sectors was positive. As the population grew and changed, new primary healthcare provisions were made available to the rank and file members of the ANC now occupying space in Lusaka, albeit as a two-tiered system. As in Zambia, health services used by the ANC in Zimbabwe were urban-based. Starting in 1982 the Zimbabwean government provided opportunities for medical staff to work in its medical facilities and for patients to be transferred to its hospitals for specialist treatment. Without a significant population in Harare, the ANC did not look for opportunities to provide primary healthcare in Zimbabwe. Instead, Zimbabwe was a location for South Africans to receive excellent, if high-priced, secondary healthcare services.

The bilateral relationship between the medical sectors in Angola and Mozambique and the ANC was markedly different from those developed with Tanzania, Zambia, and Zimbabwe. Because Angola and Mozambique were in the midst of civil war, those governments' capacity to meet the medical needs of their citizens was deficient.

Likewise, the ANC was not able to provide consistent primary health-care to South Africans in the region. However, there was cooperation between the Health Department, SWAPO, and its hosts. ANC doctors were given opportunities to work in Angolan hospitals and attend medical school. The ANC saw Angolan patients at Viana even if they had a limited capacity to provide quality care to those individuals. In Mozambique the ANC staff mainly worked as a conduit to the Maputo Central Hospital, and the hospital treated South Africans like its own citizens. In order for the ANC to establish a closer relationship with the Ministry of Health in Mozambique, Dr Naicker took up a position at the Mozambique Central Hospital but, unfortunately, the budding relationship diminished significantly after the Nkomati Accord was signed in 1984.

The ANC's role in and response to the CRPF crisis in southern Africa demonstrates some of the complexities of these bilateral relationships. The ANC's Health Department was subjected to a variety of responses to the crisis from local health ministries, exhibiting the difference in levels of authority and autonomy given to the ANC's health staff. Mozambique's government felt the threat of an unaccountable and poorly organized health program from ANC members and sought greater control and surveillance. Angola's health ministry also entered into the conversation about CRPF and responded by providing the ANC with space to perform its screening procedures. The response to the ANC from Tanzania was different from that received in the frontline states. Mazimbu and Dakawa were epicentres of the spread of CRPF and local Tanzanian authorities aided the ANC's prevention and control efforts; in keeping with the relatively well developed health infrastructure, within two years the ANC was able to use its facilities to help the region treat cases of malaria in both South African and Tanzanian residents.

The ANC's response to CRPF clearly had an impact on the ANC's response to the HIV/AIDS epidemic. The Health Department sought to absolve itself of any blame for spreading the illness while also quickly putting policies in place to screen mobile South African exiles. As was the case when dealing with CRPF, the Health Department was unable to control the actions of the military command, however, it was able to use conferences in southern Africa to show its willingness to collaborate with local efforts as well as assert itself as a department capable of some independence.

3

Exposing "Policies of Genocide": The Health Department's Role in the Anti-Apartheid Movement, 1977–1990

The vantage point of the southern African allies towards the ANC and its Health Department greatly differed from the perspective held by international audiences further afield. The ANC used the Health Department staff to elucidate the inadequacies of the apartheid medical system, and by showing that the Health Department was caring for South Africans in exile, it asserted itself as a viable political alternative. Especially in the late 1970s, this was an audacious claim. At that time the Health Department had only a handful of medical affiliates, a fledgling bureaucracy, full reliance on international donors, and virtually no contact with patients within South Africa. As a result, the South African medical association was outraged that a small collection of exiled medical staff gained international recognition as a representative for the health needs of South Africans.[1]

International financial support was not the only factor contributing to the ANC Health Department's success. The Health Department was established at a very opportune, historic moment; the WHO was in the process of setting up a concerted effort to provide global access to medical care while at the same time, general anti-apartheid sentiment was rising internationally. In addition, the growing number of South African refugees in southern Africa was a concern to hosting African governments, the UNHCR, and the WHO. The ANC's Health Department was unable to care for South Africans at home but, with the help of their hosts, was uniquely poised to care for the newly exiled South African refugees.

One of the main agendas of the ANC's Health Department was to publicize the unequal access to healthcare in South Africa, and it illuminated specific health-related injustices taking place on a daily basis in the country. Members of the department attended international conferences to spread anti-apartheid propaganda and printed material exposing some of the ways that apartheid policies contributed to the low health status of black South Africans. Their two main goals were to discredit the apartheid government and show themselves to be ready for international endorsement as the alternative department of health representing the needs of South Africans. The ANC's Health Department often met with success. In the late 1970s, the growing international anti-apartheid movement began to denounce racist health policies, and many governments and organisations in the West contributed to the Health Department's program for treating South African exiles.[2]

The ANC's strategy for gaining international credibility was by no means unique. Michael Panzer's work regarding FRELIMO's inner political workings while it fought for independence in Mozambique bears a particularly striking resemblance to the ANC's actions. Panzer convincingly argued that FRELIMO developed into a "proto-state" by creating government-like institutions while exiled in Tanzania: "Considering the circumstances of the massive refugee influx into Tanzania, FRELIMO transitioned from a Liberation Front of militant fighters into a proto-state with aspects of governmental authority."[3] He showed that FRELIMO had to "demonstrate its legitimacy," by providing for the basic needs of the Mozambican refugees in Tanzania; furthermore, he argued that the leadership carried out its protostate agenda in a relatively authoritarian manner. Primarily, Panzer referred to governmental legitimacy as a status granted by Mozambicans through their obedience to and acceptance of the increasing authoritarian FRELIMO leadership.

The political actions taken by the leaders of social movements outside of Africa show the protostate-building agenda to be a common theme of liberation movements.[4] The Black Panther movement also attempted to establish itself as a valid political entity in the United States. While the Black Panthers' militant exterior obfuscated its efforts to provide community services in the late 1960s and early 1970s the Panthers' breakfast feeding program developed for inner-city African American children was a fundamental part of its political identity.[5] The breakfast program provided a practical example of the Panthers' intention to not only protect but also to provide for poor African Americans. Underscoring this political rather than military identity, the Panthers provided African American people access to free medical care; Panther-led clinics sprang up across the country.[6] These social programs were not just designed to gain support from their patrons, they also stood as a challenge to the US government's legitimacy as political representative of African American people. Unlike FRELIMO, the Black Panthers did not establish themselves politically by seeking acceptance and obedience from their followers but by exposing the illegitimacy of the US political system.[7]

The Palestinian political organisation Hamas has had a similar political and social trajectory in their attempts to gain political power in the Palestinian territories. Hamas' provision of community social services and participation in the 2006 elections were actions taken to gain external funding; the financial support has been critical to the long-term survival of Hamas.[8] Hamas made gains locally and internationally. Hamas' initiatives in the social sphere won support for Palestinian beneficiaries, and, in addition to achieving international financial support, Hamas' provision of services met the basic needs of Palestinians and was a deliberate challenge to the governing capacity of the Palestinian National Authority.

The ANC employed a combination of these political strategies to gain international status and, in 1994, political power. Similar to FRELIMO, the ANC established state-like institutions while in exile in order to build political legitimacy, but, unlike its counterpart, the ANC was looking primarily for international rather than refugee endorsement. Like Hamas and the Black Panther movement, the ANC attempted to expose the ineptitude of South African social services while gaining legitimacy from international actors. The use of the

Health Department to this end was sometimes a conscious act on the part of the ANC leadership and sometimes a by-product of the efforts of medical staff. Unlike Hamas and the Black Panthers, the ANC was unable to challenge the NP by providing the neglected services within their home country. Instead, the ANC had to prove itself in exile.

The ANC performed state functions in order to serve its people in exile and gain international funding. Furthermore, it manipulated international support for the Health Department to bolster its military efforts. In this way, through military action, the ANC sought to build legitimacy at home. South Africans in South Africa were unable to witness the social projects developed by the ANC in exile and could only see evidence of the ANC's involvement in the anti-apartheid struggle through MK's military actions. Thus, the ANC's main target audience for their healthcare projects were people sympathetic to the anti-apartheid movement internationally. As inept as the Health Department often proved to be, its successes were internationally celebrated and, consequently, the Health Department was eventually recognized as the nucleus of the post-apartheid healthcare system.

"Health for All by 2000"[9]

The necessity for medical care and the political and financial support for bureaucratic development from Sweden pushed the Medical Committee into existence in the late 1970s. However, financial assistance was not the only factor supporting the establishment of the Health Department. It met with considerable early success because its emergence coincided with a new global emphasis on health and growing anti-apartheid support from the UN and its affiliates. The ANC's Health Department sought to broadcast its existence so that it could be closely connected with international developments in healthcare and the actions of medical associations.

In May 1974 the UN General Assembly resolved to shrink the growing economic divide between "developed" and "developing" nations. The initiative was called the "Declaration of the Establishment of a New International Economic Order."[10] The declaration was significant to the ANC; it explicitly mentioned apartheid as an obstruction to the desired "economic order."[11] The following year, in keeping with the "New International Economic Order," the WHO began a systematic investigation into the effects of apartheid on the health of black South Africans.[12] The investigation found that apartheid's racial policies were in fact extremely detrimental to the health of black South Africans and that while apartheid persisted health would be adversely affected. In a sense, this was affirmation of the 1974 declaration in the territory of healthcare. The notion that development would not be possible in South Africa under apartheid became a common theme of almost every subsequent UN study, conference, or declaration on global equality. However, in the mid-1970s, the bold declarations against racism and inequality in South Africa were not followed with practical steps for the international community to take. The 1975 WHO report on its investigation in South Africa read out by Dr Halfdan Mahler (director-general of the WHO) was yet another passionate acknowledgement that apartheid needed to end before health would be available to all South Africans, but it came up short of providing a plan of action.

In September 1977 unethical medical practices under apartheid entered into a new level of global consciousness following the controversial death of Steve Biko. Biko was a key leader of the Black Consciousness Movement in South Africa and a staunch anti-apartheid activist. In August 1977 he was arrested and handed over to the security police. Biko suffered severe head trauma while in custody – a fact confirmed by medical examinations done in hospital – but negligent follow-up assessment and treatment by the four doctors and security police involved in the case ultimately proved fatal to Biko.[13] While he was in critical condition, he was loaded into the back of a police Land Rover and driven the 1,200 kilometres to Pretoria. Approximately twenty-four hours later, Biko was dead. The case provoked a public outcry, but the doctors' actions were initially exonerated. In 1980, after the first commission of inquiry led by the South African Medical and Dental Council (SAMDC) in South Africa decided not to punish the doctors, the Medical Association of South Africa (MASA) bowed to public pressure and conducted its own investigation of the case. Its final decision was to uphold the council's not guilty ruling. As a result, in 1981 the World Medical Association expelled MASA from its ranks.

Despite the initial reaction, the World Medical Association reinstated South Africa before the end of 1981. The internal politics of the association made it possible for MASA to reenter even though the majority of countries holding membership voted against its reinstatement. This controversy ultimately led to the British Medical Association's withdrawal from the World Medical Association in 1984.[14] By 1989, Canada and all African and Scandinavian medical associations had resigned, and the WHO had severed ties with the organisation.[15] It was only in 1985 that two of the doctors were "slapped on the wrist" after being found guilty of "improper conduct."[16]

The murder of Steve Biko was not the only significant event in 1977 that had important implications for the ANC.[17] Less specific to South Africa, but nonetheless important, the World Health Assembly made the provision of healthcare for every man, woman, and child an international priority: global access to healthcare was set as a goal to be attained by the year 2000.[18] The 1977 WHO initiative, corresponding to the establishment of the ANC's Medical Committee, made the fledgling medical group relevant to the ANC's overall political goals. Later that year, the Committee of Experts on Primary Health Care in the Africa Region held a conference in Brazzaville, attended by Manto Tshabalala, to discuss the implementation of primary health care in order to achieve the WHO goals. In 1978 the WHO and United Nations International Children's Emergency Fund (UNICEF) sponsored an international conference on primary healthcare in Alma-Ata, USSR that was also attended by members of the ANC's Health Department.[19] This conference was a follow-up to the regional conferences held all over the world on primary health care and the policy recommendations had an important effect on the ANC's Health Department. It is within this context – the new global health initiative – that in 1978 the UN gave the ANC "observer status." This meant that the ANC was recognized as a worthwhile political entity and that the Health Department would be able to formally join in discussions with the WHO.[20]

South African doctors were aware of their diminishing international popularity and the ANC Health Department's growing international status. They were outraged that the untried medical sector of their political opponent could be considered a health representative in place of the NP's national Department of Health. In 1979 the *South African Medical Journal* printed an article called "WHO's Azania" that read: "The question is, why South Africa with its highly developed medical expertise has been ignored by WHO? By no stretch of the imagination can Azania (a non-existent country), and by implication the ANC and PAC, be regarded as its substitute."[21] Clearly, even prior to the 1980s, the ANC's Health Department was perceived to be a threat by the medical establishment in South Africa and the ANC department attempted to compare itself favourably against South Africa's medical system whenever possible.

The department, under the de facto leadership of Dr Tshabalala, drew heavily on international primary healthcare recommendations while planning its own policies and procedures. The Alma-Ata conference declared that health was a fundamental human right and stated that primary health "addresses the main health problems in the community, providing promotive, preventive, curative and rehabilitative services accordingly."[22] By the end of the year, Dr Tshabalala had drafted an ANC health policy with five main principles under the headings "prevention," "curative," "integration," "promotive," and "educational."[23] The draft policy was supposed to direct the Health Department's actions in exile as well as in the post-apartheid era. By mirroring the Alma-Ata values, Dr Tshabalala attempted to gain further international endorsement for her department.

In some cases, the WHO suggestions were not in line with the ANC Health Department's opinions on good healthcare practices. The department struggled to find a balance between keeping international favour by accepting the WHO recommendations and acting in the best interests of their patients. For instance, the declaration at Alma-Ata discussed the centrality of traditional healers in some societies and proposed that indigenous practitioners be incorporated into the health system.[24] Many Health Department members chafed against the suggestion of collaborating with the practitioners of traditional medicine.[25] In 1979 an ANC Medical Committee meeting stated that cadres were seeking out traditional healers, and the committee viewed this as a problem that needed rectification. While the WHO was pushing for "scientifically-guided" experimentation with traditional medicine, the ANC's Health Department, especially in Tanzania, sought to proceed with caution, clearly not wanting to endorse traditional methods.[26]

The hesitancy to fully embrace this WHO initiative was not without substance. In one incident, a medical report on the ANC's clinic at the Charlotte Maxeke crèche in Tanzania stated that, due to the influence of a traditional healer, a child was suffering from early stages of kwashiorkor.[27] A similar case was described four years later; a noticeably malnourished child who was experiencing acute fever and diarrhoea was brought to the ANC's clinic in its settlement in Dakawa, Tanzania. The child had originally been taken to a traditional healer rather than to the clinic, and, consequently, the child became acutely ill and needed to be transferred from Dakawa to Tanzania's facilities in Morogoro.[28] In another case, a child was given a blood transfusion and subsequently became infected. The mother was asked to bring the child in for penicillin every day for four days following the transfusion but, rather than return to the hospital, she took the child to a traditional healer. The child died on the fourth day after the infection was discovered.[29]

Understandably, by the end of 1982, medical staff members of the Health Department called for a well-defined policy guideline under which it could respond to patient requests to visit traditional healers.[30] The issue was politically delicate and the position taken was moderate and somewhat ambiguous. It was decided that, "the Department and [health] teams should advise of known dangers related with traditional healing. It should, however, be borne in mind that various governments and agencies supported by WHO are in the process of doing research on respective aspects of traditional healing."[31] In short, the Health Department did not want to endorse traditional healing but would not establish a policy that directly contradicted the WHO initiative.

While attempting to align their goals with those of their political and financial supporters, the ANC's Health Department seized on the opportunity for greater international recognition and support from the UN and its affiliated departments. Aside from treating South African patients, the ANC's Health Department had two main objectives: they sought to entrench the notion that the apartheid government was illegitimate and show that they were fit to step into the gap left by the NP. The health conferences were opportunities to accomplish these two goals. Dr Tshabalala directly addressed the head of the WHO Africa Region, Dr Quenum, to point out the impossibility of achieving "health for all" in the face of continued colonial oppression. This message was neither new to the WHO nor was Tshabalala trying to persuade Dr Quenum of the evils of apartheid; Dr Quenum was already in solidarity with the anti-apartheid movement. Instead, she was attempting to get Dr Quenum – and, by extension, the WHO – to take a more active role in supporting the Health Department in its fight against apartheid.

In her statement, Dr Tshabalala also argued that ending apartheid would be a step towards achieving the health goals written in the ANC's Freedom Charter. Mentioning the charter to Dr Quenum bore significance.[32] Established in 1955, the Freedom Charter flew directly in the face of apartheid policies, and it focused mostly on the need for racial equality and basic human rights for all citizens; healthcare made up a very small proportion of the document's contents. The health clause stated, "a preventive health scheme shall be run by the State; free medical care and hospitalization shall be provided for all, with special care for mothers and young children; the aged, the orphans, the disabled and sick shall be cared for by the State."[33] The Freedom Charter was a device used constantly by members of the Health Department to link themselves to the overall political goals of ending colonial oppression in South Africa. By connecting the Health Department to the more general and strongly endorsed anti-apartheid cause, Tshabalala was attempting to add legitimacy to the department and justify its need for support.

This political message continued after the reference to the Freedom Charter. Tshabalala proceeded to subtly call out the WHO for not fully committing to the "health for all" goal:

Indeed, for Africa to accede to "Health for all by the Year 2000" with the exclusion of South Africa and Namibia will be incomplete and consequently Africa would not have adequately responded to this global objective. *Failure to intensify moral and material support for the liberation movements in South Africa and Namibia, in their armed struggle* would ultimately rob these countries of a fair and valuable portion of the remaining 20 years to gear themselves in the health development programmes for their countries within the context of the Lagos Plan of Action[34] and the New International Economic Order.[35] [emphasis mine][36]

In short, healthcare for South Africans would be developed by the ANC's Health Department once the apartheid government had been overthrown and, by providing assistance to the Health Department in exile, international donors were implicitly supporting the anti-apartheid political *and military* cause.

The Health Department proposed an international conference titled "Health and Apartheid" to be held in early 1981. After months of delay, the conference – sponsored in part by the WHO – was held in Brazzaville in November. The list of participants was long and impressive: the WHO Secretariat, including Dr Mahler (director-general), Dr Quenum (regional director for Africa), and fourteen other directors or regional officers of the WHO in Africa; WHO representatives from Southeast Asia and Europe; delegates from the United Nations Development Programme (UNDP), UNICEF, United Nations Educational Scientific and Cultural Organization (UNESCO), and UNHCR among other UN organizations; Dr Kasiga, the project manager for the OAU/UN initiative to provide support for health to national liberation movements; Drs Tshabalala, Mfelang, and Dommisse representing the ANC; PAC and SWAPO representatives; two or three representatives from the ministries of health in the "Front-line States"[37] (Angola, Botswana, Mozambique, Zambia, and Zimbabwe); the chairperson from each subregion of the TCDC working groups; and an additional host of guests and observers. The attendance was indicative of the WHO's distain for the apartheid system and the growing desire to address the issue.

The conference was a major success for the ANC. Dr Quenum gave the first opening statement. He unequivocally stated that apartheid was antithetical to equal health provision in South Africa and finished his address by calling for a practical "plan for health action against apartheid." The speech of Alfred Nzo the secretary general of the ANC followed. It was plain from his address that he also wanted the conference to do more than agree to rhetorical anti-apartheid statements. He wanted "positive responses as to what each and every one of [the members present] intends to do to eliminate the unacceptable injustices [of apartheid]."[38] He emphasized that it was imperative that members act on their intentions. Dr Quenum and Alfred Nzo did not leave the conference disappointed. The conference developed a strategy that included a list of twenty-four clearly defined health-promoting and anti-apartheid actions to be taken by national liberation movements, the WHO and/or the international community at large. It also recommended increased health support for national liberation movements and the frontline states hosting them.

Despite the ANC's central position in organising the conference, "Health and Apartheid" international delegates were inclusive of all national liberation movements against apartheid including the PAC and SWAPO – both of which had sent delegates who gave opening statements to the conference. However, Alfred Nzo made sure to use his speech as an opportunity to promote the ANC's Health Department and its initiatives. Nzo drew attention to the fact that the ANC, rather than the NP, had adopted the WHO-backed primary healthcare policies. Part of Nzo's speech is worth quoting at length because it clearly conveys the self-estimation of the ANC's Health Department and the role that it envisioned for itself in the future. Further, the position received positive reception from the UN-affiliated departments and the international community. Nzo's speech included these words,[39]

> South Africa's official health delivery service is based on the Health Act No. 63 of 1977 declared by the racist Pretoria regime to be both comprehensive and community-based. We unapologetically denounce this Act as having absolutely nothing to do with the comprehensive and adequate delivery of health care, that must invariably include *promotional, preventive, curative and rehabilitation activists* ... We can see the answer to our health problem only through trust in national liberation and then through reorientation of the existing health services based on the primary health care approach. We therefore look forward to the occasion when it will be possible for us to be signatories to the Charter for Health Development for the African Region. Already we are signatories to some of the protocols for the Geneva Convention. [emphasis mine][40]

Not only did Nzo want to point out the Health Department policy of the ANC, he further went on to announce that the ANC's Health

Department, against all odds, had developed operational health teams in all regions: Nzo was pointing out that the ANC was stepping into the gap left by the NP.[41] The last words of the conference, recorded as the "Brazzaville Declaration," affirm the ANC's position and the UN, and its affiliated departments followed through on many of their initiatives. Consequently, the ANC became the beneficiary of the renewed, practical demonstration of this growing anti-apartheid sentiment.

The South African government's annoyance grew as the ANC continued to gain even more international recognition after the conference. As indicated in chapter 2, the UNHRC estimated that there were 5,000 South African "refugees" in Angola in 1981. In keeping with the "Brazzaville Declaration," it acknowledged that the ANC was strategically positioned to care for the exiles. Therefore, inciting the anger of the apartheid government, the UN division provided assistance to the ANC to care for the refugees. The 1981 UNHCR Yearbook Report included the description of a letter written by the minister for foreign affairs and information of South Africa:

> [The minister in South Africa] denied allegations made at ICARA [International Conference on Assistance to Refugees in Africa] that refugees were fleeing inhuman living conditions and persecution in Namibia and South Africa. He stated further that, while South Africa's requests for UNHCR assistance to Angolan refugees in Namibia had been ignored for political expediency, a considerable portion of funds dispensed by UNHCR and the United Nations Development Programme went to programmes executed by or benefiting the African National Congress of South Africa ... in promoting their political aims through violence and terror.[42]

The UNHCR was not concerned by the South African sentiment. Its actions displayed commitment to the proposed plan of action at Brazzaville and were a tangible indication that the ANC was an appropriate representative of South African civilians and deserved to be the beneficiaries of considerable funding.

Anti-Apartheid Health Propaganda

In dealing with the UN and WHO, the ANC Health Department strategically tapped into the momentum of the anti-apartheid movement and coupled global initiatives for health with political and military support for the ANC. The department was brand new and its foundational policies were influenced by international standards and moulded to achieve approval. This ongoing negotiation with the UN and the WHO was a core element of the department's political agenda and took up considerable time and effort. However, the ANC also attempted to use specific examples of racial injustice in the healthcare delivery system in South Africa and publicize them directly to potentially sympathetic audiences. In order to do this, the ANC had to find ways of gathering information and personal testimony about healthcare in South Africa, organize the material to appeal to an audience, and then present it to potential allies in and out of South Africa. The department hoped that this would discredit both MASA and healthcare in South Africa more generally, as well as provide a platform to advertise their own existence as an alternative representative for health in South Africa.

Medical data collection required help from within South Africa. Therefore the ANC sought to make contact with sympathetic doctors in the country. The need to establish these internal relationships was central to the Health Department's modus operandi of discrediting the apartheid regime.[43] In April 1980 ANC Drs Peter Mfelang and Ralph Mgijima travelled from Maputo to Swaziland where they met secretly with six doctors working in the Transvaal, Natal, and the Cape. The medical contingent discussed the fact that South African doctors were treating patients who had suffered from police brutality and learned that in the wake of Steve Biko's murder there was a growing number of doctors speaking out against medical injustice in the country. It was agreed that a doctor should be posted in Swaziland in order to establish regular meetings with sympathetic South African doctors in the country and keep the ANC informed of any new developments in the medical field. These reports were to be funnelled through Maputo on their way to the Health Department headquarters in Lusaka. By the end of 1980, ANC Dr Nkososana Dlamini (the first minister of health in post-apartheid South Africa) was posted to Swaziland for this task.[44]

While continually attempting to collect information from within the country, the Health Department tried to assert itself within the anti-apartheid movement already growing in the country. Because there was a strong effort being made to educate South Africans on the social determinants of health, a political presence within the country was critical for the ANC Health Department's credibility as the future health representative.[45] A pamphlet published by the ANC's medical administration in the mid-1980s demonstrates the overtly political aim. The pamphlet was titled "Doctors: where do you stand?" and disseminated in South Africa with the message that doctors operating in complicity with the apartheid government were in fact breaking the Hippocratic Oath.[46] It also reminded its intended medical audience of the Biko case alongside one other well-publicized incident of medical negligence. The ANC Health Department accused doctors in South Africa of prioritizing the interests of the South African security police over their obligation to the sick.[47] The overarching objectives of the document were to show that the underlying role of the doctor is incompatible with the apartheid system, to confront doctors about their involvement with apartheid, and to point out ways that they might be able to take an anti-apartheid stance.

Furthermore, the legitimacy of the armed struggle and its relationship to the Health Department was also a central message within the pamphlet: "The [NP] government tries to present us as communist-inspired 'terrorists'. We are, in fact, South Africans from all walks of life with a deep commitment to the future of our country. We have many doctors within our ranks."[48] The Health Department explicitly linked itself to the overarching political and military goals of the ANC and was subtly presenting its status as a government-in-waiting.

Medical staff members affiliated with the ANC's Health Department but based away from the African continent were also critical to the success of the department. These individuals took on much of the responsibility for publicizing the needs of the department and the anti-apartheid message underpinning the department's *raison d'être*. For instance, in 1979 the Canadian medical committee made up of Dr Peter Bunting, Dr Y. Mohamed, Fatima Bhyat, Enver Domingo, and Dr Fiki Radebe-Reed reported that its immediate aim was to gather information about the racist medical practices in South Africa and publicize its findings amongst Canadian medical personnel.[49]

It also promised to serve as a watchdog in Canada for medical complicity with the NP in South Africa.

The London RHT was also central to the department's international publicity efforts. The early team was made up of five members led by Comrades Mabtha and Aziza Seedat. While one report written by ANC Dr Ralph Mgijima – then located in southern Africa – indicated that the London team was still trying to figure out its identity in the anti-apartheid struggle, a different unaddressed London correspondence signed by Dr Seedat pointedly stated that the team's main job was to produce anti-apartheid propaganda and research related to the medical field.[50] Probably the most famous of the anti-apartheid medical research was conducted by Dr Seedat. Funded by the International Defence and Aid Fund for Southern Africa, Seedat published *Crippling a Nation: Health in Apartheid South Africa*, a one-hundred-page book systematically detailing the effects of apartheid on the health of South Africans.[51] Seedat's work clearly outlined apartheid's dual effect on black South African people's health. Especially in chapters 2 ("The Bantustans, Migrant Labour and Poverty") and 5 ("Occupational Health") he shows how South Africa's black-labour driven economy created a racialized and unequal health burden on blacks. In chapters 3 ("Malnutrition and Infant Mortality"), 4 ("Infectious Diseases"), and 6 ("Mental Health") he provides statistical evidence of those unequal health realities. In chapters 6, 7 ("Health Services"), and 8 ("Health Workers") he shows that in addition to bearing the brunt of these medical problems black South Africans also receive grossly substandard care. This research, and especially the statistical data, was subsequently used to promote the anti-apartheid cause.

As support grew in South Africa and abroad, the Health Department was able to benefit from the efforts of newly acquired sympathizers, and activists and issues of health in South Africa were effectively politicized to the advantage of the ANC. The Health Department's strategy to publicize *specific* policies and actions that it deemed racist and unjust is most clearly demonstrated in the ANC Health Department and Women's Section's combined campaign against the "genocidal" uses of the birth control drug Depo-Provera and other family planning policies in South Africa. The issue was a complicated one. While wishing to benefit from the international women's rights movement, the department also had to contend with its own and the ANC leadership's mixed feelings on topics like pregnancy and abortion.

"Depo Provera is a dangerous weapon"[52]

The ANC declared 1984 the "Year of the Women" and the Health Department's efforts internationally were bolstered by the ANC Women's Section and its involvement with women's reproductive rights. Together, the Health Department and the Women's Section shone a spotlight on family planning policies for black South Africans and, in particular, the use of Depo-Provera and forced sterilization. Depo-Provera is an injectable form of birth control which was introduced in South Africa in 1969 prior to its acceptance in Europe and North America. It was therefore seen by some activists as a dangerous element of the NP government's systematic attempts to control and reduce black fertility.[53] The NP's measures towards family planning and Depo-Provera were often provocatively referred to by the ANC as acts of *genocide*.

By at least 1981, the Health Department reported that it needed to "warn against the use of the injectable contraceptives – the Depo-provera."[54] Within six months of that declaration, the ANC charged the Women's Section with the task of researching into and starting a campaign against Depo-Provera. Their dual goal was to educate women about the side effects of the drug and to use "its maladministration on African women as an example of the regime's policies of genocide."[55] Once again, medical injustices were used as part of the broader project of discrediting the apartheid regime.

One of the first actions taken by the ANC was to write letters to doctors in South Africa about the use of Depo-Provera. Gertrude Shope, head of the ANC Women's Section starting in 1982, wrote to Drs Chris and Marius Barnard, the famous South African surgeons who conducted the world's first heart transplant. Identifying the surgeons as both having influence in the medical field and humanitarian leanings, Shope appealed to the men to "pay attention to the family-planning programme in South Africa, which is regarded by many of our black mothers as a kind of genocide, and in particular to the usage of Depo Provera."[56] Both letters painstakingly laid out many of the medical injustices in South Africa and focused on the use of Depo-Provera. In 1983 Gertrude Shope wrote to Kgaugelo Kgosana, an ANC medical student in Bulgaria, asking her to research and report back to the ANC on the dangers of this controversial drug. Kgonsana penned a four-page report outlining the potential side effects of using the contraceptive and providing an overview on the scientific debate about its safety. At that time, Kgonsana reported that the tests were not yet conclusive but that the drug was showing evidence of producing devastating side effects.[57]

In mid-1983 the ANC Women's Section and Health Department's campaign against Depo-Provera broadened its scope to include South Africa's aggressive policies on family planning geared to black women. Writing to Lucia Raadchelders, a member of an anti-apartheid group in the Netherlands, Gertrude Shope argued that it would be more strategic to blame apartheid and the systemic racist attitudes towards black women's fertility instead of just focusing on the use of Depo-Provera:

> [F]or the campaign to be more political and in line with the ANC policy we must launch a campaign against the whole regime's strategy of family planning and we bring up the usage of all dangerous contraceptives and highlight DP [Depo-Provera] since it the [sic] most dangerous and widely used. In this way we feel we will be able to reach out [to] even bodies like WHO, IPPF [International Planned Parenthood Federation] and others who actually distribute and defend DP. In fact as a Liberation Movement if we launch a campaign against DP in countries which host us and use this drug, we can face lots of difficulties.[58]

Despite the cautions against full condemnation of Depo-Provera, Shope also explained that the anti-Depo-Provera agenda was still ongoing; the Women's Section and Health Department were getting information from medical personnel within South Africa on the uses and abuses of the injection. It was further clear that Shope aimed to launch this awareness campaign both inside South Africa and internationally.[59]

In November 1983, financed by the WHO, the ANC Health Department sent Manto Tshabalala to the IPPF conference in Nairobi. Her unsigned handwritten report on this conference was filed in the archive.[60] Tshabalala was present with the objective of educating members of the IPPF about the aggressive and racist family planning program in South Africa, and she attempted to get South Africa removed from the federation. Her notes clearly convey the ANC's position on family planning in South Africa and her frustration with the attitudes of the people she encountered whilst at the conference:

> Does the FPA S.A. [Family Planning Association in South Africa] support [government] policy on "family planning" for black people?
> Does FPA campaign against the racist SA strategy of "family planning" and other dangerous contraceptives used by the regime. Have they asked why.
> Do they believe in overpopulation.
> Do they think also black [sic] should be their target in FP [Family Planning] because they breed like rabbits.[61]

Tshabalala returned from the meeting disappointed. Though she had pointed out that the Family Planning Association (FPA) in South Africa was racist and that Depo-Provera was being used in an unethical way, it was ruled that the FPA was abiding by the conditions set by the IPPF.

The ANC's Health Department and Women's Section remained undeterred and continued to collect evidence against the NP regarding birth control in South Africa. In July 1984 the International Contraception, Abortion and Sterilisation Campaign (ICASC) and members from three European pro-abortion campaigns held the International Tribunal and Meeting on Reproductive Rights.[62] Gertrude Shope wrote to the ICASC for financial assistance to attend the conference, justifying her attendance by saying, "Through these contact[s] we can build public opinion in other countries still supporting the racist regime which will help in isolating the regime and lead to its destruction and replacement by a government based on the will of the people which will provide health facilities for all women and guarantee reproductive rights."[63] Though Shope did not say it explicitly, she regarded her attendance at this tribunal on reproductive rights as yet another way to show the ANC to be the rightful future South African government. In a sense, the tribunal was aptly named; this was an opportunity to put apartheid on trial in front of a specific and potentially powerful interest group.

The ANC was able to send a representative, who was likely Gertrude Shope. The tribunal's by-line was "No to Population Control... Women Decide"[64] and the overall goal was to hear the diverse voices of globally marginalized women and bring them into a conversation about women's reproductive rights. Topics were listed as contraception, abortion, and sterilization; drugs; sexual politics; population control or women's control (from different countries' viewpoints); women and disability; and racism.[65] It was very likely Shope who presented the ANC's position on South African practices related to contraception, abortion, and sterilization.[66]

ICASC was an organisation founded in 1978 on the back of a growing women's movement against harmful birth control methods. This group was therefore an excellent audience for the ANC's concerns about Depo-Provera. At the tribunal, the ANC presented examples of where it was evident that racism had guided population control strategies. In particular, it outlined the racist use of birth control, sterilization, and abortion under the guise of family planning. Shope's presentation included three examples of women who had had negative experiences with Depo-Provera.[67] In all three cases, women were placed on the drug unaware of the side effects and their later concerns regarding side effects were ignored. In one of the cases, a woman reported negative side effects, was largely disregarded by medical staff, experienced severe haemorrhaging, and died shortly after making her complaints known.[68] Health authorities in South Africa denied that her death was related to Depo-Provera.

At the end of a presentation to the tribunal, which was mostly a long condemnation of the NP government, Shope used the platform to plead for international support and solidarity. She stated that she hoped those in attendance would "take action" and then quickly pointed out that the ANC had already started work against South Africa's racist policies. The message left was clear: the NP government needs to be stopped, South African women need international backing, and the ANC should be supported because it has already started to do the work.[69]

Given the international audience of the ANC at the tribunal, and the growing women's rights movement, the ANC's Health Department had to think carefully about its own policy regarding women's reproductive health in exile. The ANC leadership may have encouraged the use of condoms and birth control pills but it often held conservative views about the sexual conduct of women, pregnancy, and abortion. In order to gain international credibility with women's groups concerned with reproductive health, the Health Department and Women's Section had to tread cautiously between the values of many in the ANC leadership and the values clearly espoused in the international realm. This dilemma became evident in the debates about pregnancy and abortion amongst ANC members in exile.

Especially in the 1970s and early 1980s, the attitudes and policy towards pregnancy and abortion in exile bore some resemblance to the conservative stance taken in South Africa. There were a number of reasons for this. First, abortion was illegal in Tanzania, Angola, Mozambique, and Zambia – the countries where the ANC Health Department had developed infrastructure projects – and the ANC did not want to transgress national law. But these laws evidently reflected the views of the leadership, including some of the leadership in the Health Department until the late 1980s.

The 1981 Health Department report entitled "Child-Birth in Exile: A Problem Oriented Approach, Some Aspects of Women and Health" provides some indication of the Health Department's early negative attitudes about unplanned pregnancy and abortion. The report stated, "We are all aware of the false sense of safety flowing from the use of contraceptives. We are also equally aware that people with no scruples and a sense of pride will almost invariably indulge in random sexual life very often leading to abortions and the spread of sexually transmitted diseases."[70] It is likely that this statement was a reflection of the department's frustration over the growing number of pregnancies among students and cadres in exile, but it also betrayed the department's disapproval of abortion by linking abortion with promiscuity and STIs.

Four months after the 1984 tribunal a survey was sent by Mohammed Tikly, part of the ANC leadership in Tanzania, to seven different political bodies of the ANC in Tanzania. The survey had nine questions that considered the morality of abortion and the appropriate consequences for ANC students who became pregnant. After receiving the responses, Tikly reported that he found the level of conservatism "alarming."[71] The responses were varied. To the question "Should a pregnant student be immediately removed from school?" one individual indicated that women should be allowed to continue schooling as long as they felt able to, while another argued that, "In Africa once a student falls pregnant, she is removed from school with immediate effect. We have to retain some of our African values." In response to the question of what should be done to the male and female if an abortion is "committed," the answers indicated the view that abortion was a punishable offence: "If the male partner is not an accomplice, he must be allowed to continue with his studies … Cases must be viewed individually to ascertain that both male and female are involved in the taking of the decision … Something must be done to correct the wrong-doer."[72]

Throughout the early 1980s, in keeping with the attitudes shown in the results of the questionnaire, the ANC leadership in Tanzania sent students caught involved in procuring abortions to the Rehabilitation Section of the Dakawa Development Centre. Upon arrival at the development centre, the students filled out forms about themselves. The last question on the read "Why are you sent to Dakawa?" Answers given included "(for punishment) committed an abortion," "I was sent to Dakawa because I got pregnant and I decided to arbort," "I've done an abolion [sic]," and "I was sent to Dakawa because I responded to the president's call that there should not be pregnancy this year (1983). This brought about the two couples being involved in an abortion."[73] The responses indicated clear understanding of, and sometimes anger toward, the reason for their banishment. Despite the liberal though inexplicit position on reproductive rights presented to international audiences, the practice of sending students to Dakawa continued into 1987.[74]

Representatives of the ANC's Health Department and Women's Section avoided presenting a firm stance on abortion until the late 1980s. In the above-mentioned conference with ICASC, Gertrude Shope stated that abortion was illegal in South Africa, and she provided statistics on the number of illegal abortions procured each year. However, she did not state an opinion on abortion legalization and instead asserted that "[i]llegal abortion can thus be regarded as the fifth but unsung techniques [*sic*] used by the regime to implement its programme of population control."[75] Ending her statement on abortion with these words suggests a negative posture towards legalizing abortion but similar to the case with traditional healing, the speech does not go as far as to venture an actual contradictory opinion on the matter.

In addition to a controversial position on abortion, in at least one case the ANC's internal treatment of women had the potential to expose the Health Department and Women's Section as hypocritical at best and criminal at worst. In 1987 two female cadres, P (18 years old) and M (20 years old) became pregnant; P in Angola and M in the GDR. As was the policy, the two were told that they would be transferred to Tanzania in order to deliver and raise their babies. En route, they were stopped in Zambia where they remained for approximately one month; P and M were both between four and five months pregnant at the time. According to P's testimony, she and comrade M were taken to the clinic in Lusaka. She wrote, "I was held down by 4 women and 2 men and my mouth was covered. They used some instrument on me which caused pain and bleeding, and then gave me two injections." She was taken to the house of a member of the Health Department, comrade Daisy, who informed her that the abortion was a "favour" to her because at eighteen, she was too young to have children. The following day, while still at Daisy's house, she miscarried the baby. Gertrude Shope met her later and explained that this whole experience must be kept a complete secret. P concluded her statement by stating, "I was prepared to keep that baby. I was told I was underage. I was not given the chance to discuss the matter. I wasn't asked what I wanted to do, or given any forms to fill in."[76]

Comrade M's story was very similar. She was given an injection at the clinic in Lusaka, and when she awoke on the clinic table was bleeding and vomiting and suspected that she had been given an abortion. M recalled, "The Zambian doctor said she was told by Dr Zakes (ANC doctor) that this was a decision of the organisation, and that we were supposed to go to school and couldn't go while pregnant. Dr Zakes said to [P] she should let them do what they want to her."[77] M was given another two injections and some pills, and she, too, was sent to Daisy's house. M's recollection of her interaction with Daisy was indicative of the need for the ANC's Health Department to keep this entire affair secret. "Daisy insulted me and was saying many things. She said people will say that the organisation is aborting people, and that if I died people will say that the ANC killed me. She said I was doing the work of an agent, [by acting distressed and sick after the procedure] and tomorrow I must decide if I'm on the side of the enemy or the organisation." M miscarried the next morning. Following the whole incident, the two were sent back to Angola where they promptly told members of a horrified Angola Health Team what had happened to them.[78]

Four days after their statements were taken in Angola, P and M were invited to a meeting in Angola to discuss the events that had occurred in Lusaka. When P was asked why she thought the abortion had been performed on her, she replied that she thought it was because of the "high pregnancy rate in Angola."[79] While not immediately commented on, comrade P's statement is particularly damning in the context of the ANC's international stance on the NP's family planning program. Fear of exposure is clear throughout the rest of the meeting. One member of the ANC leadership spoke of the misconduct of P and M in this matter stating,

> [T]hey had no right to destroy a member of the NEC and head of the Women section. Could they, as young cadres of the movement go all out and say such about a leader? Where they aware of the damage they have done in Charleston [Chelston, ANC community in Zambia] … they have gone all-out to destroy a senior comrade … *If this information (abortion) could reach the enemy it will be spread not only against Mashope [Gertrude Shope] but against the ANC.* [emphasis mine][80]

The deputy head of the ANC Women's Section concluded the meeting with a reprimand to the women for spreading rumours about the conduct of the Health Department and the Women's Section and accused P and M of being "one-sided" and of telling this story in process of "cleansing themselves." This record of the 12 December 1987 meeting was the last word on the incident found in the archive. Without further evidence and testimony, it is not possible to definitively say whether P and M had been forced against their will to have abortions in Lusaka. It is clear, however, that the two women had been given abortions and were traumatized by their experiences. It is also obvious that the ANC had a lot at stake in keeping the testimonies of P and M quiet. Telling others about their experiences was seen as a treasonous act against the whole organisation. This was, in part, because this incident indicated that the ANC's Health Department was forcing family planning on unwilling women which was exactly what it was accusing the apartheid government of doing. Fortunately for the ANC, the event never received international attention.

Leading up to this case in 1987, movement of the ANC towards accepting a proabortion policy was building momentum. The changes were slowly installed, pushed by the international women's empowerment movement and implemented first in Angola due to the needs of the military. The Women's Section wanted more women to be able to continue their work as militants rather than be disarmed and sent to Tanzania to become mothers. In 1983, MK Commander Joe Modise argued that the ANC was in an "abnormal situation" and that therefore the ANC should consider exceptions to the anti-abortion policy.[81] By the late 1980s the Women's Section was publishing its stand in favour of a "woman's right to choose" and health policy documents began to echo this sentiment with clear assertions that a woman should have the right to terminate a pregnancy and should not be put under pressure in the process of making her decision.[82]

However, the Health Department's policy on abortion was not consistent across all regions. An undated late-1980s report by the Health Department outlined "selective social termination." This policy was first concerned with the military: "[T]he following comrades should be considered for social termination of pregnancy: 1) Cadres earmarked for special missions; 2) Cadres undergoing military training."[83] But in nonmilitary cases, the woman needed to prove that she had been using some kind of contraceptive at the time of conception. With these criteria in mind, a letter addressed to the health secretariat in 1988 stated,

> I hereby endorse the fact that the above mentioned [comrade] sought contraceptives from our doctors in Luanda. This measure was not provided and subsequently the [comrade] got pregnant ... This [comrade] has been given

special training and was earmarked to be sent home ... [W]
e appeal to you to render assistance to terminate [the preg-
nancy] in the interests of our struggle so that she can make
her contribution.[84]

A health secretariat progress report to the NEC in October 1987
stated that four abortions had been performed on "social grounds"
but that "[d]espite this positive attitude to social abortions, there
has been bitter reaction to the decision by certain senior members
of the movement."[85] The Health Department sought to address
the bitterness, and the desire to promote women's equality in the
military struggle pushed the issue of abortion forward. By the close
of 1987, the department advanced their liberal position and put
forward that "social abortion is a fully acceptable procedure under
present circumstances."[86]

As the conservative hold of the ANC loosened on the issue of
abortion, the Health Department asserted its new liberal stance and
made sure that its post-apartheid health policies would provide women
access to "free abortion on request."[87] This health policy, while slow
in development, was miles ahead of the laws maintained in southern
Africa. Abortion was not legalized in southern Africa in the 1980s and
in fact remains illegal in Angola and Tanzania today. The adoption
of change on the policy regarding abortion in the 1980s illuminates
the ANC Health Department's and Women Section's strong desire
to gain legitimacy with the international women's reproductive
rights movement.

The ANC Health Department's and Women Section's involvement
with international organisations interested in the issue of family
planning and contraception irradiates the politicization of healthcare for anti-apartheid ends. The campaign to publicize apartheid
family planning policies and the use of Depo-Provera were meant
to delegitimize the NP. The ANC Health Department used conferences as forums to promote itself as the future governing body that
would prioritize women's reproductive rights. However, in the early
to mid-1980s, the ANC's Health Department was unable to produce
a liberal feminist position on abortion and therefore remained quiet
about its policies on the issue. Throughout the 1980s, driven by the
needs of the military, the ANC slowly adopted a proabortion policy,

ABORTION

WHO SHOULD CHOOSE?

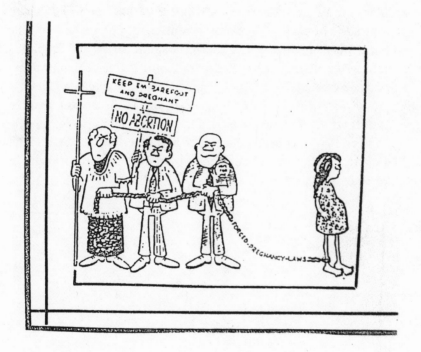

3.1 "Abortion: Who Should Choose?," no date [1989?]. The image depicts a woman, shackled to three men (one is a priest). The men carry a sign saying "No Abortion" and "Keep em Barefoot and Pregnant." The illustration conveys the message that patriarchy prevents women from being able to control their own fertility.

and the Health Department's statements in the late 1980s reveal its eagerness to announce its progressive position on this issue.

The ANC Health Department took on an important role in the ANC's international anti-apartheid campaign. It managed to find near-immediate support and success because it emerged at a politically opportune moment in the late 1970s. At that time medical practice in South Africa was put under fire because of the medical complicity in the tragic death of Steve Biko, the international anti-apartheid movement was on the rise, and the WHO launched its "health for all" campaign. As a result, the department staff met with early success. Members attended international conferences on a variety of health topics to entrench anti-apartheid sentiment, pointed out specific health-related atrocities committed in South Africa, and promoted itself as the alternative health department. The Health Department's campaign against South African reproductive health programs illumin-ates this strategy. However, it also exposes the disconnect between the department's rights-based rhetoric abroad and its predominantly conservative practices on the ground in southern Africa. The Health Department had to silence incidences of hypocrisy in the realm of reproductive health.

4

"The Ambulance is on a Safari": Primary Healthcare Delivery in Southern Africa, 1977–1990

The participation of the Health Department in the anti-apartheid struggle was politically advantageous to the ANC, and it therefore showed itself to be a relevant and important part of the liberation struggle on the diplomatic front. However, its role on the international stage should not obscure the Health Department's attempt to deliver medical services to South Africans in exile. Thousands of patients arrived at ANC facilities for medical care; some managed to receive effective treatment, but many patients were victims of a young, inexperienced, and often corrupt health department. Despite its shortcomings, the ability to treat exiles was important to the Health Department; without access to its future constituents at home, it was imperative to represent itself as an alternate medical representative of South Africa's healthcare interests by treating South Africans in exile. Disappointing to the ANC, international donors, and especially South African exiles, the department fell well short of its potential for healthcare delivery. The ANC Health Department used the favourable political climate to morally justify itself, but, much to its embarrassment, could not hide its inexperience in actually caring for the sick in a systematic, government-like manner.

One of the beneficial by-products of its international public exposure was that the ANC's Health Department gained political and financial support for its efforts in southern Africa. Proposals for massive infrastructure projects like medical training centres, clinics, and hospitals were given generous support from a variety of donors worldwide. By supporting the ANC to provide for the health needs of South African exiles, these donors were giving the ANC implicit support and recognition as a politically legitimate force in a future democratic South Africa while also serving the medical needs of refugees and MK cadres. While the ANC's political and military leadership did not often explicitly prioritize the medical sector in exile, health provision in exile cannot be divorced from politics. Furthermore, the level of funding provided by the international community was indicative of the ANC's growing diplomatic success.

Financial support from Sweden preceded the ANC medical staff's attempts to plead their case for legitimacy to the global community. By the time the Medical Committee had had its third meeting, it had already been given a substantial sum of money from the Netherlands' government.[1] Therefore, the Health Department itself was not responsible for acquiring its initial funding. Instead, the department's efforts were geared at receiving continued political endorsement and financial support from its donors.[2] The existence of the Health Department offered humanitarians a direct avenue to show their support for the liberation movement and their antipathy towards apartheid. As a result, gaining support from donors was much easier for the ANC than actually providing care for its charges.

Following its inception, the Health Department began developing plans for major infrastructure projects including clinics and hospitals in Tanzania, Angola, Mozambique, and Zambia. These received almost immediate endorsement and financial support from NGOs and national governments, particularly in Scandinavia. The projects were clear examples of the ANC's attempt to engage in statecraft.

While this chapter shows that the Health Department's infrastructure projects were examples of the ANC's practice at state-building, the detailed focus on healthcare delivery contributes to the growing body of social history dealing with the everyday experiences of people in exile. Scholars have begun to ask questions about the daily realities of living in exile and how those realities affected the exiled South African people's experience and informed their decisions.[3] This chapter follows suit; it is important to bring attention to the fact that the input of international donors and the choices of medical staff mattered to desperate patients who knocked on the newly opened doors of ANC clinics and hospitals. What follows is a series of anecdotal snapshots highlighting key health infrastructure projects and medical staff relationships. Collectively, they demonstrate the Health Department's incapacity to consistently provide basic primary healthcare to patients.

Infrastructure Projects:
Kurasini and Mazimbu

The East Africa Health Team's efforts were often very uncoordinated. This was partly due to the fact that it relied on a variety of different health facilities throughout the 1970s and 1980s and that not all of those facilities were directly under its control. The authority over health decisions was spread between the East Africa Health Team, the ANC leadership, the Mazimbu leadership, the Health Department in Lusaka, the Tanzanian government, and semi-independent foundations and donors. As a result, it was difficult to streamline medical care and adequately communicate among institutions. Unfortunately for the Health Department, the factions of health authority enjoyed their independence often at the expense of the patients.

The lack of communication was exemplified in a 1979 report written by Dr Aziza Seedat, then on the ANC Medical Committee in London.[4] Seedat arrived to inspect the Tanzanian services that he and the London medical team had been working to support. He found that due to shortages of qualified doctors drugs sent from international allies remained unpacked and essentially wasted. The ANC spent money purchasing drugs while available free drugs remained untouched and left to expire in a hot room in Morogoro. Seedat stated, "as up to now, we have had somewhat misleading reports about the Health situation here ... we have been directing our energies towards obtaining medical equipment and drugs, without being vaguely aware of the vast amount of untapped recourses [*sic*] already available."[5] Furthermore, he stated his disappointment that the materials put together by the London team for a research library were unaccounted for. As a member of the team in London actively trying to discredit the apartheid regime, Seedat wanted the Health Department to succeed so that he could report back to the international community on the ANC's smooth and effective service delivery. But the type of poor management he witnessed mired the department's efforts in Tanzania. As a result, the clinics operated in a reactive, near-crisis mode that was fiscally irresponsible, mentally difficult for staff, less effective for patients, and put a strain on the relationships between the ANC and its international donors.[6]

Kurasini

Starting in 1966 the ANC had access to the property and residence in Kurasini that would only later be used in a medical capacity.[7] The total property was 3800m[2] and included two houses that had been built in the 1950s.[8] In 1974 the Lutuli Memorial Foundation, backed by Swedish Krona, put SEK50,000 (approximately US$11,000) into a clinic.[9] This support, while crucial to opening the clinic, gave the foundation significant control over any medical or administrative decisions made at the clinic. For the next five years following that initial instalment of money, control of the property was incrementally transferred from the foundation to the Health Department. The sluggish exchange was problematic because it complicated the ability of the clinic to function effectively; it appeared that Kurasini was owned by the ANC, operated by the Lutuli Memorial Foundation, and often staffed by East Africa Health Team personnel.[10]

The majority of patients passing through Kurasini suffered from some form of mental illness (which will be discussed in more detail in chapter 5). A 1982 survey provided a breakdown of the mental health problems of the sixteen "inmates.'" According to the survey, there were

6 chronic schizophrenics – all had florid symptoms
3 alcohol and cannabis induced psychosis
3 depressions
1 anxiety neurosis

2 organic brain syndrome (one had korsakoff and the other
CVA from hypertension)
1 epilepsy[11]

Many of the patients at the residence were violent or suicidal.[12] Therefore, these patients required a specialized type of attention that was not available.[13] In fact, local Tanzanian psychiatrist J.G. Hauli observed that the staff assigned to Kurasini were negligent in their duty to implement the doctor-prescribed programs designed for ANC patients. He indicated that the ignorance of Kurasini staff to the realities of psychiatric illness was the central cause of the poor quality of patient care.[14]

Medical personnel at the residence were responsible for accompanying (and often personally driving) patients from Kurasini to Muhimbili Hospital[15] and for taking care of the sick between treatments.[16] Due to these intensive and sometimes dangerous around-the-clock demands, Kurasini was not a coveted post for medical personnel and was perpetually understaffed. At times, only one or two members of the East Africa medical staff were posted there.[17]

Consequently, the sickbay was not an ideal place to send patients. However, the facility provided ANC patients the opportunity to access Tanzanian facilities at low housing cost. It was especially crucial for patients who needed constant surveillance and more support than their daily appointments at Muhimbili afforded. Therefore, it was important for the ANC Health Department to find international support to upgrade the facility. The department managed to acquire a significant sum of money to renovate the building, but the improvements actually achieved were minimal. The international community continued to send money to the project but failed to hold the department accountable. The Health Department's unchecked incompetency resulted in the failure to develop Kurasini into a fully functional sickbay.

In 1979 Tshabalala wrote to Dr Akerele of the WHO branch in Dar es Salaam, applying for TZS36,762.65 (approximately US$4,800).[18] The WHO responded favourably and transferred money for the upgrade of the sick bay.[19] In 1981 the Health Department reported that the renovations made were minimal and that the supervisor of the project was unable to either report on the clinic's progress or offer a financial account of how the money was spent.[20] In fact, some of the materials that were purchased by WHO funding were effectively stolen by the man hired to do the renovations; this was not reported at the time, and the treasury was thus not able to successfully follow up on the mishandling of funds.[21]

The problems were not just with the physical structure. Nellie Mvulane, a staff member at Kurasini, wrote in 1981 to the ANC's administrative secretary:

> We are faced with extreme theft and assault on members of the medical team in Dar es Salaam ... Lately Kurasini has been a dumping place for comrades with anti-social behaviours due to dagga [cannabis] smoking and alcoholism. This is a sick bay for physically ill and genuinely ill mentally disturbed patients ... These [dagga smoking and alcoholic comrades] assault members of the staff and patients and also ... steal food, staff clothes, utensils and equipment from Kurasini.[22]

Without adequate oversight and support, the line between patient care and criminal restraint was blurred. In the early 1980s Kurasini was one of the frontline institutions attempting to cope with this issue.

While the patients may have presented difficulties at the sickbay, there were a number of cases when staff also proved to be an untoward challenge. In one report it was stated that medical assistant Comrade Joe Mosupye was transferred from SOMAFCO, the ANC's school in Mazimbu, to Kurasini due to his poor performance and carelessness at the Mazimbu site.[23] Mosupye came late to work and was grossly negligent. In one incident, he accompanied a critically ill patient to the hospital and, rather than waiting with the patient as his job description required him to do, abandoned his charge to an unknown nurse and left the hospital. Due to Mosupye's actions, the patient went unregistered and died in the hospital; he was only found and identified three days later. In addition to negligence, Mosupye was caught having sex with patients on more than one occasion; having sex with patients was most certainly considered unethical for medical staff due to their relative position of power. For his infractions, Mosupye was suspended from duty for one month.[24] By the end of 1981, it was reported that, "the Kurasini sick bay – which is in a mess at present and unsuitable for human habitation ... has to some extent, caused the deterioration of those affected [by physical and psychological handicaps]."[25] The conduct did not improve. In July 1985, rumours of continued negative medical staff behaviour including drunkenness and the selling of drugs in Dar es Salaam led the Regional Political Council (RPC) to unilaterally disband the entire Dar es Salaam health team. The team was suspended, blocked from future education scholarships for two years and sent to Dakawa. Indignant, the health team redeployed the individuals from Dar es Salaam to serve in Mazimbu and Dakawa; they also accused the RPC of being careless, stating that, "As a result [of the disbanding of the qualified staff] there were incidences ranging from abscesses to death of a comrade who died in the residence without even at least first-aid treatment."[26]

In late 1981 and early 1982, the ANC drew up a new proposal for the renovation and expansion of Kurasini. In their response to the proposal, donors indicated that the ANC should contribute health personnel and staff and that they, the Norwegian and/or Danish People's Relief Association (it is unclear which), would fund the renovation, "up-grade" health personnel, pay expenses, and pay health-team incentives.[27] This answer indicated that the donor was not just interested in caring for the patients; the donor wanted to provide the ANC Health Department with the finances necessary to develop staff and take self-ownership of the building. The Danish People's Relief Association raised TZS400,000 (approximately UD$43,000) for the project.[28]

Despite this promising international response, renovations were not immediately forthcoming and poor reports from the sickbay continued to be relentless and desperate. In April 1982 Manto Tshabalala reported, "Kurasini is in uninhabitable condition now. With the heavy rains, the roof leaks and the whole establishment sets [sic] flooded. The sanitary and environment situation poses a health hazard."[29] In May 1982 a third-year medical student and member of the health team, Mandla Lubanga, reported that the funds were still not yet released to the project and that Kurasini was "in aruinous [sic] state and can collapse anytime."[30] Just over a week later, Dr Tshabalala wrote to the secretary of the ANC's East Africa RHT and cc'd the ANC president, the secretary general, and the chief representative stating that the backlog on the Kurasini renovations was unacceptable and somewhat embarrassing with respect to the credibility of the Health Department with its international donors.[31] While its international presence on the anti-apartheid front was growing (as shown in chapter 3), the delays in practical health delivery in Kurasini discredited the Health Department's claim to be a functioning alternative representative of the medical needs of South Africans. As a result, patients were suffering needlessly and Tshabalala was asking for help to correct the situation.

After Tshabalala's statement, the archive is silent on the situation at Kurasini until October 1982 when yet another Kurasini renovation and upgrade plan carrying a TZ 2,179,760 (approximately US$220,000) price tag was released by the ANC.[32] Clearly the expected renovations promised earlier in the year had not yet been completed because the October planning report devised by the Morogoro Technical Committee (presumably a bureaucratic division of the ANC leadership dealing with social service development in Tanzania) stated,

> The existing premises presently accommodate a total of 15 patients ... the patients are overcrowded ... facilities are wholly inadequate. The sewage and waste disposal system is defective causing blockages as well as the periodic overflow of sewage from the existing septic tank. The roofs are leaking and extensive rot has spread through the roofing timbers. The electrical wiring is old and in a dangerous state. Conditions for patients and staff are therefore intolerable.[33]

Evidently, the anti-apartheid support in Scandinavia was strong enough to persevere despite the lack of previous action. In February 1983 the Danish People's Relief Association visited Tanzania and its report stated that DKK550,000 (approximately US$60,000) had been allocated for the Kurasini project and that new equipment was purchased for the clinic.[34]

Still no progress was made. Manto Tshabalala explained that the delay in action was caused by the ANC's reluctance to commit to a Tanzanian architectural firm's proposed plans. She also again reported on the situation in Kurasini: "Conditions ... are depressing and demoralizing both to the patients and the staff. The sewage system poses a health hazard. The environment is not conductive to introducing any rehabilitative programmes despite several offers [and] that the situation is expressed in talks such as 'Mazimbu my beginning, Kurasini my ending.'"[35] She advised that either immediate action take place or the residence be shut down altogether. On 10 April ANC President Oliver Tambo responded to Tshabalala's plea by visiting Kurasini. Tambo insisted that the project move forward. As a result, Stanley Mabizela (the ANC's chief representative in Tanzania) formed a task committee to expedite the process.[36]

In mid 1983 the Danish People's Relief Association donated a Land Rover valued at £5,040.14 (approximately US$7,600) to the sickbay. They also sent equipment for an examination room, minor theatre, and treatment room, which was supposed to arrive on 21 June 1983. As of January 1984 the Health Department in Lusaka was not sure whether the equipment had arrived and was discussing the shut down of Kurasini as a sickbay.[37] In April 1984 a National Women's Executive meeting reported that the plans for the renovation of Kurasini were still not complete and that the care was very substandard:[38] "Comrades from the West [Angola] with bullet wound[s] were reported to be simply dumped in the place with nobody to look after them. Some cannot look after themselves and nurses are very essential for Kurasini."[39] The final conclusion of the women's meeting stated "Kurashini [sic] will not be renovated. The Tanzanian government said we should do it in Mazimbu or Dakawa."[40]

As indicated in the 1984 report, the renovations for the sickbay never took place. In February 1987, Chief Administrator Tim Maseko reflecte,: "At one time the old Kurasini clinic in Dar was to have been converted into the mentally sick patients centre and it would appear that the plan was somehow shelved, and funding has been available."[41] In December 1987 renovations on the Kurasini building finally did commence; unfortunately for the Health Department, the renovations were firmly geared at housing ANC representatives and students instead of medical patients.[42]

Kurasini was clearly not a success story for the ANC in general or its Health Department in particular. The residence was an unsanitary and often dangerous accommodation that was left understaffed by the East Africa Health Team and neglected by the administration despite international support. The mismanagement of the building illuminated the lack of accountability of the bureaucracy put in place to manage funds and facilitate better services. It also showed the relative lack of power that the Health Department was able to exert over the management of money donated to its own project. The money was kept in the treasury and the broader leadership did not provide the Health Department with open access to the funds. The renovations geared to the needs of patients never materialized, and the ANC moved on, concentrating its efforts on designing a facility that could accept mentally ill patients in its own settlement in Dakawa.[43] For these reasons, the Health Department failed in Kurasini as a government-in-waiting.[44]

Mazimbu, Morogoro[45]

International support for the ANC's medical projects in the Morogoro region far surpassed the attention given to Kurasini. Part of the reason was that the ANC's two semi-autonomous ANC settlements, Mazimbu and Dakawa, were optimal opportunities for the ANC to practice its state-like social services. Because Mazimbu was the first to be developed, its infrastructure was superior to Dakawa, and it was the site of the first major hospital owned and operated by the ANC. Patients in Mazimbu suffered from the Health Department's inexperience, mismanagement of funds, and negligence of and miscommunication between medical staff members. However, Mazimbu was also a beacon of international endorsement for the ANC and a place where thousands of South African and Tanzanian patients were treated. By financing an ANC-owned hospital, international sponsors were advertising that the ANC was more than a liberation movement; it was able to semi-independently provide for some of the social needs of its constituents.

The MKA (a Netherlands-based donor) explicitly linked the ANC's capacity to provide healthcare in exile with the broader anti-apartheid effort when in 1980 it adopted the slogan: "Build a hospital and equip it, support the ANC, the liberation movement of South-Africa."[46] By that time, the organization had raised ƒ400,000[47] (approximately US$185,000) for initial construction and was set to raise another ƒ400,000 for the project.[48] MKA president Henk Odink estimated that the amount required to fund a fully equipped ANC hospital would be raised before the start of 1983. The MKA created a six-person task force to be part of the development process, and as a result it and the ANC often exchanged detailed descriptions of equipment and physical blueprints of the hospital. When the ANC proposed dramatic changes and additions to the structure, the MKA did not balk at the alterations but rather responded positively and continued to be supportive.[49] The MKA was deeply invested in the success of the Health Department because medical provision had become part of the overall liberation effort.

Although the MKA was the main donor to the Mazimbu hospital project, it was not the only one. Other NGO and government involvement was also politically important to the ANC. For instance, the Norwegian campaign to raise support for the Mazimbu hospital was witness to the growing acceptance of the ANC's government-in-waiting status. Reflecting on his time in Norway in 1979, the ANC's Dr Ralph Mgijima reported,

> Requisition for equipment for the Health Centre in Mazimbu fell out though the Foreign Ministry felt that this project would influence positively the general contribution of Norway to the African National Congress … The opening [Norwegian] rally [for ANC support] was attended by a thousand or more people and as such this was an indication that the ANC is at last being recognised by the Norwegians as the rightful representative of the people of South Africa.[50]

Despite the fact that this account was written by an ANC doctor, Mgijima's assessment of the Norwegian sentiment was likely close to accurate. Following the rally, Norway, specifically the NPA, began to provide first aid training to interested members of the ANC and took on a key role in the development of health facilities in Dakawa.[51]

In 1981, the Danish People's Relief Association also contributed DKK235,875 (approximately US$33,000) for a Land Rover and various pieces of equipment needed for the hospital.[52] Even though its financial support for the Kurasini sickbay had not produced much fruit, it, too, wanted to extend its support to the Health Department's efforts in Mazimbu. Unfortunately, much to the consternation of the

ANC leadership and Health Department alike, the building process did not begin until 1982 and the Mazimbu hospital did not open until October 1984.[53]

While the Mazimbu hospital project was still in progress, the East Africa RHT had to provide for the needs of patients, most of who were students living in Mazimbu. By 1978 the ANC had a small provisional health centre (also named the "Mazimbu clinic" or the "SOMAFCO clinic") at SOMAFCO, which was run by the newly instituted Mazimbu Team.[54] The clinic was given assistance by the Christian Council of Tanganyika to the value of TZS10,951.50 (approximately US$1,300).[55] It met with early success; staff was able to screen new secondary school students entering the area from South Africa for tuberculosis, venereal disease, and other chronic illnesses.[56] By 1980, the Mazimbu team had a medical assistant, a nurse, and a medical auxiliary to serve the clinic.[57] As previously mentioned, without a doctor the clinic partnered with the Morogoro Regional Hospital and Muhimbili Medical Centre in order to provide for the acute healthcare needs of patients.

Unfortunately, the construction of the ANC-Holland Solidarity hospital was not getting underway. As 1981 came to a close, Manto Tshabalala wrote to ANC Treasurer General Thomas Nkobi voicing her concerns at the lack of action with regards to the building process: "four years since the commitment of the funds for the Helath [sic] Centre and its equipment, there is not a single brick has been laid to mark the foundation ... to talk about the Mazimbu Health Centre has become a joke in bad taste ... it does appear that our donors are under a serious state of anxiety regarding the utilisation of the funds."[58] These construction delays were consistent with the problems that she described in her 1982 letters regarding the Kurasini sickbay. In both cases, Tshabalala presented the opinion that the ANC's international credibility was being tarnished by the lack of accountability and professionalism. Less than two months after writing her letter to Nkobi, Tshabalala wrote to Secretary General Alfred Nzo reiterating that the MKA was "expressing doubts about the utilisation of the funds donated," and she requested that the upper echelons of the party attend a (not yet planned) ceremony to celebrate the laying of a foundation stone to show leadership commitment to the project.[59] The building process began later that year, a full four years after securing the promise of funding.

The absence of a major medical facility in Mazimbu was a growing problem partly because the ANC population in the settlement was increasing rapidly. By June 1982 there were 250 secondary school students, 149 primary and nursery school children, and 129 other staff and community members at Mazimbu. In addition, the medical team was expected to provide for the needs of the 355 local workers in Mazimbu and many of the local Tanzanian people in the surrounding area. In total, it was reported that the clinic saw an average of 1,500 patients per month.[60] Without proper facilities, school dormitories were used as sickbays and in June 1982 there was no medical orderly available to consistently care for those in the dormitories.

In January 1984 Henk Odink, president of the MKA, wrote to Secretary General Alfred Nzo stating that finally the construction of the ANC-Holland Solidary Hospital was on schedule[61] and the hospital was set to open on 1 May 1984.[62] He reported that a mammoth sum of one million Dutch guilders was raised in the Netherlands, 200,000 guilders over what was promised in 1980, for the project and that the full consignment of equipment and supplies was ready to be shipped.[63] Odink further suggested that the ANC appoint a general manager as well as a full-time overseeing doctor while also offering the services of support staff such as laboratory technicians, pharmacists, x-ray technicians, and nurses.

The opening ceremony – a purely symbolic inauguration – for the hospital was an opportunity for the ANC to increase its international stature. In the face of poor management and building delays, the ceremony was a chance to improve diplomatic relationships and draw attention to the ANC's new medical success. The invitation sent to Dr A.A. Chiduo, the minister for health in Tanzania, pointed to this international focus: "this clinic reqresents [sic] a major step in the global developmental strategies of our Movement. We are confident that the clinic will contribute to the improvement of the health delivery care services in our community."[64] The array of people attending also demonstrated the significance of the event and the Department of Health's role in establishing ANC legitimacy. Guests included Dr Henk Odink, Mr Aina (representative of the OAU Liberation Committee), Mendi Msimang[65] (chair of the ANC's East Africa Regional Political Committee), Ndugu Banduka (regional secretary Chama Cha Mapanduzi) and Alfred Nzo (ANC secretary general).

With regrets, the SWAPO secretary of health was not able to attend due to flight connection difficulties. The opening speeches solidified the international solidarity for the ANC and the success of the ceremony spoke to the strength of the ANC's Health Department.

In June 1984 the health team in Mazimbu held a hospital planning meeting in which they decided that the hospital would run twenty-four hours a day, seven days a week and needed seventeen staff members in order to serve the needs of the community.[66] Evidently, the hospital was still not in use, but the staff was optimistically planning for the new building's operative opening. In July, it was becoming more urgent to finish construction and adequately staff the new hospital.

The NEC took issue with the Health Department's reliance on outside support. The NEC saw this as yet another example of incompetence and lack of planning; in short, behaviour not fitting of a future government department:

> Neither does it seem that the Department of Health at headquarters know what staff is required for the new hospital. The Department knew of the hospital almost four years ago but made no arrangements to train staff to man it. This hospital is due to open soon and there is no staff for it. It may end up a white elephant or we have to employ Tanzanians.[67]

In September the hospital was still a "white elephant." The East Africa Health Team had anticipated the hospital to be fully functional in August but as September rolled in, it was clear that the hospital was still empty.[68]

Fortunately, the delay ended in October 1984. It was reported that the hospital was finally up and running and that the MKA was in the process of collecting money for clinic equipment and supplies for use in the operating theatres, X-ray room, and kitchen. It was estimated that this, the sixth and final, container of supplies would be shipped at the start of 1985.[69] The hospital was set up with a polyclinic on one side where staff treated the patients' immediate needs and an inpatient ward on the other for cases needing overnight surveillance.

In 1987, the hospital had the fluctuating services of about twenty-six medical personnel, ten of whom were international solidarity workers, and saw between 2,500 and 3,000 people per month. Half to three-quarters of those patients were Tanzanians and between 1,250 and 1,500 of the total patients per month required a doctor's attention.[70] All twenty inpatient beds were in operation and another twenty patients were staying at home but on once-daily surveillance. Despite these achievements, the Norway coordinators' report submitted in 1987 stated that the hospital was still dangerously close to remaining a "white elephant." Notwithstanding facility design, the hospital's major surgery theatre was not yet in operation (which meant that baby deliveries had to be referred to Morogoro), equipment for diagnostic services was falling into disrepair due to the desperate need of a technician to repair and maintain the tools, and the hospital needed the help of more specialized staff to provide things like dental services.[71] Additionally, the lack of adequate drugs and supplies was an ongoing problem and even more evident within the big facility.[72] However, the Health Department worked hard to address these criticisms. By the end of the year, it was able to deliver babies on site and by the following year, was able to use the laboratory to test blood for malaria parasites and stool for intestinal parasites.[73]

It took five years from the time of the first instalment of the MKA's donation to open the hospital. The ANC leadership dragged its feet on starting the project and it took the incidence of donor disapproval to motivate the leadership to finally get going on the project. Evidently, the Health Department endeavours were not high on the ANC's priority list. However, the project brought some level of diplomatic success to the ANC and presented a physical affirmation of its legitimacy. It provided the medical staff with the opportunity to treat patients at the primary healthcare level and because it saw thousands of patients per month, the hospital clearly had a positive impact on the community as a whole. Unfortunately, the experience of the medical staff throughout this building process was less than pleasant. The negative interpersonal dynamics at the regional and "national" level (the health secretariat) were not only detrimental to the medical staff, but patients were also sometimes the victims of unprofessionalism and certain staff members' self-aggrandising behaviour.

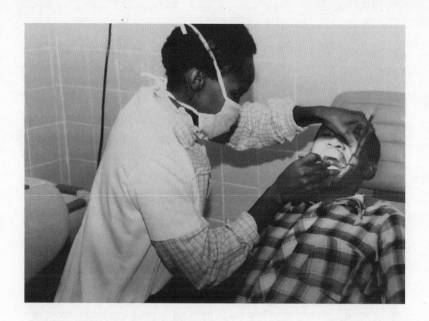

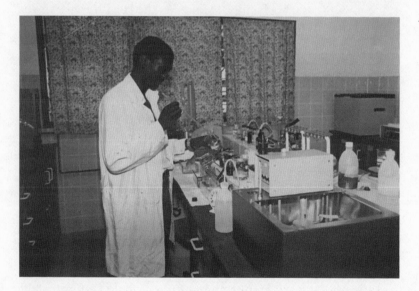

4.1 Dental services. This image shows a man receiving dental work at the ANC-Holland Solidarity Hospital in Mazimbu. Photograph, no date [1984?].

4.2 Lab equipment. This image shows some of the lab equipment, supplied by donors, that was available to medical staff in Mazimbu. Photograph, no date [1984?].

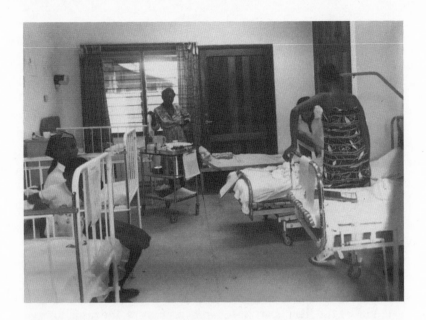

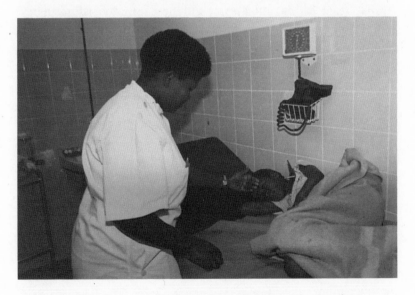

4.3 Mazimbu hospital ward. This is a photograph of a number of hospital beds in the ANC-Holland Solidarity Hospital. There are both patients and staff in this picture. Photograph, no date [1984?].

4.4 Mazimbu hospital care. This is a photograph of a medical staff worker caring for a sick child in Mazimbu. The child is huddled under a blanket. Above the child's head, there is a blood pressure machine. Photograph, no date [1984?].

Interpersonal Struggle
in Tanzania

The ANC Health Department was inexperienced at running a multiregional health operation and it struggled to establish a hierarchy of authority. As outlined in chapter 1, at the highest level of authority in the Health Department was the central leadership called the health secretariat. Manto Tshabalala, who was staying in Tanzania in the 1970s, early 1980s, and intermittently throughout the late 1980s, represented the health secretariat in the region. The next level of authority was the East Africa RHT leadership, which included between three and five individuals. Medical staff members occupying these positions rapidly changed, leaving the RHT with hardly any consistency in leadership. Under the inconsistent management of the RHT, staff in separate regions of Tanzania formed "teams" (e.g., the Mazimbu team) and these teams coordinated day-to-day services and managed semiqualified trainees. Overall, these bureaucratic tiers resembled the federal, provincial, and municipal roles that most national government structures have but this was at a microcosmic level with a limited number of qualified staff – many of who served at multiple levels in the structure.

While the Health Department had these often-confused lines of authority, it was not autonomous from other ANC political structures in Tanzania. Relative to other ANC political bodies, the Health Department was given low priority. Not only was there a general regional leadership that reported back to the NEC, there was a Mazimbu leadership body that oversaw all of the affairs of the settlement; both of these units had full authority over the medical sector. Additionally, the Women's Section was given power to advocate for the health of individual women and children under their care and at best, the Women's Section worked alongside the Health Department, but often it worked autonomously or only in tandem with the political leadership. Once again, this bore resemblance to a national government structure, but the East Africa RHT and Mazimbu health teams were often frustrated by this broader political leadership who sometimes made medical decisions without consulting medical staff.[74]

Because Mazimbu was a settlement centred on education, the political leadership in Mazimbu prioritized the student affairs at

SOMAFCO. Therefore, the Education Department's needs were given high priority in Mazimbu and their representatives often had some authority to guide the medical sector's decisions in the settlement. Additionally, much to the medical staff's dismay, the Mazimbu political leadership, Women's Section, and the Education Department acted as watchdogs and reported any poor medical performance to the health secretariat. In other words, Manto Tshabalala was constantly being informed of the undisciplined behaviour in Mazimbu.[75] Tshabalala often went to Mazimbu address the reported problems, but she was not well received by the already disempowered medical staff there.

While the early provisional Mazimbu clinic maintained a good relationship with the Tanzanian regional staff, the ANC's clinic did not continue to function well after its initial success. At least by May 1981 it was clear that the wheels were beginning to fall off the East Africa RHT as well as the Mazimbu clinic. The clinic had access to both an old ambulance and "a full complement of trained personnel"[76] but according to Tim Maseko, a member of the political leadership in Mazimbu, neither was fully functional. Maseko complained to Tshabalala:

> [I]t is no surprise lately to go the clinic and find that the ambulance is on a safari … Last Friday … [I] found that there was a child who had been sick for 3 days without the Health team showing up … Now the burning issue is the general medical treatment of students. Surely, it is not sufficient to just give them tablets and that is the end of the story and this is the pattern irrespective of the case.[77]

It was also made evident that the clinic was no longer screening or examining new students arriving in Mazimbu.[78] Clearly, the clinic was battling general negligence and indiscipline in addition to shortages of staff and equipment.

Tshabalala attempted to contact East Africa RHT members about Maseko's negative report with disappointing results. Facing no response from the RHT, the Health Department leadership pulled rank and sought to impose improvements on the situation reported by Maseko. Manto Tshabalala later defended her actions by stating,

In utter desperation and motivated by the disgruntlement of our membership, sometimes we have had to step in … and have done tasks which under normal circumstances should have been done by the teams. This has evoked a lot of criticism and has been termed as interference, but then who would set [*sic*] back and watch a house burn to ashes? That would be completely unethical.[79]

In order to address Maseko's complaints, a Health Department report in October 1981 stated that nurse Tim Naidoo – already in the area – was now head of the Mazimbu health team and a total of four members would serve the team at the clinic.[80] However, this appointment was politically contentious. Naidoo had initially been acquired by the Education Department rather than the Health Department and her involvement at the clinic represented ANC political interference into the affairs of the medical staff. Due to the animosity she felt between 1979 and 1981, Naidoo attempted to resign from the health team prior to her new appointment.[81]

After being made leader of the Mazimbu team, Naidoo clashed constantly with her own colleagues as well as other ANC departmental representatives operating in Mazimbu.[82] She insisted that the Morogoro health team[83] consult her before using the clinic facilities and that third-year medical student Mandla Lubanga (a member of the Morogoro team) show her respect as the leader of the Mazimbu team: "The fact that you [Mandla Lubanga] neither greet nor speak to me when you come to Mazimbu is not relevant, but if you want anything from the Mazimbu team or to us[e] its facilities you will have to communicate with me."[84] Naidoo's tenure finally did come to an end with her formal written resignation in early 1982.[85]

Despite the treatment of Tim Naidoo in Mazimbu, the offense taken by the regional health team was aimed mainly at Manto Tshabalala. In general, the presence of Dr Tshabalala in Tanzania and her "interference" in the region was viewed with great resentment. Tshabalala was accused of using her power and position in the Health Department to make unilateral and irresponsible decisions with regard to Mazimbu's educational courses, treatment of patients, and handling of drugs.[86] In one correspondence between Tshabalala and

Regina Nzo (the nurse at the children's nursery in Mororgoro and the RHT chair), Nzo complained about the way Tshabalala was dealing with local Tanzanian medical staff. She wrote, "Comrade Tshabalala, I implore and beg you to keep your provocation and machinations with the organisation (A.N.C.) your behavior is embarrassing us who use [M]orogoro hospital for your people."[87] Because of the stress that Nzo experienced while a part of RHT leadership, she visited a psychiatrist who reported that she had "decompensated" and needed a six-week sick leave. Part of the issue stemmed from Nzo's feeling that Tshabalala was "torturing her" by making nasty personal and professional remarks.[88] In late 1982 Regina Nzo decided to resign from her position in the RHT.[89]

Additional personal clashes abounded. A particularly nasty conflict occurred between Drs Sipho Mthembu, an ANC doctor working in a Tanzanian facility, and Manto Tshabalala. Dr Tshabalala claimed that Mthembu had not accounted for TZS10,000 given to him by the Health Department.[90] Because he did not have adequate receipts, she accused him of taking the money. He responded by claiming that Tshabalala had set him up. Demonstrating his frustration at the predicament in a tone indicative of the bitter Tanzanian regional attitude, Dr Sipho Mthembu wrote, "[T]he only thing [Tshabalala] contributed to the struggle is confusion … To date, despite repeated verbal accusations against her behaviors and attitude, she still believes in doing things single-handed … To her, other members of the Medical Team are pawns in a one-man-on-the-stage [sic] chess game."[91]

The conflict in interpersonal relationships in late 1982 and continuing in 1983 between medical staff members in Mazimbu and those in Tanzania more broadly was so extreme that the major interregional meeting – the Third Health Council – could not be held as scheduled at the end of 1982. Complaints about colleagues' behaviour, mainly aimed at Tshabalala, were vicious and constant, and the accusations were serious enough to warrant a commission of enquiry into the affairs of staff members before the council meeting could be called.[92] Yet the personnel who would lead the commission were also divisive; Health Department chair Peter Mfelang accused the commission personnel of being biased and composed of some of his "enemies."[93]

At the time leading up to the commission's investigation, the Health Department expressed its belief that the East Africa RHT was overstepping its authority by not adequately submitting to department authority. During the late 1982 Consultative Committee meeting in Lusaka, between ANC political leadership (more precisely, the Working Committee) and the Health Department, Manto Tshabalala stated, "Whatever structures are going to be created, these will have to be respected by our Movement, and in particular by the members of the department themselves. A department without control is no department at all."[94] Writing to ANC Secretary General Alfred Nzo, Tshabalala stated, "our understanding [is that] all the Health Team members should be deployed and transferred by the Health Department, and therefore are basically and technically a responsibility of the Department. The local political structures of our organisation, and any other authorized bodies will assist the Department in ensuring that the Teams carry out all the departmental programmes and activities."[95] Furthermore, the department demanded that the newly formed and essentially redundant SOMAFCO "Health Committee" be disbanded.[96] In short, the health secretariat did not have its own policing system and wanted the political leadership to defend the lines of authority necessary for a governmental department.

The commission of enquiry also sought to better understand the regional issues and address, among other things, Nzo's claim that "'there is confusion in the Health Team'; that was borne out by the fact that decisions taken by the RHT at Regional meetings are flouted immediately [by the Health Department] after meetings thus undermining the work of the Health Team."[97] In addition to discovering that the RHT members felt that their authority was questioned, the commission of enquiry also learned that the tensions between other staff and Manto Tshabalala were so high that Tshabalala and another medical colleague had actually come to physical blows.

Manto Tshabalala was not liked in the region, but it must also be stated that not all the accusations against her were well founded nor should they be cited as evidence to discount the meaningful contribution she made to the medical sector in exile. Furthermore, as the oft-made ambassador of the Health Department at international meetings and conferences, Tshabalala was probably the most deeply invested staff member in the department. Her acts of micromanagement likely stemmed from her urgent motivation to live up to her promises abroad, and she was central to the development of the

Health Department from the very beginning. The animosity aimed toward Tshabalala continued throughout the 1980s. In September 1987, she was suspended due, in part, to a mass wave of resignations from the East Africa Health Team in opposition to her position in the department. The suspension was deemed baseless and overturned in August 1989. Ralph Mgijima, then secretary for health wrote, "The unconstitutional nature in which the suspension was effected and the lack of any evidence of professional misconduct or any misdemeanour on [Tshabalala's] part has led to [her reinstatement]."[98]

Despite their desire for independence, members of the East Africa RHT clearly were in need of help and guidance, hence the complaints to Tshabalala from the Mazimbu political leadership. Many of the staff had serious drinking or behavioural problems that put patients at risk. For instance, Dr Sipho Mthembu was deemed unsuitable by the Mazimbu leadership for a position in their region. The Mazimbu leadership report stated, "he has a serious drink [sic] problem, is unstable and has anti-social tendencies."[99] In another example, in 1981 medical aid Roy Campbells was removed from his medical post at SOMFACO "for his gross lack of discipline in discharging his duties."[100] However, Campbells was still welcome to participate fully with the health team elsewhere. In late 1980 the previously mentioned Joe Mosupye was expelled from SOMAFCO due to his "misuse of the ambulance ... [and] misuse of his position on young female comrades."[101] While the SOMAFCO directorate evidently had the power to push him out of the Mazimbu clinic, he was kept on the East Africa RHT and transferred to Kurasini. The loyal East Africa RHT staff defended him by saying, "there is nobody who does not make mistakes. Patients complain about everybody."[102] Unfortunately as mentioned previously, Mosupye was not chastened by his removal from Mazimbu and continued in the same manner at Kurasini.

In another case, comrade Castro, an unqualified member of the health team, crashed an ambulance while inebriated.[103] This was neither the first nor the last time that a staff member misused the ambulance nor was his being inappropriately drunk a novel phenomenon. A 1981 report of the East Africa Health Team requested that, "Members of the team should refrain from being drunk in front of patients and on duty ... No drinks should be taken before the health team meetings."[104] Evidently drinking on the job was a serious problem across the board.

Nurse Regina Nzo, too, was thought to be "drinking excessively" at the time that the enquiry was underway.[105] But the behavioural issues were too systemic to fire all transgressors. The Health Department would have been unable to continue operations if it had let go every staff member caught for unprofessional conduct.

Negligence on the part of the medical staff was also a problem. In 1982 one letter to the East Africa RHT from Tshabalala indicated that, "The team does not seem to clearly appreciate what duties it is being charged with … there seems to be a serious lack of … commitment and also a total departure from medical ethics … there are still a number of outstanding and unresolved acts of indiscipline."[106] The rifts between Tshabalala and the regional staff were not baseless, but they were also symptomatic of the lack of clear lines of authority and communication as well as the lack of professionalism and qualified personnel on the ground.[107]

In June 1982 the Mazimbu team requested that a Swedish doctor be recruited to work in the Mazimbu clinic.[108] While still relatively small, the community's medical requirements exceeded the skills and capacity of the medical staff that in September 1982 was comprised of Nellie Mvulane (nurse), Evodia Magubane (nine-month mother/child health course graduate), Eva Ngakane (unqualified medical assistant), Moss Tshabalala (laboratory technician), and Sonia Seleke (untrained medical auxiliary).[109] The heavy reliance on Morogoro medical facilities reflected the dwindling autonomy of the East Africa RHT. The RHT begged the Health Department for the assistance of the already contacted Swedish doctor, or any doctor for that matter, but the department in Lusaka did not deem the Mazimbu clinic's needs to be great enough to warrant a full-time doctor.[110]

The Health Department was not solely responsible for this sentiment; the NEC was also growing increasingly concerned about the expectations and sense of entitlement – "the refugee mentality" – growing in the ANC communities: "Cultural standards between ANC and Tanzanians have a wide gap – they refer to ANC members as 'MAZUNGU' [white person]. It does pose a problem, for example, where we have our children taken to hospital they criticise the conditions of the hospital."[111] As a result the official position of the Health Department was that other ANC settlements and camps were in greater need of reinforcements from qualified staff. The department wrote to the RHT saying, "The deployment of our personnel has been absolutely uneven. Centres have failed to effectively utilise their personnel rationally. There is a cry for more personnel particularly in those areas [Mazimbu] that enjoy the largest number of personnel. There is no setting up of priorities and consideration of personnel/patient ratio."[112]

Despite this clear decision, even the SOMAFCO director put pressure on the Department of Health to send a doctor to the community; annoyed, the Health Department chair and secretary reprimanded the director for the request and reminded him that the community already had a) been told "no" and b) had the part-time services of local doctor, Dr Ebba Mokoena.[113] The SOMAFCO director was clearly not embarrassed by this admonishment; the following directorate meeting minutes read, "all sections women, youth, RPC [Regional Political Council], and Directorate should put pressure [on] H.Q. for a permanent doctor … if no success from the H.Q. we should request that we ourselves approach support groups."[114] This opinion was akin to a regional revolt against its state capital.

The disagreement over whether a doctor was necessary in Mazimbu was a matter of perspective and reflected the personal experience of those affected. The ANC leadership and Tshabalala were able to see the great need for doctors at the military frontline. Tshabalala had been to the MK camps in Angola on several occasions and had witnessed the bleak health conditions and unnecessary deaths that occurred there. The ANC leadership believed the Mazimbu community members were already spoiled with the provisions available to them. However, this broader perspective does not negate the experiences of people living in Mazimbu. From the perspective of Chief Representative Stanley Mabizela, SOMAFCO needed a doctor because young people were dying needlessly in the community of then about 1,000 children and 500 adults (this estimate includes Tanzanians living in Mazimbu).

In his April 1983 letter to ANC Secretary General Alfred Nzo, Mabizela describes the death of a twenty-two-year-old male.[115] The young man was examined by Dr Tshabalala and Dr Mokoena, and it was determined that he should be given an electroencephalogram. Supplies needed for the test were unavailable in Dar es Salaam and when they did arrive, there was nobody qualified to do the assessment.

During this period of delay, the boy developed a headache, went to the clinic, and found no ambulance to take him to the hospital. The Mazimbu team "bundled him into some vegetable van and rushed him to hospital, where on arrival, he was certified dead."[116] The other two deaths referred to in the letter were of babies under two years old, one of whom died from kwashiorkor. Recognizing that his letter was in opposition to the position of the upper echelons of political and health leaderships, Mabizela justified himself by saying,

> Tanzania, in so many ways, including the field of medicine, is a very sad Country; its [sic] really sad. Comrade, I am still new in Tanzania relatively speaking and I can see the stark reality of affairs; I have as yet not fallen into the Malaise of the "old-timers" here who have become conditioned and complaicent [sic]. And I, therefore, once more request that you do something.[117]

Interestingly, there were clearly two doctors involved in at least the first case, but Mabizela saw a resident doctor as an imperative for better treatment.[118]

In June 1983 the ANC leadership and Health Department capitulated. As noted above, part of the impetus for getting a resident doctor was the nearly completed hospital in Mazimbu. While the health secretariat wanted to delay acquiring a doctor until the official opening of the hospital, it was recognized that one was going to be needed in order to use the facility properly.[119] It was first suggested that Dr Sipho Mthembu take up the post, but, as desperate as the SOMAFCO directorate was, the idea was shut down on the grounds that Mthembu, as mentioned before, drank too much and was "unstable."[120] For these reasons, the Health Department then sought to send him to fill the staffing shortage in Angola[121] and then wrote to Dr Amor Moroka, who was at that time in Lusaka, to ask whether she would consider taking up the SOMFACO post.[122] With a reply pending, the SOMAFCO directorate meeting minutes stated that Vietnam offered to send a doctor if the ANC was willing to pay the airfare. It also mentioned a Cuban willing to commute from Dar es Salaam on weekends and a Swedish doctor who might be prepared to come to the community if pursued.[123] Dr Moroka turned down the request stating that she wanted to take the time to specialize in obstetrics and gynaecology rather than work in Mazimbu.[124] The subsequent health team meeting minutes do not suggest that the clinic acquired a doctor in 1983 despite the offers; they did, however, make use of the weekend assistance of Dr Fiki Radebe-Reed.

Evidence of the department's inexperience continued until the unbanning of the ANC. Reports on the function of the hospital varied dramatically based on whether the ANC leadership, Department of Health, or the Mazimbu Team wrote them. In 1985, the Department of Health, stinging from the lack of consultation from the local team, scrutinized the lack of cleanliness, organization with equipment and drugs, short hours of operation, medical application skills,[125] lack of health education courses and, of course, the lack of compliance and coordination with the Health Department.[126] Replying to the report, the Mazimbu team stated, "the Team feels that there were a few exaggerated remarks made about the ANC-Holland Solidarity Hospital" and that the report was "not a genuine report, based on the working conditions here, but rather a retaliation."[127] Furthermore the staff argued that many of the criticisms levelled against them were the fault of the health secretariat for not sending the hospital enough qualified staff. The team stated that the condemning report was "demoralising" to a team that was putting in their best effort to meet the needs of the community. Whether the issues in Mazimbu were the fault of the Mazimbu team or not, evidently the hospital still had some work to do.[128]

The Expense of Personality Clashes:
Patient MT[129]

The clinic at Kurasini and the health team coordination at Mazimbu are indicative of the way that the Health Department handled infrastructure projects and operated more generally across its other regions. While each location presented its own challenges, the department struggled to offer an efficient service and consequently the ANC often relied on local facilities for both primary and secondary care. The effects of these issues had a clear impact on patients. Most of the patients treated by the ANC were not mentioned in the archive; some patients only appear once or twice, while a handful of others are included in more than a dozen reports. The following section highlights a particular patient whose name is recorded in the archive numerous times. Typically a repeated name in the archive indicates that the patient was very sick or mismanaged. Therefore, this present case is not meant to be representative of every patient's experience but it is meant to demonstrate some of the implications of the systemic problems that were so prevalent in these facilities and between staff members. Furthermore, his story is important because he was an early casualty of the medical sector's unarmed struggle.

Between September 1982 and April 1984 patient MT's case is mentioned in the archive nearly two dozen times; his was probably the most cited patient case found in the archive.[130] MT was born in exile in Lesotho in 1980 and by late 1981, at least, he and his mother were staying at the ANC's crèche in Tanzania.[131] As residents of the crèche, the two were under the care of the Women's Section and the ANC political leadership in the region. Shortly after MT's arrival at the crèche, the medical staff working there commented that he was hydrocephalic and should be sent to a specialist for an examination.[132] Unfortunately, the child needed treatment just as the quarrel between Regina Nzo and Manto Tshabalala reached its climax and both became involved in the case. As a result, the two women used the boy's treatment and prognosis to incriminate each other. Several differing first and secondhand accounts appear in the archive and they begin to reveal how the infighting affected the child's health.

There were three different members of medical staff that claimed to be the one who referred the child to a specialist: Manto Tshabalala, Regina Nzo, and Sipho Mthembu.[133] In Tshabalala's account, she recommended that the child be taken to Muhimbili Hospital in Dar es Salaam to see whether it was too late to perform the appropriate procedure. The child was put through medical testing at Muhimbili, a fact mostly verified by Regina Nzo, and the results of the initial assessment and testing were subsequently lost. In her account of the events, Nzo included a bitter parenthesized comment about how losing medical records was a common occurrence in Tanzania.

Likely in August 1982, while the health records were lost, the child developed malaria and was taken to a local clinic (Juwata clinic) in Dar es Salaam to see a doctor from the GDR. Tshabalala reported that the GDR doctor wrongly declared that the child had conjunctivitis, and while she disagreed, she did not intervene in his treatment further at that stage. At the same time, Tshabalala reported that the child's mother was behaving in a way unbecoming of a mother with a sick child. The mother was often out drinking and dancing and did not bring her son into Muhimbili for follow-up appointments regarding his hydrocephalic condition. Nzo did not mention the mother's behaviour, but other reports noted and condemned her poor conduct.[134] Tshabalala reported that she urged the mother to take the child to Muhimbili, but instead, the mother took MT back to the GDR doctor at the Juwata Clinic in September.[135]

According to Regina Nzo, the GDR doctor indicated that the child had hydrocephalus and needed surgery within the next six months to prevent him from going blind. Regina Nzo and ANC Dr Ike Nzo immediately wrote directly to Chief Representative Stanley Mabizela of the ANC leadership in Tanzania imploring him to find the child treatment abroad.[136] As was previously mentioned, Mabizela was comparatively new to the area and was sympathetic to the plight of the sick. Nzo's communication to the political rather than health leadership exemplifies the rift between Nzo and Tshabalala specifically and of the divide between the secretariat and the RHT more generally.

Once the matter was in the hands of the political leadership, the Health Department's involvement dwindled. Furthermore, the Women's Section became an active participant in the case, which was strategically fortunate for Regina Nzo as she was a member of the group. In December 1982 three months following the GDR doctor's six-month treatment window, a member of the ANC regional leadership wrote to the Women's Secretariat voicing her concern that MT had not been transferred abroad or received treatment.[137] When Regina Nzo heard that the child was still in Tanzania, she was shocked. Following this discovery, Nzo met the mother who accused Tshabalala of actively preventing her child from receiving treatment abroad. Outraged with Tshabalala, Nzo asked the woman to record everything that was said. Nzo submitted the mother's letter as well as her own complaint to the ANC political leadership in Tanzania at nearly the same time as she tendered her own resignation from the RHT.

Reflecting on the mother's accusation more than a year later, Tshabalala claimed that the woman was unstable and had threatened her with a knife. Tshabalala recalled that the woman "would develop tantrums and swear [she, Tshabalala] would die soon."[138] The inter-action between the mother and Tshabalala is not clear; however it is likely that Tshabalala's blunt manner and conviction that the window for effective treatment had passed, clashed with the mother's feelings of anger and frustration over her son's situation. In any case, Tshabalala was angry with Nzo for reporting her to the leadership without first confronting her with the mother's accusations.[139]

The political leadership along with the Women's Section in Tanzania renewed their efforts to find a place for MT to receive treatment abroad. In mid-January 1983, the mother reported that the child was already starting to develop blindness.[140] However, on 28 January, despite the ANC's insistent pleading, the representative from the GDR reported that they were not in a position to help the boy. Only after being rejected by their international medical ally did the political leadership approach Tshabalala for assistance. By that time, Tshabalala had not been directly involved in the care of the child for weeks. Tshabalala went back to the GDR doctor at Juwata Clinic to see the medical notes and referral for treatment abroad. She claimed that the medical report necessary for the referral had not been written because the GDR doctor had always agreed that it was too "late for any meaningful surgical intervention."[141] Evidently there had either been some form of miscommunication or someone was not telling the truth about the referral abroad.

The Women's Section did not relinquish its control of the case. Tshabalala tried to explain MT's diagnosis and prognosis to the women and illuminate why she thought that treatment abroad would likely not be beneficial to the child. However, the representatives of the Women's Section mistrusted Tshabalala, and they visited the GDR doctor themselves to confirm the information. The involvement of so many people outside of the Health Department was disruptive to the now semipalliative treatment program for the child: from mid-1983 there seemed little hope for MT's recovery.[142] Furthermore, their misunderstanding of treatment options caused the boy to suffer un-necessarily. In August the Women's Section asked permission from the secretary general to fly the child to see his father, an MK cadre in Angola.[143] The child was almost immediately sent. The Women's Section still believed that MT would be transferred abroad for surgery. Additionally, they encouraged the ANC chief representative in Angola to help prepare the parents to give consent to a future surgery.[144] Throughout the late months of 1983 the child and his parents were encouraged to believe that he would soon be sent abroad, but by January 1984 the door had been firmly shut. Nobody was prepared to take MT for treatment, and the boy was not transferred.[145]

From the time he arrived in Angola, there was no medical record of MT until February 1984. Dr Sipho Mthembu found the child in an MK camp near Luanda and reported, "I found this child in Luanda now in a very serious condition. He has gone paralysed (PARAPLEGIA) on both of his lower extremeties [sic]. His health has infact [sic] gone beyond repairs. How he came to Luanda is a mistery [sic] to me."[146] While in Zimbabwe in February 1984, Tshabalala attempted to get MT transferred to Harare for treatment but there is no follow-up report in the archive to indicate whether this was accomplished. His name does not appear in the archive again.[147]

This tragic story illuminates some of the major issues with the way that medical care was provided in exile. The case was too serious to be handled in an ANC clinic, and therefore, ANC medical staff initially took over the case and sought access to secondary healthcare in local facilities. The staff did not have a lot of respect for each other. The child's mother had the ability to circumvent ANC medical opinion and involved a separate local clinic. The child's case was taken up by the ANC's political leadership and the Women's Section and effectively removed from Tshabalala's supervision. The family was constantly given the false hope of transfers abroad by people who did not fully understand the child's medical condition, and eventually the child was stuck in the ANC region with the fewest available medical provisions. In the process of trying to establish itself and its services the Health Department was not able to prevent patients from falling through the cracks.

The ANC Health Department's efforts on the ground were not in keeping with the reputation they were trying to build internationally. While the ANC insisted they were a government-in-waiting and the Health Department tried to act as a legitimate "national" department, it struggled to appropriately use the generous donor funding that they were being granted. Renovations at Kurasini were nothing short of a disaster and the construction at Mazimbu was constantly delayed. However, the money donated to prop up the Health Department's efforts in exile was a show of solidarity and an implicit political endorsement for the ANC. Every dollar given to the Health Department gave it legitimacy as an alternative health representative of the South African people. The strength of the anti-apartheid movement and the Health Department internationally provided an opportunity for the Health Department to work through its issues by providing relentless funding to its infrastructure initiatives. In this way, the Health Department in exile was a major success for the political aims of the ANC.

The medical staff's personal and interpersonal issues bridge the department's broader structural problems with its social problems. The staff was not able to work optimally in a hostile environment, the tiers of leadership were uncoordinated and the relationship between ANC departments was often unfriendly. The Health Department's inexperience and inability to adequately coordinate efforts between its own members or members of other departments directly impacted patients' medical care.

At the major Health Department meeting held at the end of 1982, Secretary General Alfred Nzo addressed the attendees. He stated, "It would have been unrealistic for the Movement to have expected that the development of the Health Department would have proceeded along unnatural lines of development. Its teething problems characterize the process of development."[148] The secretary general recognized that the department was only just starting its work and that expectations should not be placed too high. However, the "teething problems" were significant and had detrimental effects on South African patients' quality of life in exile.

5

"It Was a World of Paranoia": The Mental Health Crisis in Exile

Mental illness was pervasive in exile and had an impact on the lives of nearly every ANC or MK comrade in some way. Consequently, it was a central health concern to the ANC's Health Department. The reality of mental illness began to sink in with the ANC leadership and Health Department after 1976 when the mass exodus of students, produced by the Soweto uprising, joined the ANC at SOMAFCO or MK in military camps. The new, young demographic was particularly prone to psychological suffering for a variety of reasons, and the dramatic increase in population made it impossible for the ANC, in the late 1970s, to ignore its own undeniable mental health crisis among South African exiles. The state of exile,[1] being unable to return home, coupled with often traumatic experiences of detention and torture by the apartheid government, created a situation in which many exiles suffered post-traumatic stress disorder (PTSD), schizophrenia, depression, or severe anxiety.[2] Additionally, these illnesses often manifested in violent behaviour, drug and alcohol addiction, and suicide. Further exacerbating the problem of mental illness,

ANC cadres and refugees were subjected to the paranoia internal to the ANC itself. As became clear in the South African TRC (1996 to 1998), the ANC in exile established its own detention-without-trial system for those it believed were conspiring against the organisation. Detainees were subjected to physical as well as psychological torture. The security and secrecy dimensions of the underground revolutionary movement contributed to the inability to openly discuss issues and address patient needs. While respecting these security considerations, the ANC's Health Department was, nevertheless, forced to respond to the psychological needs of its members who were clearly suffering because, if left untreated, the ramifications of members' psychological problems negatively impacted the ANC's relationship with local citizens and governments.

The leadership's reaction was not driven entirely by internal pressure. The timing of this increasing awareness was also a reflection, in part, of new international developments in mental healthcare. The ANC was interested and involved in regional medical developments. In the late 1970s there was a new initiative to improve mental health services in southern Africa. Interregional cooperation between African governments and the WHO brought new awareness and programs intended to address the major mental health needs of southern African people. As has been shown, the ANC's Health Department was enmeshed in local facilities and, as a result, bore witness to new mental health awareness and educational programs; these efforts had an impact on the direction taken by the ANC's Health Department. Essentially, the ANC benefited from the bilateral partnership between local African governments and the WHO.

In the same way that the department was able to capitalize on the international momentum of the anti-apartheid movement and the global push for health justice, it was able to take advantage of the growing international desire to address the mental health crisis in southern Africa. It did this in order to delegitimize the apartheid government, affirm itself as a viable alternative, and better care for its own citizens in exile. However, due to the significantly debilitating effects of mental illness, so widespread among South African exiles, the problems effecting the Health Department's capacity to deliver healthcare services had mortal consequences to those individuals affected.

The ability of the department to appropriately respond to the crisis was not altogether disappointing. On the one hand, more than any other health-related issue, the ANC worked hard to provide specific services and appropriate environments for those needing psychiatric attention. Piggybacking on local efforts by the WHO, the ANC attended seminars and arranged workshops in order to better educate medical staff and their members more broadly about the realities of mental illness among their South African comrades. Additionally, staff wrote extensive and concerned reports on comrades struggling with mental illness in an attempt to better deal with these individuals. The collaborative work done between the ANC and their international allies was extraordinary under the circumstances and should be greatly commended.

On the other hand, the ANC was still hampered by all of the systemic issues already described; most particularly, the Health Department was sorely understaffed to deal with the volume of patients and the severity of their illnesses. The ANC relied on already over-burdened local services to look after patients needing acute care and was often forced to offload patients from Mazimbu, Dar es Salaam, or Lusaka on to derelict communities like Dakawa. Many patients needing serious care were neglected, which had calamitous ramifications for the patients, the ANC communities, and, more generally, efforts to destigmatize mental illness. Finally, the Health Department was dealing with a situation in which the style of treatment itself posed a security threat to the organisation. If the patients were treated by doctors not completely in support of the ANC, therapy, including taking case histories and counselling, had the potential to reveal information that put the ANC in an undesirable light internationally and that had negative effects on the organisation as a whole.

The historiography on mental health is rich and the scholarship that considers "madness" in an African colonial, anticolonial, and postcolonial context are important to this present work.[3] It has been convincingly shown that colonial societies sought aggregation of African identity rather than individualization because the construction of "the African" as a different type of citizen was central to the legitimacy of colonial capitalism.[4] As a result, attempts were made by European psychiatrists to create distinct African pathologies of mental illness.[5] During the anticolonial movement in the mid-1950s and early 1960s, colonial governments used madness as a tool to confine or imprison those influential African leaders agitating against the government and prophesying the end of the colonial regime.[6] Additionally, in some cases, colonial establishments interpreted whole revolutionary movements through a psychological lens.[7] After independence, African governments sought to redefine mental illness in the postcolonial setting; it has been shown that new frameworks attempted to balance "traditional knowledge" with Western biomedical frameworks.[8]

This chapter has the benefit of assessing "madness" within all three of these contexts. It looks at mental illness suffered by members of an anticolonial movement as defined by those also involved in the liberation effort. In addition, the local, especially Tanzanian and Zambian, medical personnel, operating within a postcolonial structure, provided the ANC with influential opinions on mental health diagnoses and treatment regimes. The facets of this dynamic were further complicated in cases where the doctors working with the patients had been trained as medical students in a host of other political or geographical regions. These other regions included Scandinavia, countries in the Communist Bloc, and North America. Ideas about mental illness adopted in these regions greatly and diversely influenced the medical opinions of the doctors who returned to southern Africa to treat the mentally ill. Therefore, contrary to previous work on mental illness in Africa, the study of mental illness in ANC communities includes and juggles the colonial, anticolonial, and postcolonial categories all at once. Mental illness that had been shaped by colonial policies in South Africa was in the process of being redefined for a postcolonial South Africa while also being used as a tool to delegitimize the apartheid regime.

The treatment of those diagnosed as mentally ill was governed by the cultural, intellectual, political, and economic structures of exile. Detailing the Health Department's response to mental illness provides a better understanding of its position in exile, its international linkages, and its ability to actually deliver meaningful healthcare to patients. Mental illness was strategically used to further the international anti-apartheid cause but also threatened the security and credibility of the movement.[9]

Mental Health in
Exile in the Early Years

Most of the South Africans exiting South Africa after 1960 did so burdened with heavy psychological baggage. They had experienced racism, persecution, political arrest, family dislocation, and a host of other indignities while living under the apartheid regime. Unfortunately, there are very few references to the mental health of South African exiles in the 1960s and early 1970s; this lack of reporting is consistent with the general lack of health-related reporting during this time.

However, there are a few accounts of exile that point to psychological distress among the first wave of MK cadres. Maurice Mthombeni, the previously discussed controversial contributor to the damning article printed in *The Black Dwarf* in 1969, wrote,

> It was rare to find a sober man in the camp. The kind of African beer that we drank was corrosive in the extreme and ruinous to our health. It was brewed by the villagers who by then contended that people from South Africa like strong drinks. This was wrong. We wanted something that would make us drunk, and quick. We wanted to forget.[10]

He also claimed that some mentally ill cadres were sent to Mirembe Psychiatric Hospital in Dodoma, Tanzania[11] and that "there were a number of attempted suicides in the camps, and particularly in Kongwa."[12] He even gives a specific example of a comrade who had recently killed himself. The article in *The Black Dwarf* has already been recognized as polemical and Maurice Mthombeni as unsympathetic toward the ANC during the time that he penned his accusations. However, his account exhibits some level of awareness of mental health issues at this early juncture and shows that the topic was, at the very least, contentious; he points the finger at poor administration and a lack of military action as causes for alcoholism and suicide.

Another early account, written by MK cadre Thula Bopela, points more indirectly to the psychological pressures of living in exile in the 1960s. Bopela, expressing the widespread frustration at not getting an immediate chance to fight against the South African Defence Force

(SADF), points to his and his fellow comrades' propensity to drink in periods of idleness. He also claims that in an angry meeting with Oliver Tambo he threatened to "womanise, do drugs and drink [him] self to the devil" if he was sent to school rather than to fight in MK.[13] Many other accounts also discuss the poor morale among the early comrades stuck in exile waiting to be deployed. Though this poor morale translated mostly into heavy drinking and sometimes violent behaviour, archival material and existing interviews do not indicate that the leadership made a strong connection between poor morale and *medical* illness at this time. The level of medical attention, never mind specifically psychiatric attention, in the 1960s and early 1970s has already been described as relatively low on the priority list.

The medicalization of negative psychosocial behaviour as well as attention paid to mental illness more generally began in the late 1970s. There were a number of important reasons underpinning this shift. First, as has been detailed in chapter 1, the bureaucratization and organisation of health-related concerns was given new priority after the second wave of mainly students from South Africa moved into exile. Creating a department to formally consider the medical needs of comrades contributed to the new emphasis on mental health. Second, the WHO began to take an interest in mental healthcare in southern Africa and brought some much-needed attention to the poor provisions for black South Africans. Just nine months after the Soweto school uprisings, the WHO investigated mental healthcare in South Africa and compiled an influential and damning twenty-two-page report on its findings.[14]

Mental Health Treatment in Southern Africa after 1977

The WHO report is worth discussing because it describes the way that mental health was both perceived and treated in South Africa and because it was an effective political stone to cast at the apartheid government – a tactic later capitalized on by the ANC in exile. Unsurprisingly, the WHO found that apartheid had negative effects on mental health, and furthermore the medical support offered to black people in South Africa was incredibly poor. A 1975 proclamation accepted by South African State President Johannes de Klerk conflated obedience of apartheid laws with mental capacity; the new definition "erases the distinctions between the penal and health care system in the African homelands and extends in a dangerous way the concept of rehabilitation."[15] Essentially, social workers were given similar power as police officers by their new ability to "arrest without warrant."

Starting in 1964 the apartheid state enlisted private companies to take responsibility for mentally ill black patients. These companies capitalized on the free labour provided by "inmates" in order to generate profit. By 1975 there were between 8,000 and 9,000 African patients in these private asylums; this constituted one third of all mental health cases seen in South Africa and the majority of the black patients who were institutionalized. Problematically, the asylums did not provide a diagnostic breakdown of the patients. In 1974/5 there was a patient mutiny in Poloko Sanatorium due to facility's deplorable conditions. Poor conditions were a widespread problem: "It seems that none of these institutions has a full-time medical officer (although some of the snatoria [sic] accommodate over 3,000 patients) and that they are only visited by a part time psychiatrist who cannot communicate directly with the patients because of the language barrier."[16] Significantly, at the time the report was written, there was not a single black psychiatrist working in South Africa.

In March 1976 a new amendment was made to the Mental Health Act, 1973 that prohibited any reporting on mental health services in the country. This shielded the often prison-like work camp conditions in the facilities from scrutiny. This is not to say that reporting prior to the amendment was very accurate. The WHO's 1977 report records an account of one nurse who had been assigned to three hundred "inmates": "Once [sic] reporter came from The Star. It was a big joke. They only took pictures of the staff, who were given orders to act like patients."[17] Treatment for patients was brutal: "Tranquilizers (Librium and calium) are extensively used for treatment. Electric shocks are given without anesthetic. Anesthetizing nonwhites is too expensive, too time-consuming, and too risky … One wonders how many people, in the midst of convulsions and without muscle relaxants, have broken arms, legs, spines, or foreheads."[18] The WHO's report also reveals that many of those said to be "discharged" in the 1970s had actually died in the facilities and were "discharged" directly into cemeteries.

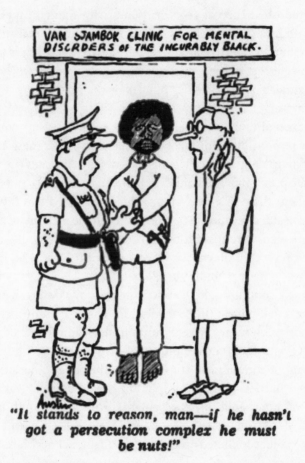

5.1 "Van Sjambok Clinic for Mental Disorders of the Incurably Black."
This cartoon was published in the "this week" column of the
weekly publication of the *New Scientist: Reed Business Information.*
The cartoon depicts a black man in a straightjacket standing
between a South African policeman and a doctor. The caption
reads, "It stands to reason, man—if he hasn't got a persecution
complex he must be nuts!" The cartoon depicts the prejudicial
treatment of black people and insinuates that many of those
institutionalized for mental illness were not ill at all.

Of course, much of the mental health services worldwide left much to be desired at the time, but the overt racism and exploitation of African patients was particularly appalling, especially when contrasted to the mental healthcare provided to white South Africans at the same time.

In the late 1970s the WHO and other international organisations such as the Red Cross and SIDA also had broader interests in mental healthcare in southern Africa. New partnerships between these organisations and state governments in the region were in an exploration phase. As a result, reports on mental health and programs for action began to emerge, and, correspondingly, services available to patients in southern African countries increased. Analyzing efforts by the ANC to cope with the mental health crisis among South African exiles must first be tempered by knowledge of the realities for treatment available in the regions in which they operated and from which they drew services, most particularly in Tanzania, Zambia, and Zimbabwe.

The developments in mental health awareness and treatment in the late 1970s and early 1980s in southern Africa had a profound impact on the ANC's treatment of its own mentally ill patients. Along with the 1977 investigative report produced by the WHO in South Africa, the WHO partnered with five sub-Saharan African countries (Swaziland, Tanzania, Zambia, Botswana, and Rwanda) in order to improve their national mental health programs. The African Mental Health Action Group was formed and, shortly thereafter, Kenya and Namibia (represented by SWAPO) joined. By 1982 Burundi, Zimbabwe, and the ANC also entered the fold to bring the total up to eight nations and two national liberation movements.

In 1981 and 1982 the WHO collaborated with the African Mental Health Action Group to investigate opportunities for African cooperation in dealing with mental illness. The resolution was called the Special Programme of Technical Cooperation in Mental Health and reports were produced yearly. For those reports each region was required to submit a survey of mental health services, and, while each region could report both positive and negative aspects of their current (1982) experiences, a similar story emerges across the board: there was not enough staff, nor facilities with inpatient capacity, transport, nor general awareness of mental health issues but there was a growing participation in new workshops and a desire to collaborate among regional services.

In Zambia the National Mental Health Coordinating Group represented the interests and endeavours of the mental healthcare sector. Yet the group existed and advocated for those with mental illness from outside of the Ministry of Health, showing mental health's very peripheral status in the country: it was, at times, referred to as the "cinderella of medicine."[19] The National Mental Health Coordinating Group reported that for the Zambian population of approximately six million people, there was only one "mental hospital," Chainama Hills, built in Lusaka in 1962. The hospital was also used for teaching and had the capacity to care for 160 long-term patients, 120 forensic patients (criminally charged individuals released from prison to the facility), 180 acute care patients, and forty children.

One solitary facility was not able to meet the mental health needs of the whole country's citizenry; therefore, the emphasis of new development was placed on decentralized primary care. Fourteen general hospitals in Zambia contained psychiatric units, providing a few beds for acute psychiatric inpatients, and it was estimated that between forty-five and fifty-two health facilities across the country had access to a mental health worker.[20] Unfortunately, treatment by a psychiatrist was not consistent; very little transport was available for psychiatrists to travel to rural areas – or for patients to come into urban areas – and there was no opportunity for new doctors to specialize in psychiatry in Zambia.[21] Without its own homegrown psychiatrists, it was difficult to coordinate a cohesive, centralized service that could accommodate regional needs. The lack of official attention to mental health meant that patients were at times cared for in police cells rather than hospital beds because hospital matrons and doctors denied patients access to the wards. While making some headway towards providing primary mental health care across the country, Zambia's National Mental Health Coordinating Group felt that in many ways, services left numerous mentally ill patients wanting.

Tanzania adopted the National Mental Health Programme in 1978 and its 1982 report focused mainly on the direction in which Tanzanian mental health provisions were headed rather than on the realities on the ground.[22] The WHO was already very involved in the creation of a cutting-edge mental healthcare model that prioritized community-centredness (using the primary facilities already in place to provide mental healthcare), training nonspecialized health workers for mental healthcare, and involving the community in support and prevention of social problems like dagga use or alcohol abuse. The central idea was to fully integrate mental health services into general healthcare. Zambia was in the process of putting this type of community-centred system into place, but, in contrast to the plan in Tanzania, it also clearly sought more national recognition, centralized authority, and large-scale facilities.

Tanzania reported on its two pilot regions (Morogoro and Moshi/Kilimanjaro), discussed how education was being diffused throughout the region and how this made an impact on the number of acute cases that needed attention. Furthermore, the WHO was sponsoring medical professionals for postgraduate work abroad because, like Zambia, Tanzania also did not have its own formal medical program in psychiatry. Muhimbili, the hospital in Dar es Salaam, often frequented by ANC members, functioned as the main referral centre and supported the healthcare efforts of the regional psychiatric units. It was not clear how many beds were available in Muhimbili because the emphasis was on outpatient treatment and care.

Due to the focus of this report on the cooperation between Tanzanian mental health initiatives and the WHO, the extent of the mental health services countrywide are hard to determine. However, it is clear that Tanzania was substantially supported by the WHO in order to improve the overall treatment of mental illness. Specifically, the WHO provided nonmedical support staff to help design and implement an efficient mental health delivery structure. Furthermore, it influenced the methods of treatment by directly advising Tanzania's National Mental Health Program leaders on programs that had proven successful elsewhere.[23]

Zimbabwe was different from Tanzania and Zambia in that the country had been independent for only two years when it joined the African Mental Health Action Group in 1982. The first report on mental health services and efforts for change indicated that Zimbabwe was in the middle of dismantling the very racialised mental healthcare system that had been in place prior to independence.[24] For instance, it was reported that at Ingutsheni Mental Hospital, built in 1908 with 720 hospital beds, major reforms to policy and infrastructure were necessary:

> [T]he compulsory shaving of heads of black male and female patients ceased, and patients were supplied with proper clothing including dresses, safari suits, shoes, underwear and nightwear and cardigans instead of prison-type garb which they had previously been forced to wear. They were each supplied with a bed, linen, and lockers; the thin felt mats on which they had been forced to sleep on cement floors in drab soulless dormitories were removed. Black and white patients were integrated.[25]

Zimbabwe's Ministry of Health had a lot of work cut out for itself to reform the system; however, it also inherited a much larger base of mental health infrastructure. The 1982 report listed that for the Zimbabwean population of eight million there were nine mental health facilities: Ingutsheni hospital (720 beds), St Francis Home (forty beds for children under sixteen), Nervous Disorders Hospital (twenty-four beds), Harare Psychiatric Unit (built in 1957, ninety beds), Parirenyatwa Psychiatric Ward Twelve (twenty-four beds, formerly a high-quality facility for white Rhodesians), Ward Eleven (twenty-six beds), Ngomahuru Hospital (240 beds, formerly a leper colony), and Mlondolozi Hospital (unknown number of beds, on the Bulawayo Prison grounds).

The level of infrastructure far surpassed the capacity of the limited expertise available. For instance, Ngomahuru was staffed by only five nurses with psychiatric training and was only visited by a psychiatrist every four to six weeks. Each of the listed facilities required serious upgrading and the patients required consistent psychiatric attention. Zimbabwe had 105 nurses with psychiatric training and eight psychiatrists operating in the public sector; four of those eight were working part-time in the public system and part-time in the private system.

The new government formed a department for psychiatric services under a deputy secretary in the Ministry of Health, and the centralized establishment was growing. The first priority was for training greater numbers of qualified medical personnel to provide psychiatric care; this was both to staff the existing facilities and also to extend services to rural areas within communities, in a program similar to the one sought after in Zambia and Tanzania.

Incidence and Treatment

The ANC's own response to mental health emerged in the middle of these regional developments and international cooperation. The ANC's first response to mental illness was most often to simply request to transfer its patients to either Tanzania (Muhimbili) or Zambia (Chainama Hills) for specialized treatment.[26] Based on its lack of medical personnel, it was much easier and more convenient to leave mentally ill patients at inpatient wards and leave treatment to hospital staff rather than develop a decentralized primary care system. In the late 1970s and early 1980s, Muhimbili Psychiatric Unit and Chainama Hills were the main referral hospitals used by the ANC for psychiatric patients. By January 1979 it was recognized that South African comrades were suffering from "anxiety syndromes," "neurosis," and, in particular, "dagga neurosis" but that the varied regional situation was "rather too fluid for the constant surveillance and follow up." [27] It was recommended that each centre's medical staff produce a survey on the mental health status of their communities. This was a well-meant suggestion and in keeping with regional efforts in Tanzania and Zambia, but these reports were more easily requested than produced; the ANC did not have access to a full-time psychiatrist and, understandably, no mental health surveys materialized in 1979.

The closest thing to a survey on mental health conditions within the ANC comes from ANC nurse Florence Maleka in Mozambique, who wrote, "Epileptics are prescribed for on the strength of their histories by clinic do[c]tors as there are no E.E.G. [electroencephalogram] technicians. Psychosis cases are also referred by clinic doctors to Psychiatric clinics ar wards [sic]. The periods between reference and examination of cases are rather long and I have to sedate patients in the interim with valium."[28] The report does not provide incidence rates on any other details about mental illness treatment, but it clearly indicates that the RHT had access to Mozambican psychiatric facilities. Unfortunately, there is no further description of these facilities in medical reports.

Still, the issue of mental illness and psychosocial disruption remained a constant problem for the ANC. Even Oliver Tambo spoke of the growing concern by publicly stating his alarm over the problem of youth suicide in exile.[29] At the end of 1979 the ANC was able to welcome Dr Freddy Reddy from Norway, a doctor considered by some to be the ANC's psychiatrist throughout the 1980s, to come and evaluate the ANC's mental health care status in all of the ANC's camps and settlements.[30] Indeed Dr Reddy wanted to be considered the sole ANC psychiatrist. He decided that he would visit southern Africa for two or three months on a yearly basis.[31] While Reddy's important contribution to the ANC was much needed and clearly necessary for the ANC's mental health program, it became evident that Reddy felt a sense of entitlement in ANC communities, visited before authorization or clearance was granted, and was often not perceived to be the most desirable option for psychiatric treatment.

Over the course of the following year there was a small number of individual patient reports describing patient treatment or requests for treatment abroad. These patients were diagnosed with depression, "combat nostalgia,"[32] or schizophrenia, and there was one reported suicide.[33] Dr Reddy offered to return to southern Africa to work in Zimbabwe and accept ANC patients there. However, he wanted the ANC to provide him with a financial incentive, something that the ANC struggled to accomplish for any of its medical staff.[34] Not much was recorded of that second visit or whether the Health Department was able to secure funding for Dr Reddy from the WHO. However, while he was in southern Africa, he reported that approximately 70 per cent of the SOMAFCO students in Tanzania needed psychological assessment and support (a percentage that remained relatively constant throughout the 1980s).[35] In March 1981 Reddy proposed to train medical personnel in mental healthcare but again stated that he would require WHO funding before attempting his proposal.[36]

The ANC Health Department looked to its international allies for support in creating a mental health program and system for treatment. The November 1981 WHO-sponsored Health and Apartheid conference described in chapter 3 was very important in this regard.[37] Mental health was specifically singled out in the Brazzaville Declaration as particularly affected by apartheid policies. It was recommended that the WHO's division in Africa, led by Dr Quenum, should pay special attention to the psychological health needs of refugees and "victims of apartheid" and create an ongoing commission to facilitate this new endeavour.[38] It was further suggested that the WHO provide South African national liberation movements (including the PAC) access to psychiatric care specialists including two psychiatrists as well as support for the movements to create a medical training and patient treatment system.[39] In initiating this process, the WHO suggested that the ANC join the African Mental Health Action Group, an action taken in May the following year.

Spurred on by the Health and Apartheid conference in Brazzaville and the May 1982 meeting for the African Mental Health Action Group, Dr Tshabalala drafted a more comprehensive plan for the ANC to conduct its own survey of mental health in ANC communities.[40] Tshabalala requested that the leader of the Tanzanian mental health initiatives and strong ally of the ANC Dr J.G. Hauli at Muhimbili Psychiatric Unit be called on to coconduct the initiative in all of the ANC communities in Zambia and Tanzania.[41] From December 1982 to January 1983, Drs Hauli, Tshabalala, and Mfelang collaborated to produce "The Psychological Effects of Apartheid: A Report on the Survey of Mental Health Problems of ANC Members in the Republics of Tanzania and Zambia."[42] This report reviews the incidence of mental illness, attitude towards mental health, available treatment for those in need, and the number of mental health personnel in each region before proceeding to propose a number of steps that should be taken towards implementing a rehabilitation program. This report offers a rare bird's eye view of the mental health status of those within ANC communities in exile and guided the department's future discussions on the direction that mental health initiatives could and should take.

This is the report's demographic context: the ANC community in Tanzania was living in Dar es Salaam, Mazimbu, and Dakawa with the vast majority residing at Mazimbu. There were an estimated total of 3,000 people, including 400 primary and secondary students as well as 250 infants. In Tanzania the ANC had access to the Muhimbili Psychiatric Unit (with Kurasini used as a sickbay for patients not kept at Muhimbili), the new Morogoro Psychiatric Unit, and the Mazimbu Dispensary. The ANC community in Zambia was estimated at 800 people roughly split between Lusaka and Chongela.[43] In Zambia the

ANC relied on the Lusaka Teaching Hospital (UTH) and Chainama Hills. The team looked at traceable in- and outpatient files of ANC members formally diagnosed with a psychiatric illness at these five centres in Tanzania and Zambia and, where possible, attempted to follow up each file with an interview.

Between 1978 and 1982 in a population of approximately 3,500 ANC members, the investigation found that there were 103 cases of people with psychiatric illness who had received formal medical attention or hospitalisation.[44] There were twenty-eight patients with schizophrenia, twenty-seven with depression, seventeen who had alcohol- or cannabis-induced psychosis, sixteen with epilepsy, thirteen with anxiety neurosis, four with intellectual disability, and eight deaths by suicide.[45] While similar specific statistics were not available from their host governments, it was mentioned on more than one occasion that Drs Hauli, Tshabalala, and Mfelang found the prevalence of mental illness to be statistically much higher than what was found in the local population.[46] Regionally, only 17 per cent of these cases were found in Zambia, and more than 50 per cent were located in Dar es Salaam. More alarmingly, Dakawa was clearly starting to become the destination for mentally ill patients; already in its first year of opening, Dakawa was home to twenty mentally ill patients. Dakawa did not have a psychiatric facility or the dedicated services of a full-time doctor and was well on its way to becoming a "dumping ground" for people deemed undesirable or inconvenient to the ANC.

The 1982 report recommended that all cases of mental illness in ANC communities across southern Africa be sent to Tanzania.[47] However, because of the large numbers of patients and the great distances between ANC settlements, plans for a variety of treatment options in various regions were being proposed instead. The Health Department sought to transform the Kurasini sickbay into an actual treatment centre (reflected in the ambitious new building proposals discussed in chapter 4), Dakawa was to develop a treatment and rehabilitation centre for nonacute cases of mental illness, there was to be a new rehabilitation centre in Harare and members of the medical staff from Angola, Lusaka, Maputo, and Dar es Salaam were to take part in a ten-day mental health workshop (budgeted at US$42,000), supported by the WHO.[48]

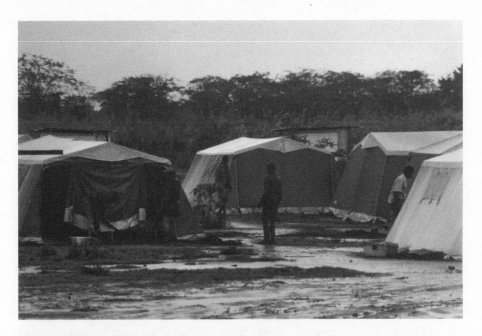

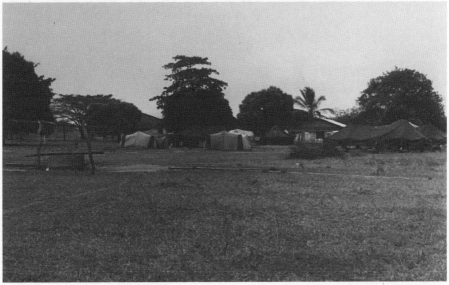

5.2 Dakawa in the rainy season. The image depicts a number of tents; likely these are not medical tents, but the image demonstrates the nonidyllic location of the camp. Photograph, no date [1983].

5.3 Dakawa in the dry season. In contrast to Dakawa in rainy season, this image shows some of Dakawa when the weather is dry. Photograph, no date [1983].

Undoubtedly, the leadership in the ANC Health Department was drawing energy and enthusiasm for mental health initiatives from its southern African collaborators and its approach was remarkable and forward thinking. Per Borgå, a Swedish psychiatrist who worked in southern Africa recalls, "From a western perspective awareness of psychiatric conditions were rather low. At the same time there was readiness [from medical staff] to deal with all kinds of problems, and an eagerness to discuss."[49] Even the type of training desired was innovative; the department wanted "intersectoral" and "multidisciplinary" approaches to mental health training for its medical personnel at all levels.[50] But once again, as suggested by Borgå, its intentions and its ability to implement its ideals were not perfectly aligned.

Kurasini limped along as a sickbay for mentally ill patients throughout 1983, but conditions steadily deteriorated, and the proposed treatment centre never came to fruition; as mentioned in chapter 4, the property stopped housing sick patients in 1984. As Kurasini was clearly in the process of crashing and burning, the Health Department saw an urgent need to redouble efforts towards completing the health projects in Dakawa.[51] Local and ANC medical staff supported the idea that ANC members with mental illness should be engaged in productive work including farming, tailoring, or other general crafting skills. The envisioned Vocational Training Centre at Dakawa was projected as a place that could possibly accomplish this, but, unfortunately, it was not used in this capacity even after finally being completed in 1988.[52] Instead, the plans for the Rehabilitation Centre in Dakawa were pushed forward and the idea of mentally ill patients working in construction was tendered. Even without the Vocational Training Centre, the Health Department thought that manual labour would be good for patients; Dakawa's slow infrastructure development provided opportunities for patients to become construction workers.

As of 1984 the ANC's own facilities for mentally ill patients were completely inadequate, and, therefore, patients in Tanzania who actually managed to find medical attention received it from Muhimbili, Morogoro, and Dodoma or were sent out of the country. Otherwise, they were "dumped" in Dakawa where there were no facilities. Some reports listed certain mental health patients as "hopeless" or suggested that they be released from the ANC altogether.[53]

Based partly on the inadequate mental health services available to the ANC and partly on deeply rooted cultural values, some patients with mental illness or epilepsy wanted to visit traditional/indigenous healers for treatment.[54] As pointed out in chapter 3, ANC medical staff were leery of alternative forms of medicine. However, the uniqueness of mental illness or epilepsy and the way that these illnesses manifest symptomatically provided slightly more flexibility for staff to accept a spiritual explanation and treatment plan. For instance, consider Regina Nzo's recommendation for her patient to receive alternative care:

> There is a need for comrade [B] to go to Lusaka [from East Africa] for psychiatric treatment through traditional medicine ... There is a definite change in modern science towards traditional medicine, especially on the psychiatric patient ... What happens to the "Amagqira", who are said by the Xhosa in Xhosa "Uyatwasa". They get traditional medicine, people make noise, they dance themselves to a fit – this is all psychiatry – this is where [comrade B] fits in. I strongly advise Headquarters to make arrangements for [comrade B's] psychiatric problem to be treated traditionally side by side with the modern medicine.[55]

It is also likely that some patients sought out traditional healers independently. Dr Borgå, interested in the role of traditional healing for mental illness, made this hypothesis: "[I]f I treat a patient in a Southern African context, I normally reckon there is likely to be a traditional colleague treating the same patient."[56] As was in the case of Nzo's patient, these patients become visible in the archive when medical practitioners recommended this form of treatment or when patients requested financial support in order to get a traditional consultation.

Hypnosis[57] and acupuncture were other treatment options that were sometimes viewed as useful to treat mental illness and addiction; in May 1984 Dr Reddy wrote a report on the efficacy of his use of acupuncture treatment.[58] While not popular for treatment in other types of illness, traditional healing, hypnosis, and acupuncture were referenced in several reports and policy suggestions discussing ways to address the high incidence of mental illness in exile.

Attitudes towards treating mentally ill patients did not just veer between so-called "traditional" or "western" approaches; there was also major controversy regarding how to distinguish between addiction, psychological disturbance, and psychiatric conditions. Individuals and departments that were affected by comrades who were under the influence of drugs or alcohol had opinions on the way that these individuals should be categorized and treated. For instance, in a special directorate meeting to review SOMAFCO student discipline, one comrade's behaviour was discussed: "The Nat[ional] Commissar understood that he [comrade M] had suffered psychological problems as a result of his suspension. Cd. Nzo said his was not a psychological but a social problem as he was a dagga smoker ... and had stolen and sold ANC property ... Such comrades should be viewed in a political manner."[59] In another case, the health team at Mazimbu was criticized for neglecting to treat patients who drank alcohol – a rather hypocritical stance to take by the team who often faced accusations of drinking on the job.[60] The less-than-compassionate feeling towards alcohol and drug users was reinforced by the government of Tanzania's clear desire to push the ANC out of Dar es Salaam because of the violent behaviour of intoxicated ANC cadres.[61]

Furthermore, as discussed in chapter 4, after Nellie Mvulane visited the Kurasini clinic in 1981 she commented that the clinic was for "genuinely ill mentally disturbed patients" rather than the dagga-smoking, alcoholic, and violent comrades who were being sent there.[62] However, she also acknowledged the blurriness of this distinction when, later in this same letter, she amended her statement slightly in commenting on one particular comrade: "YES, it can be said they [alcoholics and thieves] have psychiatric problems but comrade [O]'s problem is of excessive drinking which though he may be sent abroad for treatment it still is still him who will decide to stop drinking as he is his ultimate doctor for his treatment."[63] Mvulane stressed that, even with psychiatric problems, individuals were ultimately responsible for their decisions.

Two days after Mvulane penned her letter to the ANC administrative secretary (political leadership) in Lusaka, Tshabalala commented that a recent WHO conference held a discussion called Alcohol Consumption and Alcohol-related Problems. She indicated that there was a need for an internal ANC educational seminar regarding drug and alcohol abuse because, according to her, these problems were "some of the main causes for the increasing disability rate evidenced by the congestion in Kurasini and absentism of our students at school."[64] Tshabalala's insistence on addiction education pushed addiction back into the realm of medicine under the umbrella of mental illness but would require support from the WHO. The course, created by Regina Nzo in January 1984, underscored Tshabalala's point. The curriculum for the course pointed out that "[b]ehind all abnormal drinking is some abnormal psychological process ... a common type of alcoholic is the psychotic person who present alcoholism as one of his prominent symptoms" (emphasis in original).[65] Regina Nzo argued that alcohol was not bad behaviour as much as it was a symptom of a medical condition. Nzo herself may have been speaking from experience; as previously mentioned, in 1983 Dr Hauli observed that she was a heavy drinker and had been close to having a mental breakdown.[66]

Dagga smoking was a particularly controversial topic in relation to mental illness. By the end of 1983 the Morogoro Psychiatric Unit was no longer willing to deal with ANC drug users, and the ANC had to devise its own solution. Attempts oscillated between punishment, compassion, education, and rehabilitation.[67] In 1983 the Mazimbu political leadership (ANC directorate) called for stricter disciplinary measures against dagga users.[68] From its point of view, dagga use, not psychiatric illness, was the primary issue: "It is said that this type of action [one week of being locked into a room and three months of supervision] was not good for mental cases but in our case these cdes [comrades] primarily are dagga smokers so the question of mental illness to them is secondary to dagga smoking – so they cannot be rearly [sic] be – classified as mental cases."[69] Unfortunately, one of the two comrades put through this three-month surveillance regime tragically died by suicide shortly after "treatment."

A different approach to the issue was also put forward. The ANC's Tanzanian Regional Commissar Arthur Sidweshu called for a health education program regarding the use of dagga. In Sidweshu's proposal he states,

> [T]here is nothing one can do if the person who has this [dagga] problem is not asking for help there is nothing

much you can achieve. But as a Liberation Movement we cannot wait to see our people turning into what the National Commissar termed "vegetables". We have to take an initiative and organise ourselves and continuously fight these habits among our people. I am positive that if we had a medical doctor, a social worker, a psychiatric, this pro-gramme would be highly helpful to our community here and our people all over.[70]

Sidweshu perceived dagga use as a medical issue and, furthermore, one that would benefit from psychiatric and psychological attention.

There was a marked difference between the responses of ANC community members to mental illness in practice and the perceived ideal treatment methods. In the 1982 survey on mental health in Zambia and Tanzania, 120 students and forty-three "staff/other workers" were surveyed to determine what they thought caused mental illness and where/how it should be treated. Sixty-two per cent of students and 40 per cent of staff believed that "dagga (or other drug intoxication)" was a cause of mental illness; 87 per cent of students and only 30 per cent of staff/other workers believed that mental illness should be "handle[d] with sympathy and under-standing."[71] In the report it was indicated that the staff harboured "hidden fears on the potential violent nature of the patients." Out of all 163 interviewed only four people thought that comrades should be treated "by comrade psychiatrist," which likely referred to Dr Freddy Reddy, and 86 per cent of students and 88 per cent of staff thought patients should be treated "in hospitals locally or other frontline states." Essentially, in 1982/3 ANC students and staff members thought that mentally ill patients should not be the ANC's problem but should – according to the students – be the responsibil-ity of a compassionate, local system.

By 1984 the practice of sending all mentally ill patients from other regions to Tanzania was questioned and ultimately halted. Numerous reports note that Tanzania was overwhelmed with patients whom it was neither able to accommodate nor assist,[72] and angry letters emerged questioning why patients receiving good support in Lusaka were being transferred to Tanzania.[73] Despite the negative feedback on treatment, the situation in Tanzania was not all doom and gloom. Starting in March 1984 the ANC at the SOMAFCO clinic collaborated with the Morogoro Psychiatric Unit, and the unit sent a psychiatrist to the clinic once a month and a psychiatric nurse once a week.[74] Additionally, plans were being set for ANC members to enrol in six-month courses on psychiatric care in Morogoro; this was in keeping with the community-centred approach set out in Tanzania's African Mental Health Action Group reports.[75]

In 1984 the ANC Health Department started to collaborate closely with Zimbabwe's School of Social Work, and they had already sent Roy Campbells to take the social work course.[76] By design the benefits of the growing relationship between Zimbabwe's school for social work and the ANC was to be exported to Dakawa and Mazimbu where social work and rehabilitation services were planned for the near future. Furthermore, while the department was busy proposing candidates to be educated in Zimbabwe, two ANC students were given internships at Chainama Hills.[77] The ANC leadership and health administration saw this placement very positively as it brought the Health Department closer to the Zambian facility than it had been in the past.

In April 1984 it was decided that mentally ill comrades in Angola were to be sent to Zambia; Angola did not have the facilities to support such comrades and the frontline was decidedly not where the Politico–Military Council wanted sick cadres treated. Unrest in Angola, which culminated in the 1984 mutinies, brought slightly more attention to the issue of mental illness in the camps. Not only did the Stuart Commission point to the incidence of suicide but starting in 1984 a number of reports instigated by the Health Department began to illuminate some of the demons faced by cadres stuck in Angolan camps.[78] The reports that were written in the wake of the mutinies provide the closest look at the mental health realities in Angola. A 1987 report states,

> We may assume that the psychological strain on the members of the ANC community in Angola is even heavier than in the other regions. Military training, actual fighting and terror by the enemy, together with the poor living conditions in Angola, create stress which occasionally manifests itself in problems with alcoholism, aggression, and for some individuals in the development of serious depressions.[79]

However, those writing the report were unable to travel to Angola for "security reasons," and so it was impossible for them to do more than assume the high prevalence rate.

Meanwhile, in Tanzania there were some very positive developments as well as a growing number of psychiatric cases. When Dr Reddy was in Mazimbu and Dakawa between January and April 1985 he saw more than 120 patients with mental health issues. The most common diagnoses recorded were depression neurosis, anxiety neurosis, schizophrenia, epilepsy, acute or drug-induced psychosis, post-torture syndrome, or neurasthenia.[80] He also found that, of the 158 students he surveyed in Mazimbu, 66 per cent had worrisome psychological symptoms that needed attention. Other accounts of patients from 1985 showed that the system of surveillance and treatment was poor and that the staff was often unable to contain patients; consequently, some patients managed to obtain weapons, injure other people or "escape" Dakawa.

For instance, in March 1985 one patient staying in Dakawa stabbed a fellow comrade, stole the Land Rover, drove recklessly towards Morogoro, killed a Tanzania pedestrian on the way, and assaulted two other locals before he was stopped by the police.[81] The patient was psychotic, aggressive, and confused. At his trial he said he did not remember the incident, he believed himself to be the son of Nelson Mandela and according to witnesses, "was doing a lot of prattling." Not only were some of the reports on patient behaviour worrisome, they also suggested that the social stigma related to mental illness was still alive and well among the students and staff.[82]

The continuing updates on the efficacy of the mental health response was not consistent throughout reports from the later 1980s, but it is clear that the development of the Raymond Mhlaba Rehabilitation Centre in Dakawa and the Community-Based Rehabilitation Team headed by Roy Campbells were major milestones. Based on the success of Roy Campbells, recently graduated from the Zimbabwe Social Work Program, there was new emphasis in late 1985 on training rehabilitation workers who would be based at Dakawa. From August to October a group of ten "Community Based Rehabilitation workers" surveyed Dakawa's community plots in an attempt to identify members in Dakawa with physical and mental disabilities.[83] Furthermore, their aim was to address the needs of the community and to educate the inhabitants about mental illness and rehabilitation.

In October following the survey, the Raymond Mhlaba Rehabilitation Centre was established and able to accommodate eleven psychiatric patients.[84] By the middle of the year headway made by the team created the illusion that most of those who were "emotionally disturbed" had been transferred to Dakawa and were presumably under some level of surveillance and care by Roy Campbells' team.[85] One 1985 report states, "Since the establishment of the rehabilitation centre in Dakawa, the improvement of comrades has been remarkable."[86] The report outlines a neat system in which those from the rehabilitation centre could travel with the Rehabilitation Team to Mazimbu on Wednesday where the Morogoro Psychiatric Team assessed the patients and the hospital followed up on any physical ailments. Certainly, this was a very optimistic representation of events and alternative, less positive perspectives, are offered in the archive. However, most accounts from this period in late 1985 and early 1986 are relatively encouraging about the future of rehabilitation and reports reflect a positive attitude towards the new program.

In keeping with this theme of positivity, there was a continued effort to improve the psychosocial limitations faced by students as well. At the end of 1985 a new Social Welfare Department was added in the Morogoro region. Poloko Nkobi, a member of the Community-Based Rehabilitation Team in Dakawa, began work in one-on-one counselling with those in need. She was joined by Zola Ledjuma and Sherry McLean, an Irish social worker, and, together, they comprised the new department's Social Work Unit.[87] Nkobi took maternity leave in January 1986 and Ledjuma later in March, but the three had established a service to counsel students in need of psychological support and refer students, when necessary, to the psychiatrist in Morogoro. Patients were continually referred to Morogoro, Muhimbili, Dodoma, or Chainama Hills Hospital, but efforts for community involvement and preventative care were underway. Additionally, the department began health education initiatives among students in Mazimbu.

These efforts may have been important in dealing with the patients, but the fight against mental illness was an uphill battle. The number of reportedly mentally ill patients reached its highest point in November 1986 and the optimism evident in previous reports dimmed. Dr Reddy assessed the Dakawa and Mazimbu communities and found 143 to be in need of specialist care. The diagnoses included twenty-seven with "Schizophrenia and Paranoid States," twenty-four with "Stress and Environmental Maladjustments," twenty-three with "Neurosis and Personality Disorders," seventeen with "Mania and Hypomania," sixteen with "*Brain Fag Syndrome" (explained as involving learning problems among secondary school students), thirteen with "Depression (Endogenous and Realtive [sic] Types)," eleven with "Alcohol and Drug Abuse *(Bhangi – Psychosis)" (explained as associated with cannabis use), nine with "Epilepsy (Mainly Grand Mal type Epilepsy)," and nine with "Organic Psychosis (ACUTE CONFUSIONAL STATES)."[88] Despite efforts of the Rehabilitation Team and the Social Welfare Department, Reddy states that, upon observation, the ignorance and stigma around mental illness was a serious setback to treatment. Furthermore, there was a lack of trained personnel to deal with the number of patients and the severity of their illnesses. Medical personnel were failing to follow up with patients to ensure that they were continuing their medical program.

Part of the problem was that the Community-Based Rehabilitation Team and the Social Welfare Department did not stem from a Health Department initiative and were, therefore, not fully integrated or under the direct supervision of the Health Department. Clearly, efforts were linked, evidenced by the fact that the Social Welfare Department's office was in the Mazimbu Hospital, but more cooperation and coordination were necessary to streamline efforts to treat mental illness.[89] In 1987 an independent report from Norway observed the ANC's health infrastructure and commented on the disjuncture:

> The [Mazimbu] hospital has a number of tasks beyond its curative efforts and MCH-services. One of these is to supervise and support the minor health establishments in Dakawa. The degree to which the health team in Mazimbu is also responsible for the psychiatric rehabilitation centre in Dakawa is not clear. Since the hospital has no psychiatric expertise at its disposal, the ability to support the centre must be limited.[90]

The report also notes that Sherry McLean was not formally part of the Health Department and did not wish to become so; she preferred independence.[91] It was recommended that the Health Department clarify its position with regards to the treatment of mentally ill patients and be more directly involved in providing consistent health education and community support. It was further recommended that the department make an effort to upgrade the facilities and programs available at the rehabilitation centre in Dakawa.

Efforts in Lusaka echoed those in East Africa. By the end of 1986 the Emmasdale Clinic had acquired a rehabilitation annex. Patients were diagnosed and treated at UTH before being sent to the annex, a type of holding facility (reminiscent of Kurasini), where patients could work in a community garden.[92] But the centre was also understaffed. In 1987 it was reported that the centre had only one medical aid, and that aid had been trained on the job. The report that noted the disjuncture between the Community-Based Rehabilitation Team, Social Work Department, and health departments concluded its observations on the ANC's efforts by saying,

> Among the curative services, psychiatric care has suffered most from the lack of an elaborate strategy. The term "rehabilitation centre" now attached to the two mental institutions in operation does not reflect a clearly defined approach to the care for mental patients. The question remains: what kind of mental institutions are needed and what should be the strategy for treatment and rehabilitation?[93]

The 1987 reports and internal memos are filled with general criticism and frustration at the inability of the Health Department to deal with mentally ill cadres. Reports on the efficacy of the rehabilitation centre at Dakawa grew steadily more ominous. The entire centre staff, none of who had specialist training, were sent away due to a lack of efficiency and accusations of theft. Four new untrained staff members were found to replace them.[94] In February Tanzania's ANC chief administrator, Tim Maseko, requested that new plans for a large facility for mentally ill patients in Dakawa be drawn up due to the increasing need for infrastructure.[95] In September Sherry McLean wrote, "In my view, the situation has deteriorated considerably with the result that some of our patients are making little or no progress. The supplies and living conditions are poor, there is little or no support from the community and there are problems in supplies of drugs."[96]

In November the Dakawa health team reaffirmed McLean's assessment by stating, "We are very much appalled with the situation in Mhlaba [Rehabilitation Centre], particularly with housing ... We feel that the house is not conducive to speedy recovery but instead it is a health hazard to the patients and demoralizing to the health person [*sic*]."[97]

Similar pronouncements were made on the Emmasdale rehabilitation annex. In November 1988 the health secretariat reflected on the organisation of the facility to that point:

> The structure to deal with this important task [to rehabilitate mentally ill patients] would be the Regional Health Committee. But, as it was said earlier, the committee is defunct and the burden now falls on the clinic committee as far as community rehabilitation is concerned ... The meeting sadly noted that the clinic committee had never really taken hold of the organisation of the annex and the medical, health, subsistence and social needs of the patients were erratically addressed. Attempts in the past to organise a routine at the annex, provide good medical care and see to the economic and social needs of the patients never won the support of the clinic committee.[98]

A report in February 1989 adds that, after having recovered in Chainama Hills from the acute stage of an illness, the comrades were admitted to the annex. Of those, it was complained that, "some comrades [bring] in prostitutes who are at times entertained with the logistic supplies of the Annex which leads to tension and fights amongst the comrades [in the annex]."[99] The annex still needed qualified staff. The ANC still did not have a specific policy or program in place to deal with the mental health crisis on their hands and continued to rely on local facilities to compensate for their disappointing show of mental health infrastructure.

Starting in late 1989 the ANC became much less interested in developing a coherent strategy for dealing with mental illness in exile. Instead, a new question emerged: what will the ANC do with its mentally ill patients throughout the period of transition home? In a rather forward statement, the newly formed Social Work Unit wrote,

There has always been a dire need for the formation of the Department of Social Welfare within the ANC, but most unfortunately the necessary professionals have never been organised into a department. It is only now when our people are on the verge of being repatriated back to South Africa that the ANC seems to appreciate the important role social workers can play before and after repatriation.[100]

The immediate mandate of the department was to identify vulnerable comrades and attempt to reintegrate them into their families and communities in South Africa. In May 1990 Dr Reddy asked the health secretariat to see that the psychiatric patients treated in southern African facilities be issued with medical reports that could be used in South Africa in case of continued care.[101]

However, patients' futures were uncertain to say the least. The new Social Work Unit found cases of chronically mentally ill patients who had been supported by the networks of international and sub-Saharan solidarity for years and who were now going to be expected to pay their own medical bills.[102] According to the unit, the health secretariat's response to this conundrum was to avoid responsibility for the long-term needs of these patients.

It was impossible to trace whether the patients continued treatment at Chainama Hills, Morogoro, or Muhimbili or whether they had returned home. The Social Work Unit recommended that the young mentally ill cadres treated in Tanzania be sent home to South Africa and resettled immediately, but there was no follow-up on when, how, or if this was done. Further discussions about mental health services ignored ANC settlements and turned to post-apartheid policy discussions. The Health Department was engaged in meetings with various health bodies within South Africa and the Department of Social Welfare was determining the role that it would play in the future ANC government. The treatment for mentally ill patients in exile was at its end.

Mental Illness Politicized

Until the early 1980s major reasons cited for psychological breakdown, anxiety, dagga use and suicide concerned the ANC's inability to penetrate South Africa's borders, the "socio-economic and political conditions in South Africa exiled life," as well as the mental effects of becoming local and international charity cases and, consequently, the creation of a "psychological image of inferiority."[103] This explanation was a self-reflective admission of responsibility by the ANC and echoed the comrades' own complaints and opinions on why they were suffering.

Starting in the early 1980s there was special interest placed on how the effects of military action in exiled life affected the psyche of South Africans. Rather than looking only at the effects of boredom, poor conditions, and dramatic environmental change in exile, there was a growing awareness that symptoms of anxiety related directly to experiences of enemy attack on the front lines – later diagnosed as PTSD. This phenomenon was evident in the way that mental illness was discussed in reports. Many comrades were not given a formal diagnosis by regional staff but were declared "ill" and in need of medical attention or hospitalization due to their experiences of trauma. For instance one patient's report stated that he had "reactive anxiety" due to his capture by South African police in Swaziland.[104] Tellingly, many diagnoses were preceded with the adjective "reactive" such as "reactive psychosis," "reactive paranoid psychosis," or "reactive anxiety" to emphasize the military-related environmental causes of a patient's symptoms.[105] After experiencing enemy bomb attacks, one cadre was said to be "sick" due to his symptoms of paranoia and developed an inability to drive, and another was deemed "mentally deranged" and referred for inpatient care in Zambia.[106] This shift in diagnostic labelling was significant because it indicated a transmission of blame for mental illness from the ANC's actions to the actions of SADF and, consequently, the NP in South Africa.

By late 1981 it was evident that the blame was moving away from the ANC even further. The ANC increasingly believed that the situation in South Africa – the systemic racism and experiences of imprisonment and torture – was to blame for many of the psychological breakdowns that occurred in exile. The major reinforcement of this new emphasis came during the 1981 Health and Apartheid Conference discussed earlier. This conference specifically explored the impact of apartheid on the health of South Africans and included a small section entitled "Apartheid and Mental Health." That section declared that apartheid was to blame for many "preventable mental disorders" and many of those escaping South Africa were taxing the liberation movement's Health Department because of their experiences while living under the apartheid regime.[107] One of the conclusions is as follows: "Apartheid has created stressful social structures by its policies of forced removals, migrant labour laws, restrictions of freedom of expressions, daily harrasments [sic] and arrests etc., leading to high rates of mental illnesses and other chronic related diseases."[108] An addendum to the report takes a more measured approach and acknowledges that, "Psychological disturbances of varying degrees … are related perhaps to the situation at home that some of our comrades suffered under … Some develop outside here as a response to the new environments."[109] In other words, both apartheid and exile conditions were to blame. This was a fitting reflection of why many comrades suffered psychological distress but was also a much more strategic position to take in terms of generating international support and solidarity.

When the ANC sought money from international donors for their health-related projects, the link between apartheid and mental health was emphasized. For instance one project proposal to the WHO and UNDP states, "Health was one of the main social services to be provided at SOMAFCO, mainly because most of these young people came away from South Africa with serious traumatic and psycho-social disorders."[110] In that same proposal, the ANC discussed the injustices of apartheid and thereby justified the existence of its own Health Department and anti-apartheid movement. In another proposal for renovations to the Kurasini sickbay, a similar appeal for international legitimacy is given by saying, "The torture of South African patriots by the racist police and the severe oppression suffered under Apartheid give rise to a high incidence of psychiatric disturbance amongst our people."[111]

Linking apartheid and ill health was a successful strategy. In May 1982, directly responding to the African Mental Health Action Group conference, Manto Tshabalala reported,

The WHO Director General, Dr H. Mahler and the WHO Regional Director for Africa, Dr A.A. Quenum have further enhanced the moral credit of the world health community by reaffirming the Organization's resolute stand on the issue of apartheid and health. There is a readiness on the part of the WHO to accord as much assistance as is possible to the NLM [National Liberation Movement] to aliviate [*sic*] the health problems of the *victims of apartheid*.[112]

Further support from the WHO, in particular, was underpinned by the notion that those South Africans with mental illness in exile were "victims of apartheid" and intervention efforts were directly related to treating these victims.[113] Support was clearly more readily available for mental health when apartheid was to blame.

Additionally, the previously described 1977 report on the South African government's services available to African patients with mental illness (as well as subsequent reporting on the same issue) was used by South African-born, anti-apartheid activist Dr John Dommisse who was then practicing psychiatry in the US. In 1983 Dommisse attempted, without success, to gain support for the anti-apartheid cause from those at the World Psychiatric Association (WPA) Congress and the World Federation for Mental Health Congress. While he did not receive an immediate endorsement, he did advocate for the mentally ill in South Africa and delivered the message to some of the most significant and influential global leaders in mental health care.[114]

He was, however, rewarded for his efforts in June 1984 when an unofficial WPA Committee was created to lobby for the expulsion of South Africa from the WPA.[115] The committee, made up of ten psychiatrists, announced that "Apartheid is the greatest threat to the mental health of the majority of people in the Republic of South Africa ... We therefore call upon the international psychiatric community, in particular the World Psychiatric Association, to condemn apartheid and its effect on mental health and to sever relations with the Society of Psychiatrists of South Africa."[116] Dommisse's efforts were followed by his personal excommunication from the MASA.[117]

In July 1984 the World Federation for Mental Health did not allow South African representatives who had already arrived to attend the meeting.[118] They were subsequently told that they would not be able to join meetings for the next two years. In January 1986 John Dommisse published "The Psychological Effects of Apartheid Psychoanalysis: Social, Moral and Political Influences" in the *International Journal of Social Psychiatry* in order to more widely shame the WPA and the World Medical Association for continuing to support South Africa's participation: "[T]he World Psychiatric Association should be made to see that it had no choice, if it is to retain its integrity, but to speak out against the Society of Psychiatrists of South Africa for its relative silence on the massive government assault on the mental health of the majority of the South African people."[119] Dommisse cited the WHO's 1977 report, Peter Lambley's 1981 study "The Psychology of Apartheid," and various other independent reports, all of which attempted to illuminate the conditions of mental health and the effect of racist apartheid policies in South Africa.[120]

This new emphasis on framing mental illness as a result of apartheid policies was also increasingly reflected, and often rightfully so, in patient reports. Tim Maseko, then principal at SOMAFCO, wrote,

> Three girls suffer latent hallucinations of the sadistic torture they went through during detention by the Boers. [P]: she is a nervous wreck and her state of health disrupts the general school programme: frequent fainting and screaming at night, thereby setting the whole dormitory in tension. [Y]: Since I came here she has been literally in bed for about 4 months now. She has serious lower abdominal pains as a result of the torture!!! [C]: She literally runs amock when she has the attack. This is frequently caused by the screams of [P]. I think this makes her relive the screams she used to hear during grilling operation at John Vorster. She is, however, the less affected of the three. She is a pleasant and hard working young girl.[121]

The girls were "victims of apartheid" and not of exile and they were in need of ANC support. Dr Freddy Reddy reported that many of those who had been tortured in South Africa were angry and "usually carried within them consciously and unconsciously the revenge motive" and developed dangerous violent tendencies while helpless in exile to punish those who had tortured them.[122] Additionally, Dr Reddy believed that, when the students who had been victims of violence in the apartheid state moved into exile, symptoms of depression, anxiety, and impotency were made manifest in periods of relative calm when the adrenaline of escape and immediate action had dissipated. On a conscious or unconscious level, individuals leaving South Africa experienced psychological distress and often "acted out" in problematic ways as a result of their experiences of trauma in South Africa.

It was not only the physical violence of apartheid that was psychologically damaging. The psychological ramifications of racism, especially systemic racism, have been widely explored. This is perhaps best known in Frantz Fanon's work on the "inferiority complex" generated by colonialism and institutionalised racism against black people. In *Black Skin, White Masks*, Fanon writes,

> If he is overwhelmed to such a degree by the wish to be white, it is because he lives in a society that makes his inferiority complex possible, in a society that derives its stability from the perpetuation of this complex, in a society that proclaims the superiority of one race; to the identical degree to which that society creates difficulties for him, he will find himself thrust into a neurotic situation.[123]

This state of mind was observed by the WHO report on health and apartheid in South Africa and Dr Reddy's account of treating patients in exile. Dr Reddy reflected that

> the internalisation of this negative identification, that the white man has always told the black man for six hundred years, that you are nothing, you are dirty, you are this, somehow in the (psych) years, become a part of this aggressive attitude towards the whites, that it would explode at any time. And this anxiety thing in the black man is so great that even after twenty years, they still have difficulties to go alone into a restaurant full of white people in Europe. If they go in, they must be drunk or they must be in a gang, or things like that.[124]

The WHO report points out that the apartheid regime's racist laws and policies were a major contribution to the high incidence of psychological disturbance within South Africa.[125]

Consistent with the Health Department's strategy for international solidarity and support off the African continent, described in a more general way in chapter 3, the department politicized the causes of mental illness in order to delegitimize the apartheid regime and gain credibility for itself. This strategy was, once again, in keeping with the anti-apartheid trends already in motion; the Health Department found ways to capitalize on the momentum. Mental illness in exile was political and the Health Department proved its worth to the liberation movement once again by ensuring that it could be used beneficially. However, apartheid was not the only reason for psychological distress and trauma; the Health Department also had to contend with its comrades who had been subject to the ANC's own, often brutal, security sector.

Internal Security and Mental Illness

Undoubtedly, the situational causes for mental illness emphasized by the ANC were major factors in creating the mental health crisis in exile, and the shift of blame from itself to the NP was certainly politically advantageous. However, the major emphasis on the evils of apartheid coincided with the discovery in late 1981 of the internal network of spies in the ANC, the development of the ANC's National Department of Intelligence and Security (NAT) and the intensification of internal paranoia within the organisation. NAT was given authoritarian power to imprison and punish anyone suspected of infiltration. According to historian Stephen Davis, NAT had a wide purview of what was considered suspicious behaviour: "Spreading a rumor, crashing a car, stealing supplies or complaining about shortages, were acts of demoralization and could now get you labeled as an infiltrator."[126] Indeed, in 1981, after Dr Shangase was killed in a car crash, an unsigned letter to Andrew Masondo, the MK commissar in Angola, expressed suspicion of the driver. The letter states that "the question [is] whether this fatal accident was any less designed and purposeful than the car accidents in which our vehicles were destroyed by drivers who knew how to emerge from the crash virtually unscathed. We therefore require that the fullest investigation at the highest possible level be instituted immediately into the circumstances of the accident."[127] The increased internal paranoia coincided with increased incidences of mental illness. The ANC's 1996 submission to the TRC accounted for forty-five suicides, thirty-four of which were in Angola amongst MK cadres and thirty-two of which were during or after 1981 (the actual number was higher because the submission did not include suicides in Tanzania).[128]

The ANC's practices of internal punishment, imprisonment, and torture were contentious. This is reflected in the degree to which these practices are emphasized in literature as central to the movement. Paul Trewhela led the charge when claiming the ANC committed severe human rights abuses. He has chronicled the use of detention and torture in both SWAPO and ANC prison camps from the early 1980s.[129] He started by writing provocative accounts in the polemical publication *Searchlight South-Africa* and, more recently, has republished in his book *Inside Quatro: Uncovering the exile history of the ANC and SWAPO* some older, previously published exposés on the human rights abuses perpetrated by the ANC in exile.[130] In a similar but perhaps less punishing account, Stephen Ellis argues,

> Many cadres who fell under suspicion were sent to the MK camps in Angola and grounded there … many were left in a limbo as uncleared suspects, sometimes for years. This had a debilitating effect both on the people concerned, unsure whether they might be called for further questioning at any time, and also on the ANC as a whole, as it spread uncertainty and demoralisation. Some committed suicide.[131]

Hugh Macmillan also commented on internal security issues. He pointed out that the ANC truly did face serious infiltration risks and that security was an important and difficult task for the under equipped and "amateur" NAT.[132] He discussed some of the mistakes made by the ANC on this account, including the ill treatment of Thami Zulu who ultimately died after months of NAT detention and solitary confinement. On the subject of ANC security tactics, Macmillan states, "It is possible that the ANC itself retains a security archive … but it is equally likely that much of the documentation on both sides [NP and ANC] has been lost or destroyed. Even if these archives do exist, it may be impossible to get a clear or unequivocal picture of events that must always have seemed to be murky and obscure."[133]

Aside from the debate in the literature, the ANC conducted a number of internal commissions that gave evidence of the abusiveness of the internal security sector.[134] First, the Stuart Commission looked into the circumstances that led to the 1984 mutinies. The report, analysing camp conditions in Angola, found that in the camps, "[t]he aim of the punishment seems to be to destroy, demoralise and humiliate comrades and not to correct and build."[135] At the determination of the commission, the administration of punishments meted out for drinking, smoking dagga, or selling ANC goods killed six people; others committed suicide (the number is not included in the report). In some cases, cadres were put in locked "goods containers" for days and others were beaten and then exposed to the elements by being tied to trees. The commission found that cadres in Angola believed the security department to be "sadistic" and unaccountable for its harsh and often unwarranted actions, and, as a result, there was a generalized fear in the camp of being accused of being an infiltrator.

The Skweyiya Commission included in the ANC's TRC submission was a "report of the commission of enquiry into complaints by former African National Congress Prisoners and Detainees."[136] This report confirms that serious human rights abuses were committed by the ANC. In addition, it points out that those detained had cause to experience serious psychological distress after they had been released by the ANC:

> The mere fact that these detainees were detained for long periods of time (apart from the manner in which they were treated while in detention) constitutes, in our view, an extreme form of psychological torture. In the case of the detainees concerned, however, they have been precluded from reintegration into their own communities even though they were never found guilty of any offence. The mere fact that they had been detained by the ANC has been sufficient for them to be stigmatized as traitors to the cause of the ANC. This has resulted in ostracism and rejection.[137]

The commission found that some of the witnesses to the commission were in need of psychological support and treatment.

Directly following the Skweyiya Commission, Nelson Mandela appointed the 1993 Motsuenyane Commission, which was an "enquiry into certain allegations of cruelty and human rights abuse against ANC prisoners and detainees by ANC members" that culminated in a nearly 200-page report. Like the Skweyiya Commission, this commission also found that various MK cadres had been brutally beaten and humiliated. In one case MK cadre Mr Daliwonga Mandela "was forced to dig a grave and told that it was his own. He said that, when he was released, he 'was told not to reveal the names of the torturers to the doctor in Lusaka.'"[138] Taken together, these three commissions make it clear that the ANC's anxiety over internal threats and methods of dealing with those threats had a significant impact on its members who feared being accused of infiltration and on those who were actually exposed to detainment and/or torture.

The internal fear and suspicion within the ANC was highlighted during my interview with psychologist Dr Vuyo Mpumlwana. (As a member of the ANC, a scholarship was arranged for her to study psychology in Canada.) In the interview she explained that she travelled from Canada back to Tanzania in order to conduct her PhD research on the incidence of PTSD among students in Mazimbu and Dakawa. She had felt threatened while in Tanzania and was worried that she was going to be arrested by the security police. Dr Mpumlwana explained that it was in the nature of liberation movements to have many secrets; the ANC was not unique in wanting to keep many things away from the public eye. However, she said this did not excuse the ANC for the things that it did. In her opinion many people suffered at the hands of the ANC and then could not talk about their experiences. Furthermore, she thought it was also very possible that the ANC used mental illness and antipsychotic drugs to delegitimise the opinions or experiences of certain comrades:

> So, were the diagnoses really real or were they not, or was it a camouflage? Was it someone – I'm giving just a hypothesis here – was it someone maybe who was known as a danger of spilling the beans and therefore we should drug this person and say that they were schizophrenic? There are so many things you could say because it was a world of paranoia and a world of secrets, deep secrets. So how can you

come from a family where there is never schizophrenia and you become schizophrenic all of a sudden? I don't know. Its just a hypothesis … So if I can't kill you … and I know that you know a lot, I can drug you. And the more I drug you the more you become schizophrenic. I don't know![139]

It would be difficult, if not impossible, to prove that the ANC did, in fact, silence people in this way, but it does hint at the extreme measures that were seen as possible for the ANC to take.

As mentioned by both Macmillan and Dr Mpumlwana, the ANC *did* have a lot of trouble regarding infiltration. Part of its fear was directed towards the health sector; the ANC's NEC reported that it was afraid that "people who are mentally imbalanced find their way into the ANC. Perhaps this infiltration of drifters, ne'er-do-wells and ill people is a definite strategy of the enemy to increase the burden on the resources of the Organisation."[140] In addition, it was worried that the so-called solidarity workers were using the avenue of health – as both patients and practitioners – in order to get information about the ANC.

In 1980 there were two cases of outsiders offering desperately needed specialized psychological care to the ANC and who were denied access to comrades. The first was Dr John Dommisse, previously discussed as the agitator for anti-apartheid action in the international realm of psychiatry. Dommisse was born in South Africa, left the country as a conscientious objector to the racism in South Africa, and trained and practiced psychiatry in the US. He first offered his services to the ANC in 1980 and was set to come to southern Africa in December of that year. However, days before his arrival, Tshabalala wrote to Nzo, "we have agreed that at this stage we should only have consultations with him and we are also agreed that it would be rather pre-mature to take him on a guided tour to our projects and even to allow him to consult our psychiatric patients until we have clearance from our Headquarters."[141] Either the ANC was worried about Dommisse being an infiltrator or they were apprehensive that he would witness things in ANC communities that would subtract from his clear pro-ANC leanings.

The second solidarity worker offering to serve in the healthcare field was Pia Mothander, a Swedish clinical child/infant psychologist who had been working in Swaziland with the Swedish Save the Children Fund. As part of her duties with the organisation, she offered her services to the ANC because it was one of the groups supported by Save the Children.[142] As had already been reported by Dr Reddy, the vast majority of children and teenagers in Morogoro were in need of psychological support and the ANC chief representative in East Africa, Reddy Mazimba, sought permission from other ANC leadership for Mothander to help their community in Tanzania.[143] Pia Mothander reflected on the leadership's reception of this idea:

> I felt that I don't think they wanted to share too much infor-mation with me. Because I think that they, I got the impres-sion that they felt that I might get too much information. That I would know too much about what was really going on and I know that they had ways of disciplinary actions against teenagers and things like that that they didn't want to talk about. And that was why I was not fully invited.[144]

Mothander was only able to make a few limited suggestions to the ANC on the construction of the infant care facilities then underway in Morogoro.

In 1981, shortly after Dommissee and Mothander were restricted from ANC settlements, the Health Department issued a memo il-luminating their suspicion about new staff working in Tanzania at the Muhimbili medical centre in Dar es Salaam. New "ex-South Africans" living in Canada were to be transferred into the unit. The Health Department insisted that its patients should not be seen by these unknown new arrivals. The ANC Health Department memo states,

> Several dubious characters had sought interviews with him [likely the head of the UNHCR, the UNDP, or the head of the psychiatric unit in Muhimbili] to discuss the psychological problems of South African refugees. He had advised them, rather to approach and consult the respective Liberation Movements ... we have approached several people here in East Africa who, apparently do not realize the importance and seriousness of this situation as a safety valve contribu-tory to ensure the security of our Organisation.[145]

With great understanding, the head of the psychiatric unit recommended that the new staff be sent to a different regional centre in Tanzania that was not being used by the ANC at that time. In order to keep continued positive relations with the psychiatric unit, the Health Department suggested that the ANC help supply the Muhimbili unit with psychotropic drugs.

Furthermore, the nature of treatment meant that patients had to discuss these relatively traumatic experiences. In the case of comrade L, the ANC chief representative in Harare wrote to the ANC administrative secretary in Lusaka about his apprehensions regarding comrade L's psychiatric treatment: "We ar[e] scared the Psychiatric [*sic*] may dig into sensitive things, as he will be having every professional right to do so. Please advise."[146] The patient was then transferred to Angola where Dr Sipho Mthembu reported, "I found her rotting in the camps here with frequent relapses of her problems."[147] Two months later the patient was sent back to Mazimbu to await treatment from Dr Reddy because "doctors/comrades felt that Zimbabwe was not very safe to treat her case." [148] Her case remained contentious. Certain individuals in the medical sector were particularly agitated because it was revealed that this comrade had received funding from the UN to get treatment abroad and was being blocked from accepting the international psychiatric support.

By the end of the year, Tshabalala had to explain why this cadre was transferred back to Tanzania:

[I]n the first place, cde [L] and [J] suddenly landed in Harare unexpectedly. But when subsequently a SWAPO doctor was consulted on the matter she (SWAPO doctor) advised against treating her in Harare for security reasons. The main problem here is that if [L] has got to be handled by psychiatric specialists in Harare, it means that they will have to dig into her background. The SWAPO doctor says you need your own doctors or doctors who are sympathetic to your cause to handle such patients. Otherwise there [*sic*] a good psychiatric specialists in the area. But we cannot vouch for them politically ... In the end the SWAPO doctor recommended that she should be put on a slimming course [she was classified as obese] and be transferred to her "own community" or people ...

After a heated debate on the [L] case, the meeting resolved that cde [L] still needs treatment. The meeting therefore urged the Health Dept to pursue the matter this to be done under the supervision of SGO.[149]

The duty to provide health care had to be balanced against the constant fear of a security breach, and the nature of psychiatric evaluation and treatment does not lend itself to silence and secrecy. It appears that certain members of the Health Department had enough information about comrade [L] to worry about the political safety of allowing her to speak to an external psychiatrist.

Not only did the ANC fear what might be said in therapy sessions, patients were also afraid of saying too much in these sessions; they were afraid of being caught and accused of undermining the organisation. In Hilda Bernstein's interview with Dr Reddy in 1990, he commented on this phenomenon: "I used to give them very intensive therapy and another problem that developed was that the majority of ANC young people didn't want to tell the local psychiatrists and doctors because they were security conscious."[150] My interview with Dr Vuyo Mpumlwana reiterated this point:

So, for security reasons one could not talk about their [pause] fully about their experiences in Angola, in all the front-line areas where they were fighting … But a whole lot of things can happen to these people that they could not talk about. Because it was a secret. But in my data collection … I was not [pause] my questions were not trying to get them to talk about their experiences with the ANC. Because I knew I wouldn't get anything and I had to send all my questionnaires first to the headquarters before they could allow me to go to Tanzania in the first place. Yes. So I wouldn't be able to ask about directly okay: "tell me you were in Angola and then what." You know? [laughter] "Okay you were in the ANC jail [pause] and? [pause] for how long? And who died under that kind of treatment? And how many people died were not killed by the bullets but they were killed by other you know or the bullet didn't come from the enemy it came from within." You can't talk about those things. And the people have experiences watching their friends watching this, you know, the assassinations and you know, you don't know, they cannot tell you. Because of who is listening.[151]

Dr Mpumlwana made it clear that in her attempts to counsel people whom she had learned had had traumatic experiences, the individuals were unwilling to speak about their experiences with the ANC in exile.[152] It seems that, in many cases, the ANC had almost nothing to worry about from the psychiatric patients; the patients' fear and paranoia were adequate for keeping doctors in the dark. This was even the case when meeting with Dr Reddy and Dr Mpumlwana, two of the ANC's own people.

Officially, the main causes of mental illness in exile were apartheid policies and oppressive actions in South Africa, but after the ANC was unbanned and the human rights abuses of the ANC were more clearly illuminated, the ANC has been found culpable once more. A sober backward gaze upon the situation in exile, must consider the ANC's fear of infiltration and its internal security measures as major causative factors for psychological distress. In this way the ANC was the cause of, at least, exacerbating fear and paranoia among some of the comrades and mentally traumatizing others with its methods of punishment. In addition to the mentally damaging effects of the ANC's internal paranoia, those who were released by the ANC were expected to keep their experiences a secret. If they revealed what the ANC had done to them, they could be resuspected of wishing to undermine the anti-apartheid cause. With respect to mental health treatment practices, the ANC thought that patients in therapy would tell outsiders too much about the organisation's dubious internal activities and, as a result, sometimes prohibited possible treatment.

Other Contributing Factors to the High Incidence of Mental Illness

The general reality of living in exile, the exposure to war and violence, the psychological effects of living under apartheid and under the ANC's own internal system of fear and punishment took a major toll on the mental health of South African exiles. However, patients and psychiatrists themselves weighed in on other causes for the mental illnesses experienced in exile. Dr Reddy stressed that one problem was that students entering into exile around 1976 were children or youths from age eight to seventeen. These individuals were at or close to reaching the age of puberty, a stage of physical and mental transition, and in need of parental guidance and support. The ANC was certainly unable to meet the needs of hundreds of pubescent children.[153] Rebelliousness and independence, typical of this developmental stage, paired with internal psychological problems, led to dagga and alcohol abuse. Dr Reddy spoke specifically about male youths going through puberty without adult guidance:

> The young men were whispering about sexual arousement, pub[ic] hairs growing and so on, so that all the turmoils [sic] of becoming an adult were very, very sensitive … Their protests in terms of drinking, abusing women, girls went into prostitution, and all this had a very negative effect on these children, or young people. And of course, naturally when they were caught for these things, they were arrested, punished and this punishment was even worse because nobody knew how to tackle them there.[154]

Speaking about girls and young women, Reddy reported that girls sought comfort and developed sexual relationships with the boys or young men; many of these young women became pregnant, a situation which was punished and had serious psychological ramifications for the individuals involved.[155]

Reddy did not see these relationships as examples of "real love affairs" but there were certainly cases where the hampered ability to build and nourish love relationships in exile was the cause of mental distress. In one personal account, the cadre reports, "Though I tried my best to overcome my grief at our separation my nerves got the better of me and I had a relapse of nervous breakdown, [my boyfriend] had to be recalled from his post as the psychiatrists adviced [sic]."[156] The Stuart Commission revealed another type of relationship separation: in Angolan camps some of the young men's girlfriends were effectively taken by the leadership, leading to depression, anger, and at least one suicide attempt.[157] Male cadres were "harassed" and sometimes transferred from the area in order for men with higher military rank to seduce the now unaccompanied women.

In addition to going through puberty, the condition of being "stuck" in exile was cited as a major cause for mental illness by students, cadres, and psychiatrists alike. Young people flocked into exile in order to be trained and sent back to South Africa to "hit back," Dr Reddy explains it thus,

> [A]fter months have turned to years and with plenty of time on their hands, and with very little activity to distract them, they begin to think of the past and reflect on the future. This frustrated them and there is an overwhelming emotional reaction in the form of violent behaviour, depressions, melancholy, anxiety, insomnia, persecution complexes, nightmares, auditory and visual hallucinations.[158]

The idleness and boredom that was linked in the pre-1976 era to "poor morale" and alcoholism was now becoming explicitly linked as causes of severe symptoms of mental illness. Cadres interviewed after the 1984 Angolan mutinies said, "Our lengthy stay and conditions in exile (i.e. camps) has made some of us to lose all sense of human feeling, lose complete touch with humanity, we do not have the same resistance."[159]

In most cases the Health Department assumed that mental illness was the result of the particularly difficult or traumatic environments faced by comrades rather than the result of genetic predisposition. The hereditary element of mental illness was not totally overlooked but was not given nearly the same consideration or coverage in medical reports.[160] There was only casual mention of heredity. Reflecting on and adding to the 1982 report – which made no mention of hereditary factors – a 1983 report states, "The hereditary factors also play a prominent role, of course … There was undoubtedly a need for an indepth study of various practices in the upbringing of each person, as predisposing factors for mental disorders."[161] However, only the patient's upbringing could really be commented on in patient reports. Some comrades were reported to have developed psychiatric illnesses from a "difficult life in childhood" or the "lack of contact in early childhood … [that] has caused deep resentment and mistrust towards people."[162] Dr Freddy Reddy emphasized the role of parental abuse and estimated that 99 per cent of the patients had experienced serious abuse at the hands of their parents and this constituted some of the reason that these youths where involved in the anti-apartheid movement in the first place.[163] In detailing patient histories prior to their going into exile, Reddy states, "the situation [of physical abuse] was so agonising that one child attempted several suicides between the ages of nine and fourteen years and one attempted to kill the father by stabbing him."[164] Chaotic and abusive upbringing coupled with the movement into a challenging exile environment helped to propel mental illness to its place of influence in the ANC's overall ability to function as a liberation movement.

Mental illness was part and parcel of life in exile. ANC comrades suffered in a variety of ways in South Africa and brought the baggage of trauma into the turmoil of exile and military life. Furthermore, exiles suffered at the hands of the ANC and its military structures. It is, therefore, no small wonder that substance abuse and violence among comrades in exile was common and that records of suicide permeate the archive with relative frequency.

The mental health crisis in exile brings out the best and worst aspects of the Health Department. The department was exceptional at harnessing international favour and economic support for mental health initiatives by underscoring the impact of racism and torture on South Africans. Additionally, there were moments when the Health Department's efforts to mitigate mental health problems in southern Africa were progressive and even praiseworthy. At a time when mental health was only beginning to receive national and international attention, the ANC's Health Department attempted to survey its own communities and provide treatment for those in need. The development of the rehabilitation centres and the Department of Social Welfare in late 1985 was in keeping with cutting-edge community-based approaches to mental health advocated worldwide. The department sought to capitalize on and contribute to their hosts' mental health resources in order to serve a vulnerable and in-need patient population.

But on a practical level, the battle against mental illness was not well fought and there were decisions taken by the Health Department that should be condemned. The department, subordinate to the political and military will of the ANC, defended the propriety of the military. Comrades who had been hurt by the actions of MK commanders were unable to receive adequate psychiatric care and were forced to suffer in silence. Corruption, interpersonal squabbles, and resource shortages continued to impede proper health provision. Compounding the issue, much-needed mental health assistance offered from outside of the ANC was regarded with suspicion and often turned away. Consequently, mental illness was allowed to flourish in ANC communities. It both erupted in shows of violence and addiction and was desperately silenced behind closed doors.

Conclusion

Emerging in 1977 the Medical Committee – soon to be the Health Department – was charged with becoming "the nucleus of the post-apartheid health care system." Already, the ANC was preparing for political victory in South Africa, and it sought to have a medical sector in place when the time came for the party to take power. Officialising the medical sector served two main functions. First, the department helped to use examples of medical injustice committed in South Africa to further delegitimize the apartheid government. Furthermore, while discrediting the South African government's medical efforts, it sought to present itself as an alternative medical representative of the South African citizenry and, thereby, add credibility to the ANC's claim to be a government-in-waiting. Second, the department became a conduit for international funding geared at healthcare projects in exile. This funding, coupled with medical alliances in southern Africa, was meant to be used to provide primary healthcare to the South African exiles. With this vision in mind, the Health Department set forth. Its actions on and off the African continent had an impact on the overall liberation effort because the department helped to advance the anti-apartheid movement and the ANC politically, and because its ability – or lack thereof – to provide quality healthcare affected the daily lives and experiences of South African patients in exile.

As the Cold War ended and the political tide was turning in South Africa, the ANC redoubled its efforts to prepare new policy for its social services at home. The ANC's Health Department felt pressure to make significant changes. To this effect, at a 1990 AIDS workshop, Chris Hani stated,

> More sinister, [apartheid] is leaving behind a deeply div-
> ided society characterised by mistrust, racism and mu-
> tual suspicion. Those of us who have consistently devoted
> themselves to the attainment of the noble ideas of social
> justice, equality and peace are once more called upon to
> inherit this unfortunate legacy. As an alternative power we
> are, increasingly, called upon to make strategic interven-
> tions which [–] whilst taking the present into considera-
> tion [–] project well into the future.[1]

It was true that the apartheid legacy would push the ANC to make some massive political changes, but was the ANC's Health Department, as I've described in this book, ready to take the responsibility of facilitating the kind of change in the health sector that Chris Hani called for?

The Health Department's strength was never its ability to actually deliver consistent service to South Africans in exile. In addition to having to cope with diverse geographies and the instability of guerrilla war, the department was riddled with corruption, infighting, and a lack of accountability. The department never fully grew out of its "teething phase" and struggled to communicate and coordinate its efforts. As the ANC moved home, the rhetoric of equality and freedom, so consistently delivered in exile, was fully captured in the health policies and plans that the Health Department had for the future South Africa. But the ANC still did not have the capability of delivering the kind of system required to make meaningful and comprehensive change.

Despite its poor track record, the Department of Health in exile was the precursor to the future Ministry of Health in South Africa in the post-apartheid era. The history of the ANC's first attempt at healthcare provision paves the way for future research to examine the continuities and discontinuities of healthcare policy and provision from exile to home. There are clear indicators that the exiled Health Department had great influence on the future South African Ministry of Health. As was mentioned in chapter 1, the fledgling Medical Committee was charged with the task of creating a coherent policy for the future healthcare system in South Africa and was officially called to do that starting in the late 1980s and early 1990s. Exile experience shaped new policy. For instance, despite southern African countries' until-then legal opposition to abortion, the proposed policy for post-apartheid South Africa was to provide complete, comprehensive access to abortion. Plainly, this new policy was pushed, in part, by the evolution of thought regarding reproductive health, fostered by the international community's relationship to the ANC's Health Department, detailed in chapter 3. The new draft policy also criticized apartheid South Africa's focus on secondary and tertiary healthcare provision and placed greater emphasis on community-based primary healthcare – the same type of care that was advanced at the Alma-Ata Conference and promoted by the Health Department after 1978.[2]

Alliances formed in exile were also carried forward into the post-apartheid system. Academic Daniel Hammett has pointed out that following the demise of apartheid, 450 Cuban doctors populated health posts in South Africa, and 250 South Africans were trained in Cuba.[3] Future research might also explore the South African expatriate community of medical students who elected to stay abroad rather than return home in the immediate years following 1994.

The personnel that staffed the department in exile also took positions of authority in the National Health Service in South Africa after 1994. Dr Nkososana Dlamini(-Zuma), mentioned briefly in chapter 3 as the doctor posted to Swaziland to establish greater links with South African doctors, became the first minister of health in the post-apartheid era. She was succeeded by Dr Manto Tshabalala who became notorious for her denial that HIV developed into AIDS, a scandal that overshadowed her twenty-year contribution to healthcare efforts in exile. Certainly her personal life and struggle with alcoholism

– exposed by her controversial liver transplant in 2007 – was shaped by her difficult life in exile.[4] Manto Tshabalala's life in exile and at home is worth a study in its own right; she has proven herself to be an important and fascinating individual in South Africa's history.

As pointed out by historians Robert Shell and Carla Tsampiras, there is room to explore the epidemiology of various diseases in the context of South African repatriation in the early 1990s. Carelessness and neglect on the part of a then-preoccupied Health Department in exile evidently enabled many HIV+ patients to reenter South Africa without knowledge of their positive status.[5] The repatriation and continued care of South African patients in exile must have burdened a young and still developing public health system as well as had an important impact on both patients and their communities. This was hinted at in chapter 5 with relation to mentally ill patients but deserves a deeper analysis.

As this research is continued, it will be possible to bridge the ANC healthcare policy in exile with those scholars who have written about the continuities and discontinuities of healthcare issues before and after apartheid within South Africa. In addition to the authors of the article in *The Lancet* – cited at the beginning of this book – such scholars include Susanne Klausen's work on abortion, Rebecca Hodes' work on HIV/AIDS and abortion, and Mandisa Mbali's work on HIV/AIDS.[6]

In addition to linking this work to that considering the political transition to the post-apartheid era, there are a number of avenues related to this book that warrant greater examination and deserve future research. Specifically, the relationship between the ANC's Health Department and other liberation movements and, in particular, the collaboration between the healthcare efforts of the ANC, SWAPO, and the PAC merits further exploration. Furthermore, I looked specifically at the ANC's involvement with the WHO, but the alliance between the ANC and the OAU, UNHCR, Red Cross, or the multitude of other health associations that sought to provide assistance to the department demands a deeper analysis. With respect to the context of exile, this book hints at but does not directly address the importance of the specific and varied geographies in which the ANC operated; specifically, the ANC's military position impacted the Health Department. These geographies are potential research avenues.

Future research should most certainly explore this subject under a gendered lens. The politics of gender is a factor in the events discussed; some of the ANC leadership was trying to establish gender equity and promote women's equal place in the military and political leadership while others were harbouring patriarchal views. Furthermore, many of the Health Department staff members were women and their authority was definitely not interpreted in a gender-blind fashion; some of the interpersonal clashes between department members were fuelled at least in part by sexism.

The choice to provide an in-depth analysis of the incidence of mental illness in exile leaves future opportunities for research on other important diseases experienced by ANC exiles in southern Africa; most notably, this includes the ANC's response to the HIV/AIDS crisis in exile. Chapter 2's brief comparison between the Health Department's response to CRPF and its response to HIV/AIDS only begins to demonstrate the importance of this topic. Tsampiras' work convincingly shows that HIV/AIDS was a major concern to the Health Department in exile in the latter half of the 1980s. Her dissertation chapter on the subject details the gradual – and mostly ineffective – response to the crisis by the Department of Health and outlines the attempts of the political and Health Department leadership to put together a strategic policy to address AIDS in exile and in post-apartheid South Africa. The absence of a detailed discussion about HIV/AIDS and the Health Department's response does not reflect indifference to the subject; I did not want to subtract from the portion of this book dedicated to mental illness. Mental illness is very clearly central to the experience of being exiled, was a major concern to ANC health personnel and leadership, and has been silenced in the present academic record. Furthermore, alongside HIV/AIDS, mental illness continues to carry negative social stigma. By demonstrating its widespread incidence in exile, it is my hope that some of the shame and silence that accompanies mental illness will be mitigated.

The number of topics and avenues of analysis left to be explored only speaks to the wealth of information and the richness of sources in the archive. This present work's goal is to convey how complicated but important the role of the Health Department was in exile and give voice to the health-related experiences of South African exiles. But this book is merely the beginning of this story.

In 1978, Manto Tshabalala wrote, "It is clear ... that much still remains to be done ... the bulk of the responsibilities has been left in too few hands."[7] At the dawn of the new post-apartheid era, her words still rang true. The department was woefully short staffed and ill equipped for the magnitude of the challenge ahead of them. However, as political victory for the ANC drew near, members of the department were eager to take up their elevated positions in the official South Africa government. In 1994 the Health Department's trial run in exile was over; ready or not, it returned to South Africa to begin its work at home.

CONCLUSION

Notes

Introduction

1 For instance, the history of disease in South African mines during apartheid or the post-apartheid era denial that HIV caused AIDS. See Marks, "The Silent Scourge?" For an engaging analysis of Mbeki's stance on HIV/AIDS, see Hoad, "Thabo Mbeki's AIDS Blues."

2 Coovadia et al., "Health System of South Africa," 829–32.

3 WHO, "Bridging the Gap in South Africa."

4 The effect of colonialism and apartheid on health has been the subject of much discussion in academic literature. It has also been the subject of considerable reporting in the medical profession and by anti-apartheid activists, historians, and international organisations concerned with health. Significant research includes Swanson, "The Sanitation Syndrome," 387–410; Marks and Andersson, "Typhus and Social Control," 257–283; Packard, *White Plague*; McCulloch, *Asbestos*; Jochelson, *The Colour of Disease*; Jones, *Psychiatry*; Monamodi and Soboko, *Medical Doctors*; Searle, *Towards Excellence*; Potgieter, *Professional Nursing Education*; Tobias, "Apartheid and Medical Education"; WHO, *Health and Apartheid Part 1 & II*; Jewkes, *The Case for South Africa's Expulsion*; Rubenstein and London, "The UDHR," 160–75; Benatar, "Detention without Trial," 140–5; Nightingale et al., "Apartheid medicine," 2097–102; Dommisse, "The State of Psychiatry," 749–57; Lonsdale, *South Africa in Question*; Klausen, *Abortion Under Apartheid*; Susser and Cherry, "Health Care under Apartheid," 455–75; De Beer, *The South African Disease*; Baldwin-Ragaven, London, and De Gruchy, *An Ambulance of the Wrong Colour*.

5 Coovadia et al., "Health System of South Africa," 829–32.

6 Carla Tsampiras pointed out the gap in literature regarding the ANC's healthcare availability in exile in her chapter and article on

reproductive health and HIV/AIDS in exile. By focusing particularly on HIV/AIDS, she demonstrates the importance of looking at the ANC's healthcare intervention in exile in order to locate continuities between the health provision in exile and those put in place in the post-apartheid era. Tsampiras, "Politics, Polemics, and Practice"; Tsampiras, "Sex in a Time of Exile," 637–63.

7 Documents in the archive refer to the ANC's formalized medical sector interchangeably as "Department of Health" and "Health Department." This book follows suit.

8 Scott Couper has extensively detailed Albert Luthuli's opposition to armed struggle. Couper, *Albert Luthuli*; Couper, "Emasculating Agency," 564–86.

9 The history of the ANC in exile is captured in a robust literature. The works listed by Hugh Macmillan, Tor Sellström, Arianna Lissoni, Maria Suriano, Sean Morrow, Brown Maaba, and Loyiso Pulumani, Rachel Sandwell, and Carla Tsampiras were of particular importance. Macmillan, *The Lusaka Years*; Ellis, *External Mission*; Bundy, "Cooking the Rice Outside the Pot?"; Shubin, *ANC*; Suttner, "The (Re-) Constitution," 43–68; Davis, *Cosmopolitans in Close Quarters*; Houston, "Post-Rivonia ANC/SACP"; Magubane et al., "The Turn"; Simpson, *Umkhonto We Sizwe*; Cherry, *Spear of the Nation*; Ndlovu, "The ANC in Exile"; Lissoni, "Transformations in the ANC," 287–301; Ellis, "Mbokodo," 279–98; Trewhela, *Inside Quatro*; Onslow, *Cold War in Southern Africa*; Schmidt, *Foreign Intervention in Africa*; Sellström, *Sweden and National Liberation Vol II*; Sellström, *Liberation in Southern Africa*; Sellström, *Sweden and National Liberation Vol I*; Sellström, "Some Factors behind Nordic Relations," 13–46; Eriksen, *Norway and National Liberation*; Morgenstierne, *Denmark and National Liberation*; Soiri and Peltola, *Finland and National Liberation*; Lodge, *The ANC After Nkomati*; Callinicos, "Oliver Tambo," 587–62; Morrow, et al, *Education in Exile*; Morrow, "Dakawa Development Centre," 497–521; Hassim, *The ANC Women's League*; Williams, "Practicing Pan-Africanism"; Lissoni and Suriano, "Married to the ANC,"129–50; Sandwell, "'Love I Cannot Begin to Explain,'" 63–81; Tsampiras, "Sex in a Time of Exile," 637–63.

10 For a more detailed account of the ANC political changes in the 1950s, the turn to violence, and the move into exile by the ANC

and MK see Karis, Carter, and Gerhart, *From Protest to Challenge*; Simpson, *Umkhonto We Sizwe*.

11 For the sake of clarity, I will use "Tanzania" throughout this book. However, the country was called "The United Republic of Tanganyika and Zanzibar" from independence until October 1964 when it was renamed "The United Republic of Tanzania."

12 In 1960 Harold Macmillan delivered a famous declaration to the Houses of Parliament of the Union of South Africa. The "wind of change" was referring to the wave of independence movements occurring across Africa. For a more detailed analysis of this speech and its context see Butler and Stockwell, *The Wind of Change*.

13 The ANC was first referred to as a "government-in-waiting" in Sellström, *Sweden and National Liberation Vol II*, 421. This idea was subsequently drawn upon by Michael Panzer in his assessment of FREMILO, a study influential and important to this work. Panzer, "Building a Revolutionary Constituency," 5–23; Panzer, "Pragmatism and Liberation," 323–42.

14 Primary care refers to the prevention and treatment of routine illnesses and injuries by general medical staff whereas secondary care includes specialized medical service for patients who cannot be treated by primary healthcare providers.

15 These cataloguing issues are further contextualized and explained in Stapleton and Maamoe, "An Overview," 413–22.

16 The absence of an "Angola Mission" collection from the archive – Angola being the location of the bulk of the MK camps from the mid–late 1970s to the late 1980s and the site of greatest controversy – is a significant example of this practice of withholding of information. I have been able to partially redress this absence in the archive by looking closely at correspondence between the ANC headquarters in Lusaka and its offices in Luanda; these documents are often photocopies kept in the Zambia Mission collection. Unlike official reports, they provide details of the interpersonal relationships between Health Department members. They show letters of appeal sent from cadres or comrades to the department and disciplinary letters regarding the mismanagement of specific patients. At times, individual reports on patients are also included within the correspondence, giving insight into the diseases that afflicted cadres in Angola as well as their treatment. Thus, the files

pertaining to the Department of Health's presence in the Angolan region helps to compensate for the absence of the official Angolan collection.

Not only have major collections been (presumably) withheld from the archive, it appears as though there have been boxes and folders subsequently removed after they were originally placed in the archive. In some cases, there are older catalogues listing files and boxes related to MK, or to topics like child abuse and rape, that have been withdrawn from the archive and taken out of updated finding aids. For instance, in an older, now unavailable, finding aid for the ANC Women's Section records, "Box X Confidential" was listed and said to contain eighteen labelled folders. This box is no longer part of the ANC archive and my emailed request to view it was never answered. Unfortunately, it is impossible to accurately determine how much of the material relevant to this project has been withheld or removed from the archive. It is also unclear how much of the material will be withdrawn from the archive in the future. It is for this reason that I carefully documented the health-related files that I accessed. Through this research, I have built a small but relatively comprehensive archive regarding the Health Department and its efforts in exile.

17 In recent years a number of personal memoirs have emerged detailing individual experiences of exile and the military effort. (See for instance the memoires of Thula Bopela and Daluxolo Luthuli, Wonga Welile Bottoman, Ronnie Kasrils, Stanley Manong, James Ngculu and Barry Gilder.) Yet, while less effective at providing a global view of the "exile experience" or an understanding of the political climate within the ANC, the authors of these memoirs sometimes discuss their health status/experiences or their interactions with the medical sector. These descriptions can be important in confirming the archive's sometimes hazy or mundane details like the location of a health post, the medical supplies available, or the name of a staff member treating patients. Less mundane were their recollections of personal experience of disease. These are subjective but nevertheless extremely helpful in developing a sense of the relative importance of healthcare in ANC settlements.

Chapter One

1 This chapter is a significant extension of my 2013 master's thesis and an article that I published in 2014 in the *South African Historical Journal*. That thesis and paper specifically discuss the changing role of the Health Department with respect to the military. Armstrong, "Healthcare in Exile," 270–90; Armstrong, "Militias, Maladies and Medicine."

2 Very little documentation in the Fort Hare archive is about the health services provided in the early years of exile. Therefore, the major sources of information available were the interviews conducted with those who were in exile at that time. There were three major oral history initiatives of interest to this research. The first and perhaps most famous of those oral history initiatives was the interviews conducted in 1989 and 1990 by anti-apartheid activist Hilda Bernstein. She compiled parts of more than 100 of her nearly 300 interviews in her book *The Rift* in order to provide numerous South Africans' perspectives on the realities of exile and by so doing, illuminate the politics of apartheid. Hilda Bernstein's full transcripts are currently kept at the University of the Western Cape, Mayibuye Centre. Of the two other projects, the *Road to Democracy in South Africa* project was the wider reaching; this was mainly because the project, endorsed by former president Thabo Mbeki, was an attempt to assess the political transition from apartheid to a free and democratic South Africa. The five-volume series contains more than 5,000 pages of history on the anti-apartheid movement from 1960 to 1990 and looks at both international and African solidarity with the ANC. Relevant for this chapter, the project draws on approximately sixty interviews with those who went into exile in the 1960s and 1970s. SADET, *South Africans Telling Their Stories*. A separate less scholarly, but nonetheless important, project culminated in *The Fourth Dimension*, an in-house publication on health services used by military forces in South Africa. *The Fourth Dimension* contains one chapter devoted specifically to the ANC's medical sector. This work presumably used a combination of interviews and archival documents to form the chapter on health in exile but the

information is not cited. The writing and editing staff of *The Fourth Dimension* consisted of an impressive list of ANC political figures, many of who were present in exile. However, due to the dearth of citations and the distinctly partisan pro-ANC flavour, I have used the Bernstein interviews or SADET account when possible. Naidoo, *The Fourth Dimension*.

3 Ndlovu, "The ANC in Exile," 379.

4 Initially there were twenty-one nurses but one decided to return home before the group had even reached Tanzania. SADET, *South Africans Telling Their Stories*, 461–3.

5 Ibid.

6 Ibid.

7 South African History Online, "Dr Mantombazana 'Manto' Tshabalala-Msimang."

8 South African History Online, "Dr Nomava Eslinah Shangase."

9 "Telex to Moscow sent by Alfred Nzo," 26 October 1981, 132/271, ANCL.

10 "Application for an Acupuncture Course," 31 August 1986, 127/236, ANCL.

11 These members of the ANC were not interviewed in detail about their educational experiences in exile.

12 Dr Naicker gave a particularly moving interview to Hilda Bernstein in 1990. He talked about his relationship with his father who was heavily involved with the ANC. Their family moved to London in 1967, and his father was the editor for *Sechaba*. Dr Naicker does not discuss his path to medical school or his subsequent medical career in the interview. Bernstein, *The Rift*, 482–6.

13 "Interview with Dr Prenaiver Naicker," 105, 9/7-1631, Hilda Bernstein Interviews. His graduation date is confirmed in "Letter to University Teaching Hospital signed Alfred Nzo," 10 November 1980, 1/1ii, ANCSHD.

14 Once he reached Uganda, he was flown to London. Bernstein, *The Rift*, 46–8.

15 South African History Online, "Dr Nomava Eslinah Shangase."

16 Bernstein, *The Rift*, 25.

17 Ibid., 24–31.

18 "Interview with Dr Freddy Reddy," 9/7-1670, Hilda Bernstein Interviews.

19 Population estimates for the ANC and MK throughout the exile period are not established. ANC and MK personnel were widespread and liberation fronts necessarily have a secretive nature. The estimation of 400 to 500 cadres was given by Williams, "Living in exile," 65. This number also aligns with Maurice Mthombeni's estimate quoted later in this article, "Southern Africa: A Betrayal," *The Black Dwarf*, 26 November 1969, 3/16, Karis-Gerhart Papers.

20 Many scholars show that after the Wankie Campaign (the attempt to move cadres into South Africa through Zimbabwe in 1967) the military effort was not actively engaging the South African Defense Force (SADF) in military action: Bundy, "Cooking the Rice Outside the Pot?"; Karis, Carter, and Gerhart, eds, *From Protest to Challenge Vol. 5*. By the 1970s the Politico Military Council was making recommendations to train medical staff that could accompany guerrilla forces on missions to South Africa, but it is unclear from the records whether this was acted upon: "Interim Report of the Commission of the TRC Secretariat on the State of Affairs in MK in East Africa," April 1975, 3/23, Karis-Gerhart Papers.

21 This is made evident by a number of documents that describe the problems facing the department. See for example, "Interim Report of the Commission of the TRC Secretariat on the State of Affairs in MK in East Africa," April 1975, 3/23, Karis-Gerhart Papers. "Report on Youth & Students section to the National Executive Meeting held in East Africa in December 1972," December 1972, 3/20, Karis-Gerhart Papers.

22 "Rough Estimates of Annual Expenditure," 5 January 1972, 3/20 Karis-Gerhart Papers. SADET, *South Africans Telling Their Stories*, 210–11.

23 Williams, "Living in Exile," 63–5.

24 SADET, *South Africans Telling Their Stories*, 210–11. Naidoo, *The Fourth Dimension*, 236.

25 Williams added that there was a local doctor in Kongwa who visited the various liberation movement camps and treated cadres there for free. Williams, "Living in Exile," 68.

26 Naidoo, *The Fourth Dimension*, 236. Also mentioned less explicitly in Magubane et al., "The Turn to Armed Struggle," 422.

27 Ibid., 461–3.

28 See for example, "Circular to All Our Offices," 12 February 1976, 3/24, Karis-Gerhart Paper. "ANC Department of Health: Report on Personnel and Training," 2 April 1987, 31/11, ANCL.

29 SADET, *South Africans Telling Their Stories*, 210

30 Most of the ANC comrades, affiliated with MK, had their names changed to undercover aliases to disguise their identity. Occasionally both were used interchangeably in the archive. In this book, I use the name most frequently used in the archive. For instance, Dr Davidson Themba Masuku (alias Haggar McBerry), member of the 1986 health secretariat, graduated from medical school in the USSR in 1979. This book uses "Dr Haggar McBerry," the name used more consistently in ANC documents in order to avoid confusion.

31 Naidoo, *The Fourth Dimension*, 236.

32 Magubane et al., "The Turn to Armed Struggle," 422.

33 SADET, *South Africans Telling Their Stories*, 210–11. The ANC was also given access to a residence in Kurasini to use as a sickbay. This will be described in chapters 2 and 4. "Proposed Alterations, Additions and Equipment of the ANC Kurasini Sick Bay in Dar es Salaam," no date [1982], 112/91, ANCL.

34 These criticisms are not part of the South African Democracy Education Trust or *The Fourth Dimension* narratives.

35 *The Black Dwarf* was a socialist newspaper published in the United Kingdom between 1968 and 1972.

36 "Southern Africa: A Betrayal," *The Black Dwarf*, 26 November 1969, 3/16, Karis-Gerhart Papers.

37 "Black Dwarf Talks White Trash," 26 November 1969, 3/16, Karis-Gerhart Papers.

38 Macmillan, "The 'Hani Memorandum,'" 106–29.

39 These are the first explicitly health-related reports that I could find in the Fort Hare archives. There are only four reports, all published within a three-month period in 1969, and there are no subsequent reports with the same committee title. "Health and Welfare Department," 5 June 1969, 43/0390, OTP. "Health and Welfare Department," 23 June 1969, 43/0390, OTP. "Health and Welfare Department Committee Meeting," 17 July 1969, 43/0390, OTP. "Health and Welfare Department Committee Meeting," 23 August 1969, 43/0390, OTP.

40 The name "Barney" was not followed by a surname and was

not found in other documents from the Health and Welfare Committee. Presumably, "Barney" referred to Leonard Pitso, (MK name: Barney Mackay).

41 "Health and Welfare Department," 5 June 1969, 43/0390, OTP. "Health and Welfare Department," 23 June 1969, 43/0390, OTP. "Health and Welfare Department Committee Meeting," 17 July 1969, 43/0390, OTP. "Health and Welfare Department Committee Meeting," 23 August 1969, 43/0390, OTP.

42 Magubane et al., "The Turn to Armed Struggle," 422.

43 Shubin does not comment on the exact sum of money. Shubin, *ANC*.

44 Ibid., 27.

45 Ibid.

46 "Report on Personnel and Training," 2 April 1987, 31/11, ANCL.

47 Following these events, Chris Hani penned his complaints about the two-tiered medical system. Macmillan, "The 'Hani Memorandum,'" 106–29.

48 There is a good, concise account of the campaign in Macmillan, *The Lusaka Years*, 39–57.

49 Ellis, *External Mission*, 83.

50 Stephen Ellis shows that the details around this situation are not completely clear. However, Tanzania Foriegn Minister Oscar Kambona was later convicted as the mastermind behind the plot. Additionally, Hugh Macmillan argued that PAC leader Potlako Leballo attempted to incriminate the ANC in this plot. Ellis, *External Mission*, 84. Macmillan, *The Lusaka Years*, 97.

51 Hugh Macmillan pointed out that the "official" date of headquarters' transition to Lusaka was relatively ambiguous. The last office – the office of the ANC secretary general – under whose authority the Health Department falls, moved from Morogoro to Lusaka in 1977. The ANC sought acknowledgement from the Zambian government of their official status in Lusaka. This considered, the central ANC authority was based in Lusaka starting in the early 1970s. Macmillan, *The Lusaka Years*, 97.

52 The bulk of volume two of the SADET series assesses what the ANC and MK, alongside other anti-apartheid groups, was able to accomplish inside South Africa while in exile. The authors collectively assert that the ANC's political and military efforts were

changing. See for example Magubane, "Introduction to the 1970s," 1–35; Houston and Magubane, "The ANC Political Underground"; Houston and Magubane, "The ANC's Armed Struggle," 371–528.

53 Bundy, "Cooking the Rice outside the Pot?"

54 Davis, *Cosmopolitans in Close Quarters*, 44. Macmillan devotes two chapters of his book to the ANC's struggle to get cadres back into South Africa. Macmillan, *The Lusaka Years*, 27–56.

55 Sellström, *Sweden and National Liberation Vol I*, 249–55. For a more detailed description of the building relationship between South Africa, the ANC, and Sweden from the mid-1800s to 1973, see Sellström, "Sweden and the Nordic Countries," 422.

56 Sellström, *Sweden and National Liberation Vol II*.

57 Ibid., 399.

58 Sellström, "Sweden and the Nordic Countries," 466.

59 Ibid., 433–7.

60 Sellström, *Sweden and National Liberation Vol II*, 232–8.

61 Ibid., 240.

62 Despite the fact that Swedish contribution to other anti-apartheid groups nearly doubled over the next year, the ANC's allotment for 1973/1974 remained at SEK150,000. Sellström, "Sweden and the Nordic Countries," 401.

63 Ibid., 492; Sellström, *Sweden and National Liberation Vol II*. Monetary conversion is based on conversion charts provided by the World Bank, "Official Exchange Rate: (1990)."

64 "Letter to the Secretary General signed Max Sisulu," 22 November 1972, 13/33 ANCL.

65 "Goods Supplied to FRELIMO," 13 April 1973, 13/33 ANCL. "Letter to Menoy Msimango signed M Juma," 12 April 1973 13/33 ANCL.

66 "Letter to [T.T. Nkobi] signed M. Msimang," 17 April 1973, 13/33, ANCL.

67 Angola and Mozambique were used differently by the ANC. MK use Angola to establish training camps; Mozambique was used as a "corridor" for the military to infiltrate South Africa. Therefore, usually only trained and seasoned cadres were sent in small units to Mozambique. The situation in Mozambique was also different because in 1984 the FRELIMO government signed the Nkomati Accord with South Africa; the accord limited MK's ability to operate in Mozambique.

68 Houston and Magubane, "The ANC Political Underground," 388.

69 Sellström, *Sweden and National Liberation Vol II*, 414.

70 Houston, Plaatjie, and April, "Military Training and Camps," 48; Sellström, *Sweden and National Liberation Vol II*, 507.

71 Not all students joined the ANC/MK in exile. Thami ka Plaatjie discusses the new recruits that joined the PAC in 1976s. However, he, too, noted that the ANC was the more successful of the two parties in receiving the Soweto students. ANC often emphasizes the importance of the 1976 uprising while the event is less important to the history of the PAC. Plaatjie, "The PAC's Internal Underground Activities," and Plaatjie "The PAC in Exile."

72 Ellis, "Mbokodo," 279–98.

73 The plans for the Solomon Mahlangu Freedom College (SOMAFCO) in Mazimbu, Tanzania began in 1977 in response to the need to provide a basic education for school age children and young adults. Secondary schooling began in 1978 with an estimate of fifty students; by 1984 that number is estimated to have increased to 202 (about 450 including primary students). Morrow et al, *Education in Exile*, 20; "Report of the Commission of the NEC appointed to investigate the allocation and utilization of the financial resources of the organization in regions of the Front Line States and Forward Areas, March 1984–July 1984," 31 July 1984, 3/56/ Karis-Gerhart Papers.

74 "Circular to all our Offices," 12 February 1976, 131/267a, ANCL.

75 Sellström, *Sweden and National Liberation Vol II*, 402.

76 "Report on the Tour of Scandinavian Countries (27th April – 23rd May, 1979)," no date, 17/7, ANCM.

77 "Health Department Report Chapter I," 18 March 1981, 112/96, ANCL.

78 "Report of the East Africa Health Team Meeting," 10 May 1981, 112/96 ANCL.

79 See for example ibid.; "Minutes of the Special Health Council Meeting held in Lusaka January 24–5, 1982," 7 February 1982, 112/95, ANCL.

80 "Minutes of the Consultative Meeting to ANC," 27 August 1977, 33/8, ANCC.

81 Ibid.

82 Ibid.

83 The changing relationship between the Department of Health and the military was the focus of a previous publication. See Armstrong, "Healthcare in Exile."

84 "Minutes of the Consultative Meeting to ANC," 27 August 1977, 33/8, ANCC.

85 "Proposals to set up an administrative Machinery to direct, control and manage the affairs of the ANC(SA) in Tanzania," 20 October 1977, 96/5b, ANCL; "Structure March 1983," no date [1986], 127/236, ANCL.

86 "Medical committee ANC Secretary's Report," 2 July 1978, 37/29, ANCC.

87 Presumably, when Dr Reddy refers to the "crisis situation" he is indicating the short-staffed and under-equipped position of the Health Department in exile. "Interview with Dr Freddy Reddy," 9/7-1670, Hilda Bernstein Interviews.

88 The regional health team in Tanzania was titled the East Africa Health Team. When referring to the team, "East Africa" will be used in order to maintain consistency with the archival documents.

89 "Medical committee ANC Secretary's Report," 2 July 1978, 37/29, ANCC.

90 Ibid.

91 "Report of the East Africa Health Team Meeting," 10 May 1981, 112/96, ANCL.

92 "Medical committee ANC Secretary's Report," 2 July 1978, 37/29, ANCC.

93 "Letter to the Project Manager, Morogoro signed Manto Tshabalala," 23 August 1977, 111/89, ANCL.

94 "Letter to Manto Tshabalala signed Dr J.P. Kasiga," 4 October 1977, 111/89, ANCL.

95 "Letter to Dr Kasiga signed Manto Tshabalala," 7 October 1977, 111/89, ANCL.

96 "A Brief Memorandum on Candidates for Scholarships in East Africa," no date [1975], 96/5b, ANCL.

97 Ibid.

98 "Letter to Peter Mfelang signed Manto Tshabalala," 20 February 1981, 112/90, ANCL; "Letter to Peter Mfelang signed Cecile de Sweemer," 22 December 1980, 31/4 ANCL.

99 "Letter to Peter Mfelang signed Manto Tshabalala," 20 February 1981, 112/90, ANCL.

100 "Letter to Alfred Nzo signed Peter Mfelang," 27 January 1981, 112/90, ANCL.

101 "Letter to Manto Tshabalala signed Peter Mfelang," 6 May 1981,
112/80, ANCL.

102 "Summary Report of the ANC-SA Conference of the Health
Department held in Lusaka from 2–6 January, 1980," no date,
37/29, ANCC.

103 "Letter to Peter Mfelang signed Manto Tshabalala," 20 February
1981, 112/90, ANCL.

104 "Summary Report of the ANC-SA Conference of the Health
Department held in Lusaka from 2–6 January, 1980," no date,
37/29, ANCC.

105 "A Report on the First Aid and Instructors Course in Norway
20th August 1979 to 26th October 1979," no date, Part I Additions
69/2, ANCL.

106 This new elevation enabled the Health Department to be included
within the ANC command structure. However, the Health
Department still remained in a low position of power on the
hierarchical ANC command structure. In the ANC structure, the
National Executive Council (NEC) was superior to the Politico
Military Command and the External Coordinating Committee.
These were the most authoritative bodies for MK and the
ANC respectively, and both reported to the NEC. The External
Coordinating Committee was responsible for overseeing the
office of the president, the secretary general and
the treasurer general. The Department of Health was one of
several departments (including the Department of Education)
reporting to the office of the secretary general. "Structure March
1983," no date, 127/236, ANCL.

107 "Letter to Florence Maleka signed Manto Tshabalala," 4 January
1979, 17/3, ANCM.

108 "Medical Committee Report," [1979], 37/29, ANCC. "Health
Department Report Chapter 1," 18 March 1981, 112/96, ANCL.

109 "Report of the East Africa Health Team Meeting," 10 May 1981,
112/96, ANCL. "Health Department Report Chapter 1," 18 March
1981, 112/96, ANCL.

110 Between 1977 and 1989 some of the titles of the positions changed.
For clarity, the 1983 structure and models are used.

111 The health secretariat was elected by the health council.

112 The shortage of personnel was not the only reason why reports were inconsistent. In a letter from the later inaugurated Botswana Health Team, A. Gqabi wrote, "We must apologize for the delay in answering your letters and also for sending you untyped letters. Since we do not have a typist and none of us can type we have to depend on willing individuals to do it for us." "Letter to the Secretary for the Health Department signed A. Gqabi," 15 April 1984, Part II Additions, 6/2, ANCL.

113 See, for example, "Chairman's Remarks," no date [1982], 160/1, ANCL. "Consultative Committee Meeting between Working Committee and Health Department held from 30 November to 2nd December 1982 in Lusaka–Zambia," no date, 160/1, ANCL.

114 "Letter to Comrade Sindiso [Mfenyana] signed Manto Tshabalala," 12 May 1981, 31/4, ANCL.

115 "Chairman's Remarks," no date [1982], 160/1, ANCL. "Consultative Committee Meeting between Working Committee and Health Department held from 30 November to 2nd December 1982 in Lusaka–Zambia," no date, 160/1, ANCL.

116 "Interview with Dr Freddy Reddy," 12, 9/7-1670, Hilda Bernstein Interviews.

117 "Chairman's Remarks," no date [1982], 160/1, ANCL. "Consultative Committee Meeting between Working Committee and Health Department held from 30 November to 2nd December 1982 in Lusaka–Zambia," no date, 160/1, ANCL.

118 "Preamble," 26 March 1985, 31/11, ANCL.

119 The secretariat had six portfolios in 1983: the secretary, who headed the Department of Health and was responsible for the reports sent to the secretary general (Dr Peter Mfelang); the deputy secretary who acted in the place of the secretary where needed but also corresponded with the regional departments (Dr Manto Tshabalala); the administrative secretary, who kept the minutes of meetings and the health records (Mrs Edna Miya); the information and publicity officer, who was in charge of correspondence with health personnel in South Africa and with the creation and distribution of a health bulletin (Dr Haggar McBerry); the personnel officer, who kept a record of those who were health personnel across the regions (Dr Ike Nzo); and the health

education program officer, who planned and evaluated programs to educate ANC personnel on health related material (Mrs Khulukazi Mzamo). "Secretariat Job Description," no date [1986], 127/236, ANCL. 1983 names taken from "Report of the National Preparatory Committee (NPC)," November 1986, 31/11, ANCL. In 1986 Dr Haggar McBerry, Dr Manto Tshabalala, Dr Ralph Mgijima, Dr Pren Naicker, Dr Zakes Mokoena, Dr Bob Mayekiso, Mr Mkhulu Radebe, Mrs Winnie Nkobi, Mrs Edna Miya, Mrs Florence Maleka, and Mrs Regina Nzo were elected to become the new health secretariat. The secretariat therefore expanded to include a number of extra portfolios, one of which was designed to get a better account of drug inventory in each region. However, the new positions are not clearly allotted in the attainable record.

120 "Draft: Health Secretariat Report to the 3rd Health Council Meeting Delivered by the Secretary for Health on 29.07.86," no date, 127/236, ANCL.

121 "Secretariat Job Description," no date [1986], 127/236, ANCL. For details of office holders see "Report of the National Preparatory Committee (NPC)," November 1986, 31/11, ANCL.

122 "Draft: Health Secretariat Report to the 3rd Health Council Meeting Delivered by the Secretary for Health on 29.07.86," no date, 127/236, ANCL.

123 "Objective and Critical Analysis of the Present State of Affairs in the Health Department," 24 November 1982, 160/1a, ANCL. The council convened for the first time in 1980. "Minutes of the Special Health Council Meeting held in Lusaka January 24–25, 1982," 7 February 1982, 112/95, ANCL.

124 "Draft: Health Secretariat Report to the 3rd Health Council Meeting Delivered by the Secretary for Health on 29.07.86," no date, 127/236, ANCL.

125 "Report on the Tour of Scandinavian Countries (27th April–23rd May, 1979)," no date, 17/7, ANCM.

126 See for instance "Letter to Ndugu signed Manto Tshabalala," 28 September 1981, 112/90, ANCL. "Draft: Health Secretariat Report to the 3rd Health Council Meeting Delivered by the Secretary for Health on 29.07.86," no date, 127/236, ANCL.

Chapter Two

1 Lesotho, Swaziland, and Botswana could also be considered, but the health activities in those countries are out of the scope of this book.

2 The East Africa Health Team was the ANC Health Department's official name for the Tanzania Health Team and so it will be used throughout.

3 Those medical personnel included some of the nurses that came from South Africa in the 1960s as well as doctors such as Ike Nzo and Sipho Mthembu.

4 After independence, the facility was called "Muhimbili Hospital" but after 1976, it changed its name to "Muhimbili Medical Centre." Documents in the archive refer to the facility by either name or, alternatively, as "Muhimbili."

5 *The Fourth Dimension*, 2009. See also "The Structure of the Department of Health and its Function," 3 October 1986, 127/236, ANCL.

6 "Report of the Commission of the National Executive Committee appointed to investigate the allocation and utilization of the financial resources of the organization in regions of the Front Line States and Forward Areas, March 1984–July 1984," 31 July 1984, 3/56, Karis-Gerhart Papers. The use of Temeke as a transit residence for cadres from Angola and Mozambique is also reported in "Letter to the Chief Representative signed W. Mwaipyana," 9 May 1981, 95/5a, ANCL. "Letter to the Secretary General signed Reddy Mazimba," 14 May 1981, 95/5a, ANCL. "Regional Health Team (East Africa) Tanzania Quarterly for period July to September 1983 Report," no date, 160/1b, ANCL.

7 "Proposed Alterations, Additions and Equipment of the ANC Kurasini Sick Bay in Dar es Salaam," [1982], 112/91, ANCL. "Kurasini Medical Centre Report on Proposed Extension and Conversion of Existing Buildings," 21 October 1982, 84/17, ANCL.

8 "The Present Situation in East Africa Needs Serious Attention," 24 August 1981, 3/40, Karis-Gerhart Papers.

9 Ibid.

10 The ANC wrestled with the notion of "refugee." The leadership felt that the "refugee mentality" of many ANC members in exile was creating a culture of entitlement and laziness. Instead, the leadership

wanted to establish a strong work ethic and create a system of self-sufficiency in Tanzania. "Report of the Commission of the National Executive Committee appointed to investigate the allocation and utilization of the financial resources of the organization in regions of the Front Line States and Forward Areas, March 1984–July 1984," 31 July 1984, 3/56, Karis-Gerhart Papers.

11 The desire for nonpermanency had to do with the agreement between the ANC and the Tanzanian government. The government supplied the ANC land in order for South Africans to be contained outside of Tanzanian cities; therefore, Dar es Salaam was only to be used by ANC officials and not the rank and file of the liberation movement. "Letter to the Secretary General signed Reddy Mazimba," 14 April 1981, 95/5a, ANCL.

12 Morrow, et al, *Education in Exile*, 10.

13 A detailed account of the development of Mazimbu and SOMAFCO is provided by Morrow et al., *Education in Exile*.

14 "Medical Committee ANC Secretary Report," 2 July 1978, 37/29, ANCC. "Letter to Nkobi signed Hans Heuvelmans," 21 March 1979, 112/94 ANCL. "Letter to Comrade Thomas signed Manto Tshabalala," 26 December 1981, 112/94, ANCL. "Summary Report of the ANC-SA Conference of the Health Department held in Lusaka from 2–6 January, 1980," no date, 37/29, ANCC.

15 "Minutes of the ANC(SA) Medical and Health Committee Meeting," no date [1978/01], 112/95, ANCL.

16 "Report of the Commission of the National Executive Committee appointed to investigate the allocation and utilization of the financial resources of the organization in regions of the Front Line States and Forward Areas, March 1984–July 1984," 31 July 1984, 3/56, Karis-Gerhart Papers.

17 "Report and Minutes of the Meeting of the Health Secretariat," 3 July 1984, Part II Additions, 33/1, ANCL. (Folder contained in ANCL, 161.)

18 Ibid.

19 "Summaries from Speeches at Official Opening of the ANC-Holland Solidarity Hospital," 1 May 1984, 8/22, ANCSHD.

20 Malaria accounted for more than half of the total patients seen. "Regional Health Report for the Year 1985," no date, 161/3b, ANCL.

21 "The Physicians Forum," *Bulletin*, Fall 1985, 2/1iii, ANCSHD.

22 Sean Morrow provided an important article and book chapter on Dakawa. Morrow's research focus was the education system, particularly SOMAFCO, and his publications on Dakawa reflect this focus. However, he also managed to convey the overarching negative atmosphere of the settlement. This and chapter 5 continue to build on Morrow's account by discussing Dakawa from a health perspective. Morrow, "Dakawa Development Centre," 497–521; Morrow et al., *Education in Exile*, 143–55.

23 "The Present Situation in East Africa Needs Serious Attention: Bring of people in Tanzania," 24 August 1981, 3/40, Karis-Gerhart Paper.

24 "Mr Chairman/Chairwoman," no date [1982], 85/22, ANCL. "Statement Made by the Treasurer General Thomas Nkobi to our Chief Representatives, Milan," March 1982, 3/42, Karis-Garhart Papers.

25 "Seminar on the Development of Dakawa held from 28th July to 1st August 1982 at SOMAFCO, Morogoro, Tanzania," no date, 86/34, ANCL.

26 Due to the fact that the ANC had the full commitment of the Medisch Komitee Angola (MKA), a Netherlands-based donor, to fund the Mazimbu Hospital, it was agreed that the money donated by Dansk Folkehjelp could be used elsewhere. "Letter to Thomas Nkobi signed Manto Tshabalala," 18 November 1981, Part II Addition, 42/87, ANCL.

27 "Letter to the Health Department signed Regina Nzo," 19 April 1982, 112/91, ANCL. "Special Directorate Meeting with Invited Members to Discuss Suspensions and Disciplinary Actions taken Against Students from SOMAFCO," 18 April 1982, 127/228, ANCL.

28 "Special Directorate Meeting with Invited Members to Discuss Suspensions and Disciplinary Actions taken Against Students from SOMAFCO," 18 April 1982, 127/228, ANCL.

29 "Letter to the Health Department signed Regina Nzo," 19 April 1982, 112/91, ANCL. "Special Directorate Meeting with Invited Members to Discuss Suspensions and Disciplinary Actions taken Against Students from SOMAFCO," 18 April 1982, 127/228, ANCL.

30 This estimate of 1,000 patients was the only estimate available for the post at the time, and it was likely an exaggeration because the later May 1984 report stated that the health post only saw 404 patients: "Seminar on the Development of Dakawa held from 28th

July to st August 1982 at SOMAFCO, Morogoro, Tanzania," no date, 86/34, ANCL. "Health Report to the Directorate," May 1984, 9/31, ANCSHD.

31 There were over 16,000 Tanzanians in the "Magole Ward" (near to where Dakawa was) according to the 1987 census. "ANC Development Centre, Dakawa Tanzania: Norplan, Volume 1," September 1984, 108/70b, ANCL.

32 "East Africa Health Team Meeting held in Mazimbu," 22 January 1983, 160/1, ANCL.

33 See for instance "Regional Health Team Report for the Year 1985," no date, 161/3b, ANCL.

34 "Minutes of the Directorate Meeting," 29 January 1983, 118/126, ANCL.

35 Ibid.

36 "Letter to the Health Department signed Regina Nzo," 19 April 1982, 112/91, ANCL. "Minutes of the Health Committee Meeting," 25 March 1983, 8/22, ANCSHD.

37 "Confidential Report to the ANC," 19 May 1983, 118/126, ANCL.

38 "RE: Comrade [redacted]," 21 January 1983, 8/21, ANCSHD.

39 Each of these zones housed between ten and 150 comrades (totalling more than 400 comrades), each housing a different demographic of the population. For instance Ruth First was for students upgrading their education so that they could attend SOMAFCO; Raymond Mhlaba was for those in need of mental or political rehabilitation; Elias Motsawledi was for MK combatants waiting for medical attention or reassignment; and Lillian Ngoyi was for secondary school graduates waiting for assignment. "ANC-SA Development Centre – Dakawa Health Report up to and Including 6 April 1985," no date, 9/31, ANCSHD.

40 Evidently the long awaited second health post had been erected, though the archive is mainly silent on its development. Both doctors were new graduates staying at Lillian Ngoyi and awaiting assignment.

41 Turiani Mission Hospital (two hours drive) was also used as a referral hospital. However, this hospital was not often well equipped, and ANC medical staff member Mandla Lubanga reported patients returning to Dakawa untreated. "Unaddressed letter signed Mandla Lubanga," 28 December 1982, 160/1, ANCL.

42 "ANC-SA Development Centre – Dakawa Health Report up to and Including 6 April –1985," no date, 9/31, ANCSHD. Understandably, in May 1985 Peter Mfelang asked the ANC treasurer general to financially prioritize small incremental health goals rather than put off support due to the inability to start a grandiose hospital project. He sought more health posts (with an examination room, treatment room, and five beds with mattresses), the availability of cold storage for drugs, and a regional physiotherapy department. "Letter to Treasurer General T.T. Nkobi signed Peter Mfelang," 8 May 1985, 161/3b, ANCL.

43 "ANC-SA Development Centre – Dakawa Health Report up to and Including 6 April –1985," no date, 9/31, ANCSHD.

44 More than once Chongella was described as a community similar to Dakawa in Tanzania, and it was felt that the community was similarly neglected in terms of health provision. By the end of 1982, the farm had no medical facilities and Health Department members at the Consultative Committee Meeting suggested that auxiliary nurse Isaac Salele be seconded to Chongella to help with the health needs of a growing community at the farm. Relative to the developments in Lusaka, reporting on medical provision at Chongella was thin. However, some manner of medical clinic or health post was established at Chongella in 1983/1984 and the Health Department attempted to keep at least one medically trained staff member based at the farm at all times. This health post provided for primary health-care needs when possible and referred patients to Lusaka when their facility was unable to adequately treat the patient. "The Psychological Effects of Apartheid: A Report on Survey of Mental Health Problems of ANC Members in the Republics of Tanzania and Zambia," 13 December 1982, 17/8, ANCM [additionally found in ANCL, Part II Additions, 42/88, and ANCL 161/3d]. "Notes for Record WHO-ICP/ BSM/002 – Lusaka Antenna Technical Support to ANC Activities in Zambia," 20 April 1983, 90/86, ANCL.

45 Macmillan, *The Lusaka Years*.

46 This was also the case in Tanzania.

47 "Housemanship" is a term used in Zambia to refer to an internship. Housemanship can mean different things in different regions depending on the medical school's requirements. In this case, a new doctor was licensed but not yet allowed to practice without

supervision. Naicker described his housemanship period: "I had to do my house jobs. That consisted of doing three months service in four major areas of medical care, that was obstetrics and gynaecology, general surgery, internal medicine and paediatrics." "Interview with Dr Prenaiver Naicker," 105, 9/7-1631, Hilda Bernstein Interviews.

48 "Medical Committee ANC Secretary Report," 2 July 1978, 37/29, ANCC.

49 "Letter to the Superintendent of UTH signed Alfred Nzo," 10 November 1980, 1/1ii, ANCSHD. "Letter to the Superintendent of UTH signed Alfred Nzo," 15 February [1982], 1/1ii, ANCSHD.

50 These frontline states included Angola, Botswana, Mozambique, and, after 1980, Zimbabwe.

51 The dispensary was not an effective storage space because it was so small. "African National Congress National Consultative Conference June 1985. A. NEC Reports. A2 & A3: NEC (Secretary General and Treasurer General) Reports," June 1985, 3/61, Karis-Gerhart Papers.

52 "Minutes of the ANC(SA) Medical and Health Committee," no date [1979/01], 112/95, ANCL.

53 "The Psychological Effects of Apartheid," 13 December 1982, 17/8, ANCM.

54 "Confidential Report to the ANC," 19 May 1983, 118/126, ANCL.

55 "Interview with Dr Prenaiver Naicker," 105, 9/7-1631, Hilda Bernstein Interviews.

56 Ibid.

57 "Consultative Committee Meeting between Working Committee and Health Department held from 30 November to 2nd December 1982 in Lusaka–Zambia," no date, 160/1 ANCL.

58 "Letter to the Secretary of the Lusaka Health Team signed E.N. Miya," 11 February 1984, 160/1c, ANCL.

59 "Letter to the Health Secretariat signed A. Pemba," 8 November 1984, 106/53, ANCL [also in, Part I Additions, 9/28].

60 "Discussion Paper: Problems Affecting the Health Care Activities of the Regional Health Team (Zambia)," no date [1986], Part II Additions 31/38, ANCL.

61 The 1987 Hippe and Pedersen report claimed that the clinic was "built and equipped through funds raised from 'the general coffers'

of the ANC," and it further claimed that there was no external donor. However, letters from 1984 suggest that the ANC was provided with equipment from the Norwegian Medical Association, Danish Medical Association, and the WHO; with that support, progress was made on the development of the clinic in the district of Emmasdale in Lusaka. Hippe and Pedersen, "Health Care in An Exile Community: Report on Health Planning in the ANC," 1987, p. 72, 31/8, ANCL. "Letter to the Secretary General Alfred Nzo signed John Matjwe," no date [1984/05], 161/3a, ANCL. "African National Congress National Consultative Conference June 1985. A. NEC Reports. A2 & A3: NEC (Secretary General and Treasurer General) Reports," June 1985, 3/61, Karis-Gerhart Papers.

62 Ibid.

63 "Letter to ANC Headquarters, Secretary General signed Sipho Mthembu," 1 February 1985, 106/53, ANCL.

64 Ibid.

65 "Letter to the Military Head-Quarters, signed Edwin Mmutle [?]," 12 November 1986, Part II Additions 9/39, ANCL.

66 Hippe and Pedersen, "Health Care in An Exile Community," 1987, p. 69, 31/8, ANCL.

67 "Clinic Report for Quarter Ending Dec. '86 – For Meeting held 1st–5th April 1987,'" no date, Part II Additions 41/70, ANCL.

68 Hippe and Pedersen, "Health Care in An Exile Community," 1987, p. 73, 31/8, ANCL.

69 The problem of confidentially persisted for years. "Discussion Paper: Problems Affecting the Health Care Activities of the Regional Health Team (Zambia)," no date [1986], Part II Additions, 31/38 ANCL. "Response to issues raised in the Zambia RHT Report," 11 October 1987, Part II Additions, 42/103, ANCL. "Circular to all ANC Branches," 17 October 1988, Part II Additions, 6/8a, ANCL.

70 "The Running of the Clinic," no date, [1988?], Part II Additions, 41/74, ANCL. "Discussion Paper: Problems Affecting the Health Care Activities of the Regional Health Team (Zambia)," no date [1986], Part II Additions, 31/38 ANCL.

71 Hippe and Pedersen, "Health Care in An Exile Community," 1987, p. 77, 31/8, ANCL.

72 "Zambia Health Report – Period July–Aug–Sep," no date, [1987], Part II Additions, 42/72, ANCL.

73 "Preparation for Health Education Programme within the Primary Health Care System," 16 March 1988, Part II Additions, 41/63 [also in Part II Additions, 41/82], ANCL.

74 Hippe and Pedersen, "Health Care in An Exile Community," 1987, p. 71, 31/8, ANCL.

75 "Letter to Zambia Health Team signed Manto Tshabalala," 20 February 1986, Part II Additions, 6/8, ANCL.

76 "East Africa Regional Health Team Meeting held on 24/07/83 at Mazimbu Clinic," no date, 112/93, ANCL.

77 "Letter to Dr Comlan A.A. Quenum (WHO) signed Manto Tshabalala," 26 September 1983, Part II Additions, 11/49, ANCL.

78 "Visit to Harare, Zimbabwe from 25.01–01.02.84," 5 February 1984, 160/1c, ANCL.

79 Ibid.

80 "Report on Activities in Harare (01–04.04.84)," 10 April 1984, 161/3a, ANCL. "Letter to The Chairman of the ANC Health Team in Zimbabwe signed E.M. Miya," 4 October 1984, 161/3a, ANCL.

81 "Report, Formation of Medical Committee," 25 September 1984, 161/3a, ANCL. Population breakdown is not given in this document, but it is clear that the population was indeed small: "Report of the Commission of the National Executive Committee appointed to investigate the allocation and utilization of the financial resources of the organization in regions of the Front Line States and Forward Areas, March 1984–July 1984," 31 July 1984, 3/56, Karis-Gerhart Papers.

82 For instance Dr Sandile Mfenyana, Dr Abel Maminze, nurse Rebecca Mogale, and Dr Zinto Hashe all applied to be posted in Harare between January and March of 1985. "Letter to the P.M.C. signed Dr Mfelang," 11 February 1985, 161/3b, ANCL. "Letter to the Health Secretariat signed Rebecca Mogale," 9 January 1985, 160/3c, ANCL. "Letter to Peter Mfelang signed Dr Zinto Hashe," 6 March 1985, 161/3b, ANCL. Students were trained in a range of health-related fields including, but not limited to, physiotherapy, laboratory technology, prosthetics, medicine, and social work. "Letter to the Permanent Secretary in the Ministry of Health, Harare signed Peter

Mfelang," 30 July 1985, 161/3b, ANCL. "Visit to Harare, Zimbabwe from 25.01–01.02.84," 5 February 1984, 160/1c, ANCL.

83 "Zimbabwe Regional Health Team Report," 8 October 1987, Part II Additions, 42/89, ANCL.

84 "Reorganising for a Healthier Revolutionary Movement Report of ANC Health Department Seminar, 8–12 October 1987 Lusaka," no date, Part II Additions, 42/89, ANCL. "ANC Department of Health: The Zimbabwe regional Health Team Harare, Project Proposal for the year 1988," 30 October 1987, Part I Additions, 20/5, ANCL.

85 "ANC Department of Health: The Zimbabwe regional Health Team Harare, Meeting with the Regional Treasurer," 29 October 1987, Part I Addition, 20/5 ANCL. "ANC Department of Health: The Zimbabwe regional Health Team Harare, Expenditure on Health for the year 1986," 30 October 1987, Part I Additions, 20/5, ANCL.

86 "ANC Department of Health Finnida Project Proposal for 1989–1990, Zimbabwe," no date, 6/8, [also in ANCL, Part II Additions, 42/86], ANCF.

87 "Minutes of the Health Secretariat Meeting," 15 August 1990, 118/131, ANCL.

88 "Minutes of the ANC(SA) Medical and Health Committee," no date [1979/01], 112/95, ANCL.

89 Also spelled "Katenga."

90 "Interview with Dr Gwendolyn Sello (Tanzania 1989)," 4, 9/7 –1682, Hilda Bernstein Interviews. "Angolan Diaries of Prof. Jack Simons', incomplete manuscript of unpublished book by (and about) Jack Simons, Chapter 3," 9, 14 February 1979, 3/34, Karis-Gerhart Papers.

91 Cuban doctors were important to the ANC's medical care in Angola but that relationship is out of the scope of this book. "Angolan Diaries of Prof. Jack Simons', incomplete manuscript of unpublished book by (and about) Jack Simons, Chapter 3," 9, 14 February 1979, 3/34, Karis-Gerhart Papers.

92 "Medical Requisite to MPLA," 13 May 1977, Part II Additions, 42/99, ANCL. "Receipt of Medicaments from MPLA," 21 May 1977, Part II Additions, ANCL. "Packing list as per our Forwarding Advice as I dated 24.1.1978 consignment of medicaments and dressing material for the African national congress (SA) Luanda/Angola," 24 February 1978, Part II Additions, 42/99, ANCL. "Medicines

from Rumania," 19 August 1978, Part II Additions, 42/99, ANCL. "Medicines from the G.D.R.," 19 August 1978, Part II Additions, 42/99, ANCL. "Medicines received from Fraternal Organisation Secours Populaire francais," 20 August 1978, Part II Additions, 42/99, ANCL.

93 "Interview with Dr Gwendolyn Sello (Tanzania 1989)," 1–4, 9/7 –1682, Hilda Bernstein Interviews. "Angolan Diaries of Prof. Jack Simons', incomplete manuscript of unpublished book by (and about) Jack Simons, Chapter 3," 18, 14 February 1979, 3/34, Karis-Gerhart Papers.

94 Bopela and Luthuli, *Umkhonto We Siswe*; 173.

95 "East Africa Regional Health Team Meeting held on 24/07/83 at Mazimbu Clinic," no date, 112/93, ANCL.

96 The number of cadres in exile has been the subject of some debate in the literature. Speaking directly to this conflict, scholar Marin Saebo comments on the UNHRC estimates in her master's thesis and argues that most of these refugees were likely part of MK. She defends her argument by pointing out that Angola was a military zone and she posits that the demographic data on these refugees reflects MK's military demographic distribution. Saebo does not provide a specific ratio of cadres to refugees. I agree that a significant number of the South Africans in Angola had some involvement with MK. However, some of these refugees recorded by the UNHCR were not MK; instead they were family members, children of MK men and Angolan women, or people generally attempting to escape the apartheid government. The discrepancies between ANC population estimates and the published UNHCR numbers support this. Additionally, Hugh Macmillan argues that by 1987, "there were less than 2,000 MK cadres, including about 350 trainees, in the Angolan camps." MK cadres were leaving the area by that time, but as stated in the text it is not likely that 3,000 MK cadres had already left the area. Saebo, "A State of Exile," 107; Macmillan, *The Lusaka Years*, 174.

97 UNHCR, "Report of the United Nations." Adepoju also stated that in 1977, there were 10,000 Namibian refugees. This number grew to 35,000 by the end of 1979. Adepoju, "The Dimension of the Refugee Problem," 28. According to the UNHCR, that number increased to 70,000 by 1981. UN, "Yearbook of the United Nations," 1032.

98 "Interview with Dr Gwendolyn Sello (Tanzania 1989)," 4, 9/7 –1682, Hilda Bernstein Interviews "Angolan Diaries of Prof. Jack Simons', incomplete manuscript of unpublished book by (and about) Jack Simons, Chapter 3," 9, 14 February 1979, 3/34, Karis-Gerhart Papers.

99 The Women's Section was constantly pushing for more women to join MK and lamented that women were grossly underrepresented in the army. See for example "African National Congress Women's Second National Consultative Conference September 1–6, 1987," no date, 92/13, ANCL.

100 Sellström, *Sweden and National Liberation Vol II*, 363.

101 It has been estimated that in the mid-1980s there were approximately 35,000 Namibian exiles at Kwanza Sul. Williams, "Exile History," 44.

102 Sellström, *Sweden and National Liberation Vol II*, 363.

103 Ibid., 365.

104 "Report on the Secretary's Trip to Angola from the 27th July to August 13, 1980," 10 September 1980, 31/4, ANCL. The second half of this report was found in 112/90, ANCL.

105 In June 1985 it was curiously reported that contrary to Tshabalala's report, ANC doctors were in fact not registered. This statement may have been legally true, but it was not consistent with the practices on the ground. ANC doctors certainly worked in Angolan facilities at that time. "African National Congress National Consultative Conference June 1985. A. NEC Reports. A2 & A3: NEC (Secretary General and Treasurer General) Reports," June 1985, 3/61, Karis-Gerhart Papers.

106 "List of Annexures [Consultative Committee Meeting, 1982/11-12]," various dates, 105/45, ANCL.

107 "Report on the Secretary's Trip to Angola from the 27th July to August 13, 1980," 10 September 1980, 31/4, ANCL.

108 "Report on ANC in Angola for the Year Beginning January 1984 to 8 January 1985," no date, 32/2, ANCL. "Letter to Peter Mfelang signed Manto Tshabalala," 9 April 1985, 2/1iii, ANCSHD. "Finnsolidarity RY ANC Viana Centre," 25 September 1986, 6/9, ANCF.

109 "Report on the First Aid Instructors Course (NORSK-Dansk Folkehjelp, ANC-SWAPO) run in Denmark, Norway and Kwanza-Sul," August 1982, 160/1, ANCL.

110 Hippe and Pedersen, "Health Care in An Exile Community," 1987, 57–60, 31/8, ANCL.

111 Ibid., 57–60.

112 UN, "Yearbook of the United Nations," 1032.

113 *The Fourth Dimension* claimed that Florence Maleka did not begin work until sometime in the early 1980s. However, it is evident from the reports sent out of the region in the late 1970s that she arrived earlier than this estimate. Furthermore, in May 1979 Maleka wrote that she arrived in October 1978. "Letter to Chief Representative signed Florence Maleka," 4 May 1979, 17/3 ANCM.

114 1979 was the final year that Mozambique used the Portuguese currency "escudos." The amount listed was 4,000 to 5,000 escudos. The conversion: World Bank, "Official Exchange Rate: (1979)."

115 "Maputo Clinic Report," no date [December 1979], 17/7, ANCM.

116 "Letter to the Chief Representative, Maputo [missing pages]," 9 December 1980, 17/3 ANCM.

117 "Report of the Special Health Council Meeting January 24-25, 1982 – Lusaka," 3 February 1982, 112/95 [also in ANCL, 112/96], ANCL.

118 "Letter to Alfred Nzo signed Manto Tshabalala," 19 April 1982, 112/91, ANCL.

119 Ibid.

120 "Interview with Dr Prenaiver Naicker," 105, 9/7-1631, Hilda Bernstein Interviews.

121 "Report on the 35th World Health Assembly Geneva. May 3–15, 1982," 29 May 1982, 17/8, ANCM. "Quarterly Report addressed to Manto Tshabalala signed Prenaven Naicker," 3 April 1983, Part II Additions, 41/61, ANCL.

122 ANCM, "Quarterly Report addressed to Manto Tshabalala signed Prenaven Naicker," 3 April 1983, Part II Additions, 41/61, ANCL.

123 Ibid. The account of Pren Naicker's deployment to Mozambique provided in *the Fourth Dimension* (which coincides with the interview that Naicker gave to Hilda Bernstein) deviates slightly from the timeline provided in this chapter. *The Fourth Dimension* account stated, "In his quest to investigate the reason why so many cadres were falling ill, Dr Pren discovered through clinical observation that chloroquine-resistant malaria was the culprit." From my research, Naicker may have been sent to better understand the disease pattern in the region, but it is less likely

that CRPF was the issue at that initial stage. Naidoo, *The Fourth Dimension*, 268. "Interview with Dr Prenaiver Naicker," 105, 9/7-1631, Hilda Bernstein Interviews.

124 "Letter to Aunt Edith signed Pren Naicker," 20 May 1983, 17/3, ANCM.

125 "Visit to Nampula – A Follow up on the Chloroquine-Resistant Malaria, July 21–28, 1983, by Solomon Molefe and Manto," 8 August 1983, 160/1b, ANCL.

126 Ibid.

127 This was yet another of the ANC's attempts at self-sufficiency, but the project itself is beyond the scope of this book. "Visit to Nampula – A Follow up on the Chloroquine-Resistant Malaria, July 21–28, 1983, by Solomon Molefe and Manto," 8 August 1983, 160/1b, ANCL.

128 Ibid.

129 "Minutes of Special Directorate Meeting on new Arrivals from Mozambique etc.," 17 April 1984, 118/126, ANCL. "Religious Affairs Department," 20 September 1984, 107/54b, ANCL.

130 Malaria is a disease caused by the blood-borne parasite *Plasmodium*; there are four species of *Plasmodium* that infect humans: *P. falciparum*, *P.ovale*, *P.vivax*, and *P.malariae*. The species of primary concern to the ANC was *P. falciparum*, the most aggressive of the four strains and the most common in southern Africa. If *P. falciparum* malaria is left untreated, the victim becomes anaemic and often dies. Additionally, it is possible for someone suffering from *P. falciparum* malaria to develop "cerebral malaria." The process of this development from malaria to cerebral malaria is not completely predictable or understood but the longer an individual is ill, the greater the chance of development. H.C. van der Heyde, "A Unified Hypothesis for the Genesis of Cerebral Malaria: Sequestration, Inflammation and Hemostasis Leading to Microcirculatory Dysfunction," *Trends in Parasitology* 22, no. 11 (n.d.): 5. The ANC Health Department's slow response to treat infected individuals meant that some cases did develop into cerebral malaria; cerebral malaria is often deadly or the cause of lasting psychotic effects.

131 In his book *The Making of a Tropical Disease*, Randall Packard discussed some of the social and biological factors that enabled the spread of the first instances of CRPF on the Thai–Cambodian

border in the 1960s. His case study bears a striking similarity to the ANC's situation in exile. He stated that labour migrants came to Palin, a Cambodian mining city, in order to supplement their agricultural income. This labour came from regions where malaria was less prevalent and as a result, these labourers – like the South African exiles – had no immunity to the parasite. The environment that was well-suited to mosquito breeding in combination with the high number of nonimmune migrants staying in close quarters created the perfect conditions in which *P. falciparum* malaria could spread widely. Unfortunately, starting in 1955 miners were given chloroquine prophylactically in amounts inadequate to kill the parasites in the blood. The constant influx of new nonimmune and highly transient workers who took noncurative doses of chloroquine enabled the rapid spread of new chloroquine-resistant strains of malaria in the region. Packard concluded the case study by arguing that chloroquine resistance was not an inevitable global phenomenon but instead a result of a specific set of environmental, economic, and social circumstances in the region. I found a similar set of circumstances facing the ANC's Health Department in exile, and I think that these specific factors also contributed to the rapid spread of CRPF in sub-Saharan Africa. Packard, *The Making of a Tropical Disease*, 31.

132 Wellems and Plowe, "Chloroquine-Resistant Malaria," 770–6.

133 Wernsdorfer and Payne, "The Dynamics of Drug Resistance," 102

134 Due to malaria's relative treatability and the fact that it was not the cause of strain between host governments and the ANC, malaria prior to CRPF does not seem to be a preoccupation of the Health Department. It was also likely that this silence reflected the mundane, if insistent threat of malaria; malaria fever was not nearly as internationally sensational as those diseases that were attributed to the policies of apartheid, like for instance mental illness.

135 Heyde, "A Unified Hypothesis," 5.

136 Packard, *The Making of a Tropical Disease*, 31

137 Wernsdorfer and Payne, "The Dynamics of Drug Resistance," 102.

138 "Letter to Aunt Edith signed Pren Naicker," 20 May 1983, 17/3, ANCM.

139 "Interview with Dr Prenaiver Naicker," 105, 9/7-1631, Hilda Bernstein Interviews.

140 "Report on the Health Situation of Mazimbu from Jan–April 1983," 3 June 1983, 9/31, ANCSHD.

141 ANCSHD, 8/22, "Minutes of the Health Committee Meeting," 20 April 1983, 8/22, ANCSHD.

142 "Report on the Health Situation of Mazimbu from Jan–April 1983," 3 June 1983, 9/31, ANCSHD.

143 This account of the two patients was explained in a single correspondence: "Re: Chloroquine-Resistant Strains of Plasmodium P[f]alciparum," 13 May 1983, 112/92, ANCL.

144 "Letter to the Secretary General signed Sipho Mlambo," 17 July 1983, 112/92, ANCL.

145 "Initial Report on Chloroquine-Resistant Malaria (Maputo)," 12 July 1983, 112/96, ANCL.

146 Ibid.

147 The need for quinine was particularly concerning because of quinine's extensive side effect profile. Extended use can result in blindness.

148 The ANC also claimed that the security police in South Africa interrogated anyone treated for malaria in a South African hospital, suspicious that those with malaria were ANC/MK infiltrators. They were, in 1983, worried about the implications of a future discovery of CRPF in South Africa. "African National Congress," 15 September 1983, Part II Additions, 42/73, ANCL.

149 "Initial Report on Chloroquine-Resistant Malaria (Maputo)," 12 July 1983, 112/96, ANCL.

150 "Meeting with the Minister of Health Maputo," 10 August 1983, 17/5, ANCM.

151 "Visit to Nampula – A Follow up on the Chloroquine-Resistant Malaria, July 21–28, 1983, by Solomon Molefe and Manto," 8 August 1983, 160/1b, ANCL.

152 "Meeting with the Minister of Health Maputo," 10 August 1983, 17/5, ANCM.

153 "Meeting of the Regional Health Team with the National held at Mazimbu Clinic," 15 August 1983, 8/20, ANCSHD.

154 The relationship was viewed by the ANC Health Department as indispensible: "Letter to Pren Naicker signed Manto Tshabalala," 29 September 1983, 17/3, ANCM.

155 Robert Shell and Patricia Oaga make a similar argument about the ANC and MKs transmission of disease. In their study, they look at the

transmission of HIV/AIDS from exile back to South Africa. Shell and Qaga, "Trojan Horses," 24–7.

156 "Initial Report of the Results of Chloroquine Investigation of our People (Caxito and Viana)," 5 October 1983, 160/1b, ANCL.

157 "Report on the Malaria Programme August 16–30 1983, Angola," no date, 17/7, ANCM.

158 "Meeting with the Minister of Health Maputo," 10 August 1983, 17/5, ANCM.

159 "Report on the Malaria Programme August 16–30 1983, Angola," no date, 17/7, ANCM.

160 Ibid.

161 Ibid.

162 "Letter to Comrade Nkokheli [?] signed Manto Tshabalala," 11 September 1983, 160/1b, ANCL.

163 "Initial Report of the Results of Chloroquine Investigation of our People (Caxito and Viana)," 5 October 1983, 160/1b, ANCL.

164 "ANC Department of Health, Report – Health Department January 1983–December 1983," January 1984, 161/3d, ANCL.

165 "Initial Report of the Results of Chloroquine Investigation of our People (Caxito and Viana)," 5 October 1983, 160/1b, ANCL.

166 "Regional Health Team (East Africa) Tanzania Quarterly for period July to September 1983 Report," no date, 160/1b, ANCL.

167 "Letter to the Secretary of the East Africa Health Team signed Manto Tshabalala," 1 November 1983, 160/1b, ANCL.

168 "Letter to the Secretary of the Health Department signed Victor Maome," 1 August 1984, 161/3d, ANCL.

169 "Letter to Manto Tshabalala signed Pren Naicker," 6 October 1984, Part II Additions, 6/5, ANCL.

170 "Report on TCDC Meeting Held in Mauritius, 18–22 March, 85," 26 March 1985, Part II Additions, 42/106, ANCL.

171 "ANC Department of Health, Report – Health Department January 1983–December 1983," January 1984, 161/3d, ANCL.

172 "Letter to Joe Nhlanhla signed Manto Tshabalala," 24 May 1984, 161/3a, ANCL. "ANC Department of Health, Report – Health Department January 1983–December 1983," January 1984, 161/3d, ANCL.

173 ANCL, 161/3a, Letter to Dr Quenum signed Manto Tshabalala, 1984/08/08.

174 Presumably, the budget cuts referred to her 9,000 refugee proposal. "Report on the 34th Regional Committee of the World Health Organisation = held in Brazzaville in September, 1984," 6 October 1984, 106/53, ANCL.

175 "Untitled Report by the PMC," no date, [1984], 128/245, ANCL.

176 "Report on ANC in Angola for the Year Beginning January 1984 to 8 January 1985," no date, 32/2, ANCL.

177 "Mazimbu Health Report for the Ending of Fabruary [sic] 1984," no date, 9/31, ANCSHD.

178 "Assessment of the Sensitivity of P. Falciparum to Chloroquine using the in Vivo and in Vitro methods at ANC Settlement in Tanzania," no date, [1984/01], 160/1c, ANCL.

179 "Letter to Dr Tshabalala signed Professor W.L. Kilama," 11 January 1984, 160/1c, ANCL. Payment for these tests became a source of embarrassment and frustration. The ANC advanced a cheque to the National Institute for Medical Research in Tanzania but it bounced and created strain between the department and the institute. "Letter to the Treasurer General Thomas Nkobi signed Manto Tshabalala," 28 June 1984, 161/3a, ANCL.

180 "Letter to the Head of the SOMAFCO Clinic signed Manto Tshabalala," 9 March 1984, 1/1, ANCSHD.

181 "Preamble," 26 March 1985, 31/11, ANCL.

182 "Re: Problems and matters for clarification," 1 August 1984, 161/3a, ANCL.

183 "Religious Affairs Department," 20 September 1984, 107/54b, ANCL.

184 "Regional Health Report for the Year 1985," no date, 161/3b, ANCL.

185 "Report on a visit to East Africa from 7th July to 10th August 1985," no date, 2/1iii, ANCSHD.

186 "Letter to the Director (Mazimbu) signed Manto Tshabalala," 15 July 1985, 161/3b, ANCL.

187 In the 1985 yearly regional health report for ANC communities in Tanzania, it was shown that of the 16,738 patients seen at ANC medical facilities, a total of 9,346 people (3,898 ANC and 5,448 local Tanzanians) were treated for malaria, the bulk of which were resistant to chloroquine. Of the reported ten deaths, four were caused by malaria "Regional Health Report for the Year 1985," no date, 161/3b, ANCL.

188 "Letter to the Treasurer General signed E.M. Miya," 29 January
    1985, 161/3b, ANCL.
189 "Last Assignments to the Angola Health Team," 25 March 1985,
    161/3b, ANCL.
190 "Letter to Manto Tshabalala signed Dr Pren Naicker," 11 May 1985,
    Part II Additions, 6/5, ANCL.
191 Five examples of daily breakdowns were provided in the archive,
    during these five dates, average percentage of malaria patients
    ranged from 24–60 per cent and was the number one cause
    for attendance each day: "A.N.C. Holland Solidarity Hospital
    Mazimbu. Analysis of Disease," 5 June 1986, 7 June 1986, 12 June
    1986, 13 June 1986, 19 June 1986, 7/16, ANCSHD. See also "Clinic
    Report for Quarter Ending Dec. '86 – For Meeting held 1st–5th
    April 1987,'" no date, Part II Additions 41/70, ANCL. Other reports
    also confirm the high incident rate of malaria: "Secondary Division
    Report; Health Division of SOMAFCO, Nursery Division," no
    date [1986?], 128/239, ANCL. However, there are some instances
    where other diseases become more prevalent, especially during
    dry seasons: "ANC Development Centre – Dakawa Health Team
    Report," no date [September 1986], Part II Additions, 41/69, ANCL.
    However, as soon as the rainy season started, malaria cases return
    to the top of the list: "African National Congress of South Africa
    Development Centre – Dakawa Health Monthly Report," 30
    October 1986, 25/40, ANCSD.
192 See for instance "Health Report to the Directorate, Mazimbu/
    Dakawa, Nov–Dec 1986," no date, 9/31, ANCSHD. "Health Council
    Meeting: Malaria," 3 February 1986, 127/236, ANCL.
193 "Report of the National Preparatory Committee (NPC)," November
    1986, 31/11, ANCL.
194 "Malaria, 3rd Health Council Meeting," 1986, 127/236, ANCL.
195 "Minutes of Directorate Meeting held 1 March 1986," no date, 8/22,
    ANCSHD.
196 "Clinic Report for Quarter Ending Dec. '86 – For Meeting held
    1st–5th April 1987,'" no date, Part II Additions 41/70, ANCL. "ANC
    Development Centre – Dakawa Health Team Report," no date
    [September 1986], Part II Additions, 41/69, ANCL.
197 "Annual Regional Health Report East Africa from 1/1/86 to 27/3/87,"
    no date, Part II Additions, 41/64, ANCL. "Directorate Meeting,

8th November, 1986, Re= Health Report of A.N.C. Hoalland [*sic*]
S. Hosp and Dakawa," 9 November 1986, 9/31, ANCSHD.

198 "Annual Regional Health Report East Africa from 1/1/86 to 27/3/87,"
no date, Part II Additions, 41/64, ANCL.

199 Hippe and Pedersen, "Health Care in An Exile Community," 1987,
36, 31/8, ANCL.

200 "Project Proposal Document for a Malaria Workshop," 4 January
1985, 161/3a, ANCL.

201 Tsampiras, "Sex in a Time of Exile," 637–63; Tsampiras, "Politics,
Polemics, and Practice."

202 "Clinic Report for Quarter Ending Dec. '86 – For Meeting held
1st–5th April 1987,'" no date, Part II Additions 41/70, ANCL.

203 "Towards Comprehensive Intervention Strategies for the
Prevention and Control of HIV/AIDS infection," 1990, Part II
Additions, 42/104, ANCL.

204 Ibid.

205 Ibid.

206 "Response to Issues Raised in the Zambia RHT Report," 11 October
1987, Part II Additions, 42/103, ANCL.

207 "Reorganising for a Healthier Revolutionary Movement Report of
ANC Health Department Seminar, 8–12 October 1987 Lusaka," no
date, Part II Additions, 42/89, ANCL.

208 "Response to issues raised in the Zambia RHT Report," 11 October
1987, Part II Additions, 42/103, ANCL.

209 "Progress Report on the Work of the Department for the NEC,"
October 1987, Part II Additions, 41/69, ANCL.

210 This notion was posited in previous work: Tsampiras, "Politics,
Polemics, and Practice."

211 "Response to issues raised in the Zambia RHT Report," 11 October
1987, Part II Additions, 42/103, ANCL.

212 "Angolan Region- Progress Report on 'AIDS PROJECT,'" 15
November 1989, Part II Additions, 42/102, ANCL.

213 See for instance, work by Shell and Qaga on the spread of HIV in
South Africa by the movement of MK cadres, untested or unaware
of their HIV status: Shell and Qaga, "Trojan Horses," 24–7.

214 "Towards Comprehensive Intervention Strategies for the
Prevention and Control of HIV/AIDS infection," 1990, Part II
Additions, 42/104, ANCL.

Chapter Three

1 See for instance "WHO's Azania," *South Afrikaans Medical Journal*, 965, 9 June 1979, 7/3 ANCM.

2 The historiography of the international anti-apartheid movement is deep. A sample of this work includes Sapire and Saunders, *Southern African Liberation Struggles*; Nixon, "Apartheid on the Run," 68–88; Murray, "The Sports Boycott and Cricket," 219–49; Fieldhouse, *Anti-Apartheid*; Thörn, *Anti-Apartheid*; Williams, "Anti-Apartheid," 685–706; Skinner, *The Foundations of Anti-Apartheid*; Skinner, "The Moral Foundations," 399–416; Nesbitt, *Race for Sanctions*; Saul, "Two Fronts of Anti-Apartheid Struggle," 135–51. Significant work underpinning this study includes the *National Liberation in Southern Africa: The Role of the Nordic Countries* project, which was coordinated by historian Tor Sellström at the Nordic Africa Institute cited previously. The series provides rich detail of Sweden, Norway, Denmark, and Finland's contributions to the Southern African liberation effort, including the Anti-Apartheid Movement (AAM) and its involvement with the ANC. Another important collection was introduced in *Volume Three: International Solidarity* of the Road to Democracy in South Africa project; this edited volume is divided into two parts and includes chapters from more than twenty-five authors.

3 Panzer, "Building a Revolutionary Constituency," 6.

4 Other examples include Eklind and Angenfelt, "From Bullets to Ballots"; Robinson, "Hamas as Social Movement," 112–39; Early, "'Larger than a Party,'" 115–28; Johnson, "Non-State Health Care," 735–58; Stokke, "Building the Tamil Eelam State," 1021–40; Nelson, *Body and Soul*.

5 Jones, *The Black Panther Party*; Bloom and Martin, *Black against Empire*, 179–98.

6 Nelson, *Body and Soul*, 49.

7 The US government felt that the Panthers' use of social programs in African American communities was threatening to the security and stability of the nation. President Nixon used his counterintelligence unit to stop the breakfast program and the Panthers' medical initiatives.

8 Bhasin and Hallward, "Hamas as a Political Party," 75–93.

9 WHO, *Health and Apartheid: Part 1 & Part II*; United Nations Centre against Apartheid, Halfdan, and WHO, "Health Implications of Apartheid."

10 "Declaration on the Establishment of a New International Economic Order," 1 May 1974, 3201 (S-VI), United Nations.

11 Ibid.

12 WHO, *Health and Apartheid: Part I & Part II*.

13 For a detailed account of the litigation process see Baxter, "Doctors on Trial," 137–51.

14 Mji, "The World Medical Association in South Africa," 351–3.

15 Dommisse, "World Medical Association," 1280.

16 Baxter, "Doctors on Trial," 137–51.

17 An additional 1977 development was the WHO's investigation of mental health provision in South Africa.

18 WHO, "Executive Summary."

19 "Medical Committee ANC Secretary Report," 2 July 1978, 37/29, ANCC. WHO, "Primary Health Care."

20 The granting of observer status was discussed in the July 1978 ANC Medical Committee meeting: "Medical Committee ANC Secretary Report," 2 July 1978, 37/29, ANCC.

21 "WHO's Azania," *South Afrikaans Medical Journal*, 965, 9 June 1979, 7/3 ANCM.

22 WHO, "Primary Health Care."

23 "Draft Policy of the ANC(SA) Medical and Health Committee," 30 December 1978, 17/2, ANCM.

24 WHO, "Primary Health Care."

25 "Minutes of the ANC(SA) Medical and Health Committee," no date [1979/01], 112/95, ANCL.

26 "African National Congress (S.A.) Solomon Mahlangu Freedom College, EA Regional Joint, Medical Team Meeting held on the 26/27.1.80," no date, 20/8, ANCSHD.

27 Kwashiorkor is a type of malnutrition caused by protein deficiency. "Monthly Report of Charlotte Maxeke Clinic for December 1983," no date, 160/1b, ANCL. "Minutes of Directorate Meeting Held 3rd December 1983," no date, 118/126, ANCL.

28 "Dakawa–Mazimbu Health Team Reports," November 1987, 14/19, ANCSD.

29 "Minutes of Special Directorate Meeting on new Arrivals from Mozambique etc.," 17 April 1984, 118/126, ANCL.

30 "Consultative Committee Meeting between Working Committee and Health Department held from 30 November to 2nd December 1982 in Lusaka- Zambia," no date, 160/1, ANCL.

31 Ibid.

32 In her message to Dr Quenum, Tshabalala said, "For us, a prerequisite for this social objective is the overthrow of the existing state in South Africa, and its replacement by a democratic one, based on the will of the people. In short it means the seizure of political power, political commitment to ensure social well-being to all and the development of health policies which would guarantee an adequate level of health for all with the full participation, commitment and collaboration of our communiteis [*sic*] in achieving the health goals enshrined in the Freedom Charter." It should be stated that Dr Tshabalala recorded her comments to Dr Quenum in a report given to the ANC leadership. Therefore it is impossible to say whether this was what she actually said to Dr Quenum. "Report on our Visit to the Republic of Zimbabwe From November 14 to 19th to Negotiate with the Government of Zimbabwe to host an International Conference on "Health and Apartheid" in 1981," no date [November 1980], 112/96, ANCL.

33 "The Freedom Charter: Adopted at the Congress of the People at Kliptown, Johannesburg, on June 25 and 26, 1955," AD1137, FSAW.

34 Prompted by perceived economic stagnation in Africa, the Lagos Plan of Action was a twenty-year (1980–2000) plan to improve the economic situation continent-wide. The plan emphasized the need for African solidarity and African self-sufficiency. The plan outlines a series of initiatives in various government sectors including food and agriculture, science and technology, transport and communications, women and development. Healthcare is not a separate sector in the plan of action but it is a common theme throughout all of the sectors. OAU, "Lagos plan of action," 1980.

35 In May 1974 the UN General Assembly resolved to shrink the growing economic divide between "developed" and "developing" nations." "Declaration on the Establishment of a New International Economic Order," 1 May 1974, 3201 (S-VI), United Nations.

36 "Report on our Visit to the Republic of Zimbabwe From November 14 to 19th to Negotiate with the Government of Zimbabwe to host an International Conference on "Health and Apartheid" in 1981," no date [November 1980], 112/96, ANCL.

37 Lesotho and Swaziland were not yet recognized as frontline states but together they sent six representatives to the conference.

38 WHO, *Health and Apartheid: Part I & Part II*.

39 Nzo was absent from the conference and somebody (unmentioned) read the speech aloud on his behalf.

40 WHO, *Health and Apartheid: Part I & Part II*, 10–12.

41 Ibid., 12.

42 UN, "Yearbook of the United Nations,"1039.

43 "How to Strengthen Link with Health Personnel at Home," 1986, 127/236, ANCL.

44 "Memorandum to the Secretary-General from the Health Department," 21 July 1980, Part II Additions, 6/7, ANCL. Records relating to subsequent meetings that she had with sympathetic doctors were not kept with the rest of the Mozambique files, and I was not able to locate them elsewhere in the archive. It is clear however that Dlamini was not always in Swaziland. For example, in November 1982 Swaziland's medical support for South African people in the region went from four to two. Two nurses, Lindelwa Guma and Khumbuzile Phungula, reported a need for donor support and more staff; they were both working their regular shifts at Swazi facilities and then treating ANC members after hours. "Medical Department Swaziland, Report on the above committee," 3 November 1982, 17/7, ANCM.

45 One important contribution to anti-apartheid literature in the health field, produced in South Africa, was *Critical Health* (1980–1990?). This publication included submissions from many different academics and activists. *Critical Health*, issues: 1980, December 1984, May 1985, September 1986, December 1986, August 1988, November 1990, 31/8, ANCL

46 "Doctors: Where Do You Stand?," no date [1986?], 3/76, Karis-Gerhart Papers.

47 The doctors' negligence assisted in the death of Steve Biko and prolonged the suffering of Marcus Thabo Motaung before the police killed him.

48 "Doctors: Where Do You Stand?," no date [1986?], 3/76, Karis-Gerhart Papers.

49 At the time of the report, the Health Department in Lusaka was unaware of the Canadian "medical committee" and, while pleased by the support, asked that the Canadian group coordinate more closely with Dr Manto Tshabalala. However, correspondence between this team and the administration in southern Africa was sporadic, and so by the 1980s, the Canadian team operated relatively independently and might be considered a supportive anti-apartheid group rather than a direct department member. "Medical Committee Report," no date [1979], 37/29, ANCC. "Letter to the Canadian Medical Committee signed Sindiso Mfenyana," 20 March 1979, 4/55, ANCC.

50 "Report on the Tour of Scandinavian Countries (27th April–23rd May, 1979)," no date, 17/7, ANCM. "Brief Report on the Medical Situation in Dar es Salaam and Morogoro area," 8 March 1979, ANCL.

51 Seedat, *Crippling a Nation*; Lonsdale, *South Africa in Question*.

52 "Letter to Dr Marius Barnard signed Gertrude Shope," 10 January 1983, 6/60, ANCW.

53 For a discussion on the politics of contraception and population control see Brown, "Facing the 'Black Peril,'" 256–73; Klausen, *Abortion Under Apartheid*, 200–1.

54 "African National Congress (S.A.) Health Department: Child-Birth in Exile, A problem Oriented Approach, some aspects of women and health," July 1981, 156/41, ANCL.

55 "African National Congress (Women's Secretariat) Draft Programme of Action," 22 February 1982, 10/51, ANCL.

56 "Letter to Chris Barnard signed Gertrude Shope," no date [1983], 6/60, ANCW. "Letter to Dr Marius Barnard signed Gertrude Shope," 10 January 1983, 6/60, ANCW.

57 "Letter to the ANC(SA) Women's Secretariat [Gertrude Shope] signed Kgaugelo Kgosana, with enclosed report on Depo Provera," 24 August 1983, 62/11, ANCW.

58 "Letter to Lucia Raadschelders signed Gertrude Shope," 19 July 1983, 154/23b, ANCL.

59 In Botswana health authorities were offering Depo-Provera as a birth control method. At the Botswana commemoration of the

30th anniversary of the Federation of South African Women, the use of Depo-Provera sparked debate between representatives from the Botswana Ministry of Health and the ANC women attending the conference. The women from Botswana defended the use of Depo-Provera as a legitimate drug given after the patient is made aware of the consequences. The commemoration report stated that the discussion on family planning was heated and would have to be postponed. "Report on the Commemoration of the 30th Anniversary of the Federation of South African Women by the Women's Section of the African National Congress (S.A.) (Botswana)," no date [19 April 1984], 62/10, ANCW.

60 "To see Dr Simwanza and Introduce ANC and interest in IPPF," no date [November 1983], 44/17, ANCW. "Letter to Dr Tshabalala signed E.A Duale (WHO)," 26 October 1983, Part II Additions, 11/49, ANCL.

61 "To see Dr Simwanza and Introduce ANC and interest in IPPF," no date [November 1983], 44/17, ANCW.

62 The group operated from London. In 1984 the ICASC changed its name to the Women's Global Network for Reproductive Rights (WGNRR). Crane, "The Transnational Politics of Abortion," 252.

63 "Letter to the International Contraception Abortion and Sterilisation Campaign signed Gertrude Shope," 2 April 1984, 154/23c, ANCL.

64 The tribunal was also called the fourth International Women and Health Meeting (IWHM). Women's Global Network for Reproductive Rights, "History."

65 Dufour, Masson, and Caouette, *Solidarities Beyond Borders*, 111.

66 "Untitled Document regarding contraceptives, abortion and sterilization practices in South Africa," no date [July 1984], 44/17, ANCW.

67 Ibid.

68 Haemorrhage is not specifically associated with the administration of Depo-Provera. What is important in this example is that Depo-Provera is used by the ANC to illustrate a political point about racism in South Africa.

69 Ibid.

70 "African National Congress (S.A.) Health Department: Child-Birth in Exile, A problem Oriented Approach, some aspects of women and health," July 1981, 156/41, ANCL.

71 "Circular from the Director – 21st. November 1984. Subject

– Pregnancies/Abortions/Miscarriages," 21 November 1984, 7/11, ANCSHD.

72 "Solomon Mahlangu Freedom College General Staff Meeting, 29/11/84," 29 November 1984, 7/11, ANCSHD.

73 "African National Congress (SA) Dakawa Development Centre Rehabilitation Section Registration forms," November 1983–29 February 1984, 37/112, ANCSD.

74 This was not the only response to abortion. Following the 1981 ANC Women's Conference, the National Executive Council charged the Health Department to consider abortions "not on demand, but when necessary and under specified circumstances." "Response of the Working Committee of the NEC on Recommendations of the Conference of ANC Women held in Luanda People's Republic of Angola on September 10–14, 1981," no date, 153/22a, ANCL. "Gynecological Report from 11.4.86 to 24.3.87 signed Dr Claudia Randree," no date, 9/31, ANCSHD.

75 "Untitled Document regarding contraceptives, abortion and sterilization practices in South Africa," no date [July 1984], 44/17, ANCW.

76 "Statement by Comrade [redacted]," 8 December 1987, 6/60, ANCW.

77 Ibid.

78 "Letter to Pren Naicker signed Dr Haggar McBerry, Florence Maleka and Dr Bob Mayekiso," 9 December 1987, 6/60, ANCW.

79 "Meeting with comrades MaNjobe [?] (deputy head of ANC women section), Thembi, [redacted] and [redacted]," 12 December 1987, 61/4, ANCW.

80 Ibid.

81 "Minutes of Special Directorate Meeting Held 7/8/83," no date, 118/126, ANCL.

82 "Report of ANC Health Department Seminar, 8–12 October 1987 Lusaka," no date, Part II Additions, 42/89, ANCL.

83 "Memorandum on Unplanned Pregnancies," no date [October 1987?], 6/60, ANCW.

84 "Letter to the Health Secretariat signed [?]," 10 November 1988, Part II Additions, 9/29, ANCL.

85 "Progress Report on the Work of the Department for the NEC," October 1987, Part II Additions, 41/69, ANCL. "Report to the NEC, from the N.H. Secretariat," no date [1987], Part II Additions, 42/103, ANCL.

86 "ANC Department of Health Annual Report to the ECC for the Year 1987," February 1988, Part II Additions, 41/65, ANCL.

87 See for instance: "Abortion – A Woman's Right to Choose," no date [1989?], 59/212, ANCW. "Commission on Health and Social Welfare," no date [1992?], 74/22, LH. "ANC Additions to the Women's Health Section of the National Health Plan," no date [1993?], 48/27, LH.

Chapter Four

1 By 1978 the MKA (an NGO in the Netherlands) was already engaging in talks to financially support a new ANC hospital in the Tanzanian region. "Medical Committee ANC Secretary Report," 2 July 1978, 37/29, ANCC.

2 The third task set out by the Medical Committee in 1978 was to "collect and disseminate information on the medical and health conditions and needs of our people in and outside South Africa." "Medical Committee ANC Secretary Report," 2 July 1978, 37/29, ANCC.

3 Davis, "Training and Deployment," 1325–42; Davis, *Cosmopolitans in Close Quarters*; Williams, "Living in exile"; Sandwell, "'Love I Cannot Begin to Explain,'" 63–81; Tsampiras, "Sex in a Time of Exile" 637–63; Lissoni and Suriano, "Married to the ANC," 129–50.

4 "Brief Report on the Medical Situation in Dar es Salaam and Morogoro area," 8 March 1979, ANCL.

5 Ibid.

6 Another clear example of miscommunication between the staff in Dar es Salaam and Morogoro was its constant "blind" transfer of patients. The patients were sent between cities without patient reports and were sometimes sent back without treatment. "Minutes of the ANC Medical and Health Committee," 26 January 1979, 112/89, ANCL.

7 "Section 6: Publication and Communications: the Role and Needs of Publication and Communication," 22 June 1979, 3/30, Karis-Gerhart Papers. Other documents suggest different dates of occupancy. For instance, "Building Project, Plot 28 – Kurasini: Report from the Project Coordinator signed A. Mekki," 15 September 1987, 41/20, ANCT. However, it is likely that the ANC

had access to the plot in the 1960s, purchased the property in the early 1970s, and only really put the accommodation to use in the mid–late 1970s. The ANC-commissioned account in *the Fourth Dimension* of the medical service provided to MK devotes a short three-paragraph description of the clinic. The account presumably made use of the archive at Fort Hare but does not cite any of the documents that it might have used in constructing its narrative. There are very few details regarding the clinic and the account presents Kurasini as a useful and unproblematic site of ANC health provision. According to the documents that I found, this ANC account does not accurately depict the health provision at the Kurasini sickbay. Naidoo, *The Fourth Dimension*, 237.

8 "Building Project, Plot 28 – Kurasini: Report from the Project Coordinator signed A. Mekki," 15 September 1987, 41/20, ANCT.

9 The Lutuli Memorial Foundation was established by the ANC's National Executive Committee in 1968 to commemorate the political work of Albert Lutuli. SEK220,000 was donated to the foundation by the Swedish government, which was consequently partly controlled by Sweden and partly controlled by the executor of Albert Luthuli's will, Gatsha Buthelezi. Tor Sellström provides a more detailed description of the history of the Luthuli Memorial Foundation in Sellström, *Sweden and National Liberation Vol II*, 522.

10 "Medical committee ANC Secretary's Report," 2 July 1978, 37/29, ANCC.

11 "The Psychological Effects of Apartheid: A Report on Survey of Mental Health Problems of ANC Members in the Republics of Tanzania and Zambia," 13 December 1982, 17/8, ANCM.

12 "Letter to the Secretary General signed Mandla Lubanga," 14 June 1982, 112/91, ANCL.

13 "The Psychological Effects of Apartheid," 13 December 1982, 17/8, ANCM. "Letter to the Secretary General signed Mandla Lubanga," 14 June 1982, 112/91, ANCL.

14 "Confidential Report to the ANC," 19 May 1983, 118/126, ANCL.

15 Most of the documents state that patients were taken to Muhimbili Hospital, which catered to the ANC's people suffering from mental illness. However, it can be assumed that some patients were taken to other hospitals in Dar es Salaam or were sent abroad for treatment.

16 "Letter to the Secretary General signed Regina Nzo and Mandla Lubanga," 8 April 1982, 112/91, ANCL.

17 "Report of the Commission of the National Executive Committee appointed to investigate the allocation and utilization of the financial resources of the organization in regions of the Front Line States and Forward Areas, March 1984–July 1984," 31 July 1984, 3/56, Karis-Gerhart Papers. There were also times where unqualified members of the ANC were operating as medical assistants. For example, Jabu Maphumulo failed to complete the Medical Assistants Course in the USSR but came back to Tanzania and worked full time in Kurasini as medical personnel. "Letter to Henry Makgothi signed Manto Tshabalala," 23 January 1984, 1/1, ANCS.

18 "Letter to Dr Akerele signed Manto Tshabalala," 12 March 1979, 17/3, ANCM.

19 Also in that year, another US$5,000 was provided by Medico International (based in Frankfurt), but this money was not immediately released to the East Africa Health Team. "Memo on Kurasini," 28 February 1983, 160/1, ANCL.

20 "Health Team Report on East Africa," 6 October 1981, 111/89, ANCL. "Report of the East Africa Health Team Meeting," 10 May 1981, 112/96, ANCL.

21 "Letter to Comrade Reddy signed Manto Tshabalala," 20 October 1981, 112/90, ANCL.

22 "Letter to the Administrative Secretary signed Nellie Mvulane," 17 October 1981, 111/89, ANCL.

23 "Confidential Report," 2 January 1981, 112/96, ANCL.

24 Ibid.

25 "Health and Apartheid in South Africa," November 1981, 51/67, ANCW [also in ANCL, 156/41].

26 "Letter to Ben Mhlathi signed Amor Moroka and E. Maseko," 17 July 1985, 3/33, ANCW. The situation in Dar es Salaam after 1985 was a disaster and of major concern to the Mazimbu team who relied on its ability to refer patients to Muhimbili Medical Centre. "Regional Health Report for the Year 1985," no date, 161/3b, ANCL.

27 "Proposed Alterations, Additions and Equipment of the ANC Kurasini Sick Bay in Dar es Salaam," [1982], 112/91, ANCL.

28 "Letter to the Treasurer General signed Manto Tshabalala,"

30 April 1982, 112/91, ANCL. "Minutes of the Regional (Tanzania) Treasury Meeting," 5 May 1982, 84/17, ANCL. "Memo on Kurasini," 28 February 1983, 160/1, ANCL. Additionally, at least part of the US$5,000 sent from Frankfurt in 1979 was also transferred into the ANC's East Africa regional treasury. Presumably, the ANC had financial accounts in each of the regions that it operated.

29 "Letter to the Treasurer General signed Manto Tshabalala," 30 April 1982, 112/91, ANCL.

30 "Unaddressed letter signed Mandla Lubanga," 14 May 1982, 112/91, ANCL.

31 "Letter to the Secretary of the East Africa Health Team signed Manto Tshabalala," 22 May 1982, 112/91, ANCL.

32 The proposal was drafted by Spencer Hodgson from the ANC Morogoro Technical Committee; the committee was presumably a bureaucratic division of the ANC leadership dealing with social service development in Tanzania. "Kurasini Medical Centre Report on Proposed Extension and Conversion of Existing Buildings," 21 October 1982, 84/17, ANCL. Monetary conversion: World Bank, "Official Exchange Rate: (1982)."

33 "Kurasini Medical Centre Report on Proposed Extension and Conversion of Existing Buildings," 21 October 1982, 84/17, ANCL.

34 It was unclear from the archive whether this US$60,000 donation was in addition to the $43,000 already given or whether it was a new total calculated by the ANC; it is likely that this was a new total raised by the organisation: "Report on Visit with Danish People's Relief Association, 5–13 February, 1983," no date, 112/92, ANCL.

35 "Memo on Kurasini," 28 February 1983, 160/1, ANCL.

36 "Unaddressed letter signed Stanley Mabizela," 24 April 1983, 32/24 ANCL.

37 "Report – Health Department for 1983," January 1984, 161/3d, ANCL.

38 "The Report of the National Women's Executive Committee held in the Libala Offices of the Women's Secretariat from the 5th to the 8th April, 1984," no date, Part I Additions, 71/13, ANCL.

39 Ibid.

40 "Meeting of the NEWC with Members of the NEC in the Libala Office," 2 April 1984, 154/23c, ANCL.

41 "Letter to Ralph Mgijima signed T.K. Maseko," 10 February 1987, Part II Additions, 9/28, ANCL.

42 "Building Project, Plot 28 – Kurasini: Report from the Project Coordinator signed A. Mekki," 15 September 1987, 41/20, ANCT. "Agreement on the Kurasini Project, Dar es Salaam, Tanzania, signed Toril Brekke (Norwegian Council for Southern Africa (FSA)) and T.T. Nkobi," December 1987, 41/20, ANCT.

43 Sean Morrow provides a good general account of the community. Sean Morrow, "Dakawa Development Centre," 497–521.

44 It is important to note, however, that the ANC Health Department continued to receive international financial support for its proposed building renovations until the ANC decided to terminate the initiative. Despite all the shortcomings of the department, donors staunchly funded medical initiatives, which demonstrated the success of the ANC's bid for political legitimacy in the anti-apartheid struggle.

45 Morrow et al. provides a basic but informative four-page account of the Mazimbu clinic. After stating that the ANC created a Health Committee, the account briefly mentions the major components: Scandinavian aid, clinic facilities available, and internal staff issues (including a mention of Tim Naidoo). Morrow's discussion invites a more detailed history of the clinic, which is provided in this section. Morrow et al, *Education in Exile*, 24–8.

46 "Letter to Manto Tshabalala signed Henk Odink," 25 November 1980, 112/94, ANCL.

47 The Dutch guilder was replaced by the euro in 2002.

48 The conversion was more complicated because the Dutch guilder was ƒ1.99 per one dollar US in 1980 but ƒ3.21 per one dollar US in 1984 when MKA's last monetary instalment was made. It was estimated that the MKA ended up raising ƒ1,000,000 Dutch guilders by May 1, 1984, but because this was not paid at one time, it was not possible to accurately calculate what this amounted to. For later figures see: "Letter to Alfred Nzo signed Henk Odink," 31 January 1984, 112/94, ANCL.

49 "Letter to Alfred Nzo signed Henk Odink," 6 July 1981, 112/90, ANCL. "Letter to Manto Tshabalala signed Henk Odink," 23 July 1981, 112/94, ANCL.

50 "Report on the Tour of Scandinavian Countries (27th April – 23rd May, 1979)," no date, 17/7, ANCM.

51 Eriksen, *Norway and National Liberation,* 147–55.

52 It is not clear whether this is the same Land Rover that was donated by the Danish People's Relief Association to the Kurasini clinic. The two Land Rovers are mentioned in correspondence from different years and in relation to separate clinics and so it is likely that they were two separate vehicles. "Letter to the ANC c/o Manto Tshabalala signed Kurt Hansen and Birthe Jeppesen (Dansk Folkenhelp)," 16 March 1981, 111/89, ANCL. "Letter to the ANC c/o Manto Tshabalala signed Birthe Jeppesen (Dansk Folkenhelp)," 11 November 1982, 111/89, ANCL.

53 "Health Supply in the Tanzania Region," no date [1987?], 31/8. ANCL. One report suggests that building the hospital actually started at the beginning of 1980, but it is likely that this was a political deception rather than accurate statement: "Summary Report of the ANC-SA Conference of the Health Department held in Lusaka from 2 – 6 January, 1980," no date, 37/29, ANCC. "Letter to Oswald Dennis signed Henk Odink," 24 October 1984, 112/94, ANCL.

54 "Medical Committee ANC Secretary Report," 2 July 1978, 37/29, ANCC. It should also be stated that the lines between the East Africa Health Team and the Mazimbu team were often blurred. Medical staff worked at Mazimbu but might be called elsewhere in Tanzania. Alternatively, a member of the broader team might be called to work in Mazimbu. Doctors working at local Tanzanian institutions are sometimes clearly members of the ANC whilst others are merely ANC sympathizers who helped out when necessary. Additionally, multiple departments reported on health issues in Tanzania. Unlike in any other region, healthcare at Mazimbu was seen as the business of the Mazimbu health team, the regional health team, the Department of Health, the Department of Education, the SOMAFCO directorate, and the Women's Section. Consequently, all of these departments reported, critiqued, and made demands. Often their accounts conflicted with one another, which added to the confusion in authority and disaster of interpersonal relationships. While there were clear clashes between the East Africa team, the Mazimbu team, and the Health Department, these might be seen as personality differences

rather than as fights between three autonomous and separated teams. See for example, "Report of the East Africa Health Team Meeting," 10 May 1981, 112/96, ANCL.

55 "Medical Committee ANC Secretary Report," 2 July 1978, 37/29, ANCC.

56 Ibid.

57 "Letter to the Secretary General signed Peter Mfelang," 7 August 1980, 111/89, ANCL.

58 "Letter to Comrade Thomas Nkobi signed Manto Tshabalala," 26 December 1981, 31/4, ANCL.

59 "Letter to Alfred Nzo signed Manto Tshabalala," 22 February 1982, 112/91, ANCL.

60 "East Africa Health Team Report to the Secretary General," 14 June 1982, 112/91, ANCL.

61 There were internal doubts as to whether the construction of the facility and acquirement of staff and equipment would be in place for the 1 May deadline. See for example: "Letter to Administrative secretary Edna [Miya] signed Manto Tshabalala," 10 February 1984, 160/1c, ANCL.

62 "Letter to Alfred Nzo signed Henk Odink," 31 January 1984, 112/94, ANCL. In March the ANC attempted to revise this date to 26 May 1984, but the new date was unacceptable to the Dutch representatives who had already booked holidays in southern Africa following the grand opening. The date was reinstated to 1 May. "Letter to Henk Odink signed Alfred Nzo," 8 March 1984, 160/1c, ANCL. "Letter to Oliver Tambo signed Henk Odink," 13 February 1984, 112/94, ANCL.

63 "Letter to Alfred Nzo signed Henk Odink," 31 January 1984, 112/94, ANCL.

64 "Letter to Chiduo signed Alfred Nzo," 17 April 1984, 130/265, ANCL.

65 In the document bearing the summaries of the speeches given at the opening ceremony, the participant is listed as "Maindy Msimang," however the name likely should have read "Mendi Msimang." "Summaries from Speeches at Official Opening of the ANC-Holland Solidarity Hospital," 1 May 1984, 8/22, ANCSHD.

66 "Planning and Organisation Meeting for the ANC-Holland solidarity Hospital held on 13/06/[19]84 – 18/06/[19]84," no date, 8/20, ANCSHD.

67 "Report of the Commission of the National Executive Committee appointed to investigate the allocation and utilization of the financial resources of the organization in regions of the Front Line States and Forward Areas, March 1984–July 1984," 31 July 1984, 3/56, Karis-Gerhart Papers.

68 "Letter to Tikly re Mrs Mzamo's arrival in Mazimbu signed Edna Miya," 7 September 1984, 161/3a, ANCL.

69 "Letter to Oswald Dennis signed Henk Odink," 24 October 1984, 112/94, ANCL.

70 Hippe and Pedersen, "Health Care in An Exile Community: Report on Health Planning in the ANC," 1987, 26–7, 31/8, ANCL.

71 One December 1986 report stated that the hospital did manage to complete sixteen circumcisions. "Health Report to the Directorate, Mazimbu/Dakawa, Nov–Dec 1986," no date, 9/31, ANCSHD. Hippe and Pedersen, "Health Care in An Exile Community," 1987, 5, 31/8, ANCL.

72 See for example: "Letter to Chief Representative Stanley Mabizela," 8 September 1987, 19/133, ANCL. Hippe and Pedersen, "Health Care in An Exile Community," 1987, 33, 31/8, ANCL.

73 "Report of the ANC-Holland Solidary Hospital – Oct–Dec. 1987," no date. ANCSD, 14/19, "Health Report to the Mazimbu Directorate March 1st–31st 1988," no date, 9/31, ANCSD.

74 "Appropriate Political and Administrative Structures are the Basic Requirements for Progress at Mazimbu," November 1980, 85/22, ANCL. "Letter to SOMAFCO Director signed Manto Tshabalala and Peter Mfelang," 19 January 1983, 112/92, ANCL.

75 "Report of the East Africa Health Team Meeting," 10 May 1981, 112/96, ANCL.

76 While the letter states that there were trained personnel at the clinic, the number and qualifications of staff is not clear. ANCL, 84/17, "Transport Report (Tanzania)," 30 June 1980, 84/17, ANCL. "Letter to Manto Tshabalala signed Tim Maseko," 9 June 1981, 112/90, ANCL.

77 "Letter to Manto Tshabalala signed Tim Maseko," 9 June 1981, 112/90, ANCL.

78 "Health Team Report on East Africa," 6 October 1981, 111/89, ANCL.

79 "List of Annexures [Consultative Committee Meeting, 1982/11–12]," various dates, 105/45, ANCL.

80 "Health Team Report on East Africa," 6 October 1981, 111/89, ANCL.
Before being appointed to the head position of the Mazimbu health
team, Tim Naidoo had been acquired to work as the SOMAFCO
nurse. Her role in the Mazimbu community (and the department she
was accountable to) was often ambiguous. "Minutes of the Special
Meeting between Directorate and Members of Women's Comm.
Medical Team held at Mazimbu," 17 April 1982, 112/95, ANCL.

81 "Unsigned letter for Tim Naidoo," April 1982, 1/1ii, ANCSHD.
"Report of the East Africa Health Team Meeting," 10 May 1981,
112/96, ANCL.

82 See for example, "Minutes of the Special Meeting between
Directorate and Members of Women's Comm. Medical Team held
at Mazimbu," 17 April 1982, 112/95, ANCL.

83 The imposition at Mazimbu highlighted authority clashes between
the East Africa Health Team and the microcosmic teams in
Mazimbu and Morogoro. Morogoro seemed to have a separate,
arguably redundant team. In 1982 the team had four members:
chair Roy Campbells and comrades Isaac Salele, Mandla Lubango,
and Meisie Martins. "Report of the Special Meeting held by the
East Africa Health Team," 8 April 1982, 31/4, ANCL.

84 "Letter to Mandla Lubango signed Tim Naidoo," 17 November 1981,
1/1ii, ANCSHD.

85 "Minutes of the Special Meeting between Directorate and Members
of Women's Comm. Medical Team held at Mazimbu," 17 April 1982,
112/95, ANCL. "Letter for Tim Naidoo," April 1982, 1/1ii, ANCSHD.

86 "Health Commission Findings," 4 December 1983, 105/45, ANCL.
"Joint Commission of Enquiry – Chief Representative's Office and
the SOMAFCO Directorate East Africa – on the Resignation of
Comrade Regina Nzo from the Health Team of the ANC SA East
Africa," 4 December 1983, 105/45, ANCL.

87 "Letter to Manto Tshabalala signed Regina Nzo," 19 January 1983,
153/22b, ANCL.

88 "East Africa Health Team meeting held in Mazimbu," 22 January
1983, 160/1, ANCL.

89 "Letter to the Secretary General signed J.G. Hauli," 17 January 1983,
160/1, ANCL.

90 "Letter to Doodles Gaboo signed Manto Tshabalala," 23 March
1983, 160/1 ANCL. 160/1, "Letter to the Treasury Department signed

Connie," 19 March 1983, 160/1, ANCL.

91 "Letter to the Chief Representative and Secretary General signed Sipho Mthembu," 31 May 1982, 160/1a, ANCL. This claim about Tshabalala's propensity for acting independently can also be seen in "Directorate Meeting," 4 June 1983, 118/126, ANCL.

92 Establishing the commission was an example of the ANC's practice at statecraft. Hugh Macmillan wrote that the ANC, for all its faults, "was unique among Southern African liberation movements for its level of self-criticism." For this reason, letters, reports, and commissions flood the archive pointing to the department's flaws; if the ANC wanted to be considered a government-in-waiting, it needed to hold departments accountable for their mistakes and show the international community that it was more than an authoritarian liberation movement. Furthermore, it was evident that the Health Department was struggling to keep its regional leadership from leaving southern Africa. Despite the problems between members, the department could not afford to lose qualified medical staff. Macmillan, *The Lusaka Years*, 166.

93 "Unsigned letter to the Chief Representative," 16 March 1983, 1/1ii, ANCSHD.

94 "List of Annexures [Consultative Committee Meeting, 1982/11–12]," various dates, 105/45, ANCL.

95 "Letter to Alfred Nzo signed Manto Tshabalala," 18 March 1983, 160/1, ANCL.

96 "Letter to the SOMAFCO Director signed Mfelang and Manto Tshabalala," 24 January 1983, 160/1, ANCL.

97 "Joint Commission of Enquiry – Chief Representative's Office and the SOMAFCO Directorate East Africa – on the Resignation of Comrade Regina Nzo from the Health Team of the ANC SA East Africa," 4 December 1983, 105/45, ANCL.

98 "Letter to James Stuart signed Zakes Mokoena," 20 September 1987, Part II Additions, 33/1, ANCL. "Memo to the Heads of all Regional Health Teams," 31 August 1989, Part II Additions, 9/30, ANCL.

99 "Directorate Meeting," 4 June 1983, 118/126, ANCL.

100 "Health Team Report on East Africa," 6 October 1981, 111/89, ANCL.

101 "Confidential Report," 30 December 1981, 112/96, ANCL.

102 "Report of the East Africa Health Team Meeting," 10 May 1981, 112/96, ANCL.

103 Ibid.

104 Ibid.

105 "Confidential Report to the ANC," 19 May 1983, 118/126, ANCL.

106 "Letter to East Africa Health Team signed Manto Tshabalala," 15 July 1982, 1/2, ANCSHD.

107 The issues did not abate after the joint commission. Instead, the friction remained relatively constant. See for example, "Letter to the Treasurer General signed [Victor Maome?]," 4 January 1984, 160/1b, ANCL.

108 "ANC Regional Health Team – need for a doctor in Mazimbu," 18 June 1982, 96/5a, ANCL.

109 In cases of emergency, the clinic could call on the services of three medical students in the area as well. "Report by the Commission on Enquiry into the Accident on the August 1982," 10 September 1982, 128/239, ANCL.

110 "Consultative Committee Meeting between Working Committee and Health Department held from 30 November to 2nd December 1982 in Lusaka–Zambia," no date, 160/1 ANCL.

111 "Report of the Commission of the National Executive Committee appointed to investigate the allocation and utilization of the financial resources of the organization in regions of the Front Line States and Forward Areas, March 1984–July 1984," 31 July 1984, 3/56, Karis-Gerhart Papers.

112 "Consultative Committee Meeting between Working Committee and Health Department held from 30 November to 2nd December 1982 in Lusaka–Zambia," no date, 160/1 ANCL.

113 "Letter to Joe Nhlanhla signed Peter Mfelang and Manto Tshabalala," 21 February 1983, 160/1, ANCL.

114 "Directorate Meeting," 26 March 1983, 118/126, ANCL.

115 "Letter to the Secretary General signed Stanley Mabizela," 22 April 1983, 108/71, ANCL.

116 Ibid.

117 "Letter to Secretary General Alfred Nzo signed Stanley Mabizela," 4 December 1983, 112/92, ANCL.

118 For other similar examples, see: "Letter to Makgothi signed the Primary School Mazimbu Staff," 25 May 1983, 1/1ii, ANCSHD. "Letter to Henry Makgothi signed Mohammed Tikly," 30 May 1983, 112/92, ANCL.

119 "Meeting of the Regional Health Team with the National held at Mazimbu Clinic," 15 August 1983, 8/20, ANCSHD.

120 "Directorate Meeting," 4 June 1983, 118/126, ANCL.

121 The Department of Health did not state that the reason for sending Mthembu to Angola was his unsuitability for SOMAFCO. Instead, they diplomatically wrote, "Whilst recognising the desires and pleasures of our population in Mazimbu, we never-the-less consider that Angola and other forward areas should be given the priority … the presence of a doctor in the hospital in Luanda would not only be contributing to the development of this country but also help in clearing some of the referred patients." "Letter to the Secretary General signed Mfelang and Tshabalala," 13 June 1983, 1/1ii, ANCSHD.

122 "Letter to Amor Moroka signed Manto Tshabalala," 20 June 1983, 112/92, ANCL.

123 "Minutes of Directorate Meeting," 9 July 1983, 118/126, ANCL.

124 "Letter to Manto Tshabalala signed Dr A. Moroka," 31 August 1983, 160/1b, ANCL.

125 Specifically, the problem of injection abscesses was raised; the leadership called for an in-service training course to make sure staff was sterilizing the needles correctly. "Meeting with Mazimbu Health Team," 7 July 1985, 161/3b, ANCL.

126 "Report on a visit to East Africa from 7th July to 10th August 1985," no date, 2/1iii, ANCSHD.

127 "Regional Health Report for the Year 1985," no date, 161/3b, ANCL.

128 There is a similar case between a solidarity worker Dr September Williams (who worked in Mazimbu for approximately six months) and the Mazimbu team. Upon her return home, September Williams gave an interview on her experience in Mazimbu; this was done, in part, to raise money for pharmaceutical drugs for the hospital. The Mazimbu team believed that Williams embellished the incompetency of the health team and the hospital: "It wass [sic] absurd, and again a nagative [sic] image of the A.N.C., a good propaganda for the Boers to destroy the stature of the A.N.C. in ezile [sic], and how it runs its health services. While we criticise the health services rendered by the regime to our people in South Africa." They then lamented the lack of screening personnel when recruiting non-ANC people from abroad. From documents

in the archive, Dr Williams' statements were not an outlandish embellishment of the situation but the paternalistic tone in which the interview was written certainly hit a nerve with the health team. "Letter to Robert Manci signed E. Maseko," 27 January 1986, 2/1iii, ANCSHD. "The Physicians Forum, *Bulletin*," Fall 1985, 2/1iii, ANCSHD.

129 At times, the child's treatment course does not seem to make medical sense. However, without a complete medical record, it is impossible to develop a coherent clinical picture and fully appreciate the strictly medical decisions made on behalf of this child. This example demonstrates the way that infighting, and miscommunication affected patient care.

130 The child's surname did not remain consistent throughout the documents. However, the letters and reports cited here are definitely discussing the same child.

131 "Report on the Treatment of [redacted] in East Africa," 9 March 1984, 160 (held in box 161)/53, ANCL.

132 Ibid.

133 Ibid.; "Report signed by R. Nzo, missing page one," no date [1983], 112/92, ANCL; "Medical Report," 22 February 1984, 160/1c, ANCL.

134 "Special Directorate Meeting held on the 29th April, 1983," no date, 118/126, ANCL. "Meeting of the Regional Health Team with the National held at Mazimbu Clinic," 15 August 1983, 8/20, ANCSHD.

135 It is possible that the child was actually taken to the clinic in October.

136 "Report signed by R. Nzo, missing page one," no date [1983], 112/92, ANCL.

137 "Letter to the Women's Secretariat signed Jane Dumase," 7 December 1982, 118/131, ANCL.

138 "Report on the Treatment of [redacted] in East Africa," 9 March 1984, 160 (held in box 161)/53, ANCL.

139 Ibid.

140 "Letter to Stanley Mabizela signed Mohammed Tikley," 10 January 1983, 112/92, ANCL.

141 "Report on the Treatment of [redacted] in East Africa," 9 March 1984, 160 (held in box 161)/53, ANCL.

142 "Meeting of the Regional Health Team with the National held at Mazimbu Clinic," 15 August 1983, 8/20, ANCSHD.

143 "Letter to Alfred Nzo signed Gertrude Shope," 15 August 1983, 154/23C, ANCL.

144 "Letter to Uriah Mokeba signed Simon Makana," 3 October 1983, 118/131, ANCL. "Letter to Wilfried signed [redacted] and [redacted]," no date [December 1982], 118/131, ANCL. "Letter to Wilfried Morke signed Uriah Mokeba," 7 October 1983, 118/131, ANCL.

145 "Letter to Alfred Nzo signed Uriah Mokeba," 15, January 1984, 32/2, ANCL.

146 "Medical Report," 22 February 1984, 160/1C, ANCL.

147 "Report on the Treatment of [redacted] in East Africa," 9 March 1984, 160 (held in box 161)/53, ANCL.

148 "Consultative Committee Meeting between Working Committee and Health Department held from 30 November to 2nd December 1982 in Lusaka–Zambia," no date, 160/1 ANCL.

Chapter Five

1 The "State of Exile" is the title of Tom Lodge's 1987 article. In contrast to what is described here regarding the individual's experience of exile, Lodge argued that the ANC's position in exile was advantageous to the collective development of the ANC as a political movement. Lodge, "State of Exile," 1–27.

2 An excellent chapter on the trials and tribulations of living in exile can be found in the first chapter of Hugh Macmillan's account of the ANC in Zambia. Macmillan, *The Lusaka Years*, 1–12.

3 Considerable scholarship was spurred on, in part, by Michel Foucault's 1965 publication of *Madness and Civilization* – which proposed that the definition and treatment of madness was a reflection of society and its cultural, intellectual, and economic structures – historians also looked at madness not as a timeless condition but as a shifting historical category. Foucault, *Madness and Civilization*.

4 Vaughan, *Curing Their Ills*, 8–12.

5 McCulloch, *Colonial Psychiatry*; Keller, Colonial Madness; Parle, *States of Mind*; Vaughan, *Curing Their Ills*.

6 See for instance, Edgar and Sapire, *African Apocalypse*.

7 Mahone's account suggests pathology of mass revolution. Mahone, "The Psychology of Rebellion," 241–58. Mahone also points to

psychiatrist J.C. Carothers' report "The Psychology of Mau Mau."

8 See for example, Jackson, "The Place of Psychiatry," 38–71; Packard, "Post-colonial Medicine," 97–112; Dousemetzis, *The Man Who Killed Apartheid*; Jones, *Psychiatry*.

9 This chapter also draws on examples of patients with epilepsy. Health reports diagnose patients with "hysterical epilepsy," a diagnosis consistent with the time period's understanding of the causes of epilepsy. One description of a patient was particularly revealing: the patient was said to have the "hysteric form of epilepsy with concealed depression – poor emotional control." This was thought to be caused by the experience of being in exile. "ANC Health Report to Directorate," May 1984, 9/31, ANCSD.

10 Maurice Mthombeni, "Account of experiences while training as a guerrilla for the ANC of S. Africa," [1969?], 3/16, Karis-Gerhart Papers.

11 The use of Mirembe in the 1960s was confirmed by patient histories produced in the 1980s. See for instance "Letter to Manto Tshabalala signed Dr J.G. Hauli," 20 March 1981, 112/90, ANCL.

12 "Southern Africa: a Betrayal", *The Black Dwarf*, Nov. 26, 1969," 26 November 1969, 3/16, Karis-Gerhart Papers.

13 Bopela and Luthuli, *Umkhonto We Siswe*, 34.

14 "Apartheid and Mental Health Care," 22 March 1977, 8/25, ANCSHD.

15 Ibid., 16.

16 Ibid.

17 Ibid., 20.

18 Ibid.

19 "African Mental Health Action Group – Regional Reports," 7 May 1983, Part I Additions, 84/8, ANCL.

20 "African Mental Health Action Group: Fifth Meeting," 8 May 1982, Part I Additions, 84/8, ANCL.

21 Ibid.

22 "African Mental Health Action Group – Regional Reports," 7 May 1983, Part I Additions, 84/8, ANCL. "African Mental Health Action Group: Fifth Meeting," 8 May 1982, Part I Additions, 84/8, ANCL.

23 Ibid.

24 Ibid.

25 Ibid.

26 See for instance, "Letter to the Secretary General signed Stanley Mabizela," 10 December 1977, 96/5b, ANCL.

27 "Minutes of the ANC Medical and Health Committee," 26 January 1979, 112/89, ANCL.

28 "Maputo Clinic Report," no date [December 1979?], 17/7, ANCM.

29 "President's Draft Report," 5, May 1979, 3/30, Karis-Gerhart Papers.

30 "Letter to Freddy Reddy signed Manto Tshabalala," 11 February 1983, 160/1, ANCL. "Letter to Freddy Reddy signed Manto Tshabalala," 30 March 1983, 112/92, ANCL. "The Psychological Effects of Apartheid: A report on survey of mental health problems of ANC members in the Republics of Tanzania and Zambia," 13 December 1982, 17/8, ANCM. "Meeting of the Regional Health Team with the National," 15 August 1983, 8/20, ANCSHD. "East Africa Regional Health Team Meeting held at Mazimbu Clinic," 11 September 1983, 160/1b, ANCL. Personal correspondence with Dr Per Borgå, 2 October 2016.

31 "Summary Report of the ANC-SA Conference of the Health Department held in Lusaka from 2–6 January, 1980," no date, 37/29, ANCC. "Interview with Dr Freddy Reddy," 12, 9/7-1670, Hilda Bernstein Interviews.

32 "Depression" and "Combat Nostalgia" were the labels used by the patient herself; Mayford Ngqobe (part of the Lusaka health team) does not specify the patient's diagnosis. However, it is likely that both labels were given to the comrade, and she included them in her personal plea to visit her parents in Botswana as part of her rehabilitation process. "Letter to the Secretary General signed Mayford Mgqobe with enclosed letter from patient," 8 November 1980, 130/126, ANCL.

33 See for instance, "Memo regarding [redacted]," 21 November 1980, 31/4, ANCL. "Letter from Comrade Makopo re [redacted] signed Joe Nhlanhla," 31 January 1980, Part I Additions, 1/4, ANCL. "Psychiatric Finding on [redacted] signed Freddy Reddy," 23 July 1980, 111/89, ANCL.

34 "Report on the Secretary's Trip to Angola from the 27th July to August 13, 1980," 10 September 1980, 31/4, ANCL.

35 "Letter to the Secretary General signed Reddy Mazimbu," 3 December 1980, 96/5a, ANCL.

36 "Letter to Sindiso Mfenyane signed Freddy Reddy," 6 March 1981, 111/89, ANCL [and 112/90, ANCL].

37 WHO, *Health and Apartheid Part 1 & II.*

38 Ibid., 36.

39 The WHO did offer the help of a consultant psychiatrist who was a member of the Bulgarian Communist Party, but there is little evidence in the archive of this man working for the ANC. It may be that he was not cleared by security or simply that he did not write reports back to the ANC on his work with patients. "Letter to Alfred Nzo signed Manto Tshabalala," 27 December 1981, 112/90, ANCL; WHO, *Health and Apartheid Part 1 & II*, 37.

40 "Letter to Ndugu Chiduo signed Alfred Nzo," 28 June 1982, 160/1, ANCL; "Aide-memoire: Implementation of the recommendations and the plan of action of the Brazzaville Conference on Health and Apartheid," 17 May 1982, 112/91, ANCL.

41 Including outsiders to such a degree of involvement was considered a security hazard and would require permission from a number of people in the leadership. It is interesting to note that Dr Hauli and not Dr Reddy was selected for this important role. ANCL, 112/91, "Letter to Secretary General Alfred Nzo signed Manto Tshabalala," 17 May 1982, 112/91, ANCL; "Letter to Secretary General Alfred Nzo signed Manto Tshabalala," 21 June 1982, 160/1, ANCL; "Letter to Tanzania Minister for Health Ndugu Chiduo signed Alfred Nzo," 28 June 1982, 160/1, ANCL.

42 "The Psychological Effects of Apartheid: A Report on Survey of Mental Health Problems of ANC Members in the Republics of Tanzania and Zambia," 13 December 1982, 17/8, ANCM.

43 The report estimates 800 ANC members in Zambia but curiously accounts for only 600 of these in its regional breakdown. Further, it is hard to assess how much this report reflected the realities on the ground. It should be considered a reference point rather than a perfect representation.

44 The investigation did not include infants in the analysis.

45 Suicide in the military frontline states appeared to be much higher than the rate recorded in Zambia and Tanzania. Additionally, there was good reason to believe that many mentally ill patients were not reported.

46 Zimbabwe's 1983 report to the African Mental Health Action Group showed that its community nurses saw approximately 2,700 patients per month in a population of more than 7.5 million people. "African Mental Health Action Group- Zimbabwe Report; Sixth Meeting,

Geneva," 7 May 1983, Part I Additions, 84/8, ANCL.

47 "The Psychological Effects of Apartheid," 13 December 1982, 17/8, ANCM. "ANC Department of Health, Report – Health Department January 1983–December 1983," January 1984, 161/3d, ANCL.

48 "Project Proposal to WHO for Extrabudgetary Funding – Mental Health and PHC Workshops," 1983, 11/34, ANCSD.

49 Personal interview with Dr Per Borgå, 2016/10/02.

50 "Recommendations of the ANC Primary Health Care Workshop," 30 December 1983, Part II Additions, 9/28, ANCL.

51 "ANC Department of Health, Report – Health Department January 1983–December 1983," January 1984, 161/3d, ANCL.

52 Morrow, "Dakawa Development Centre," 511.

53 For instance, "Minutes of the Health Committee Meeting," 20 April 1983, 8/22, ANCSHD. ANCL, 34/24, "Letter to Secretary General signed Stanley Mabizela," 31 May 1983, 34/24, ANCL.

54 See for Example, "Patient Report [redacted]," 8 May 1984, Part II Additions, 9/28, ANCL.

55 The patient was sent to a traditional healer in Dar es Salaam instead of in Lusaka, and there was no accompanying report on whether the treatment was helpful to the patient. "Continuation of Adjourned Meeting of Directorate," 16 July 1983, 118/126, ANCL. "Letter to H. Makgothi signed R. Nzo on behalf of the East Africa Health Team," no date [1982], 112/91, ANCL.

56 Personal interview with Dr Per Borgå, 2 October 2016.

57 "Report of the National Preparatory Committee (NPC)," November 1986, 31/11, ANCL.

58 "ANC Health Report to Directorate," May 1984, 9/31, ANCSD.

59 "Special Directorate Meeting with Invited Members to Discuss Suspensions and Disciplinary Actions taken Against Students from SOMAFCO," 18 April 1982, 127/228, ANCL.

60 "Report of the East Africa Health Team Meeting," 12, 10 May 1981, 112/96, ANCL. For examples of accusations against the medical staff see "Directorate Meeting," 4 June 1983, 118/126, ANCL. "Report of the East Africa Health Team Meeting," 10 May 1981, 112/96, ANCL.

61 "The Present Situation in East Africa Needs Serious Attention," 24 August 1981, 3/40, Karis-Gerhart Papers.

62 "Letter to the Administrative Secretary signed Nellie Mvulane," 17 October 1981, 111/89, ANCL.

63 Ibid.

64 It is unclear which specific conference she is referring to. "Letter to the Secretary of the Regional Political Committee in East Africa signed Manto Tshabalala," 19 October 1981, Part II Additions, 42/87, ANCL.

65 "The Menace of Alcoholism," 29 January 1984, 7/11, ANCSD.

66 "Letter to the Secretary General signed Dr Hauli," 17 January 1983, 160/1, ANCL. "Confidential Report to the ANC," 19 May 1983, 118/126, ANCL.

67 "ANC Second Seminar on Dakawa Development Centre 17–19 November, 1983," no date, Part I Additions, 79/37, ANCL.

68 "Directorate Meeting," 26 March 1983, 118/126, ANCL.

69 "Letter to the Secretary of Ed Makgothi signed Victor Maome," 1 August 1984, 161/3a, ANCL.

70 "Health Education Program Proposals signed Arthur Sidweshu," September 1983, 7/16, ANCSD.

71 "The Psychological Effects of Apartheid," 9, 13 December 1982, 17/8, ANCM.

72 "Letter to National Health Secretary signed Victor Maome," 20 April 1984 161/3a, ANCL. "Report on the Special Extended Meeting of the Secretary General's Office to Discuss the Pressing Problems of the Department of Health, 29th Nov–2 Dec 84, Lusaka," no date, 106/53, ANCL.

73 See for instance, "Letter to the Medical Department Lusaka signed Sipho Mthembu," 12 March 1984, 160/1c, ANCL [also in: ANCL, Part II Additions, 7/16, ANCL].

74 "Minutes of Special Directorate Meeting on Adult Education," 27 March 1984, 118/126, ANCL.

75 "Letter to the Secretary/Deputy Secretary for Health signed E. Maseko," 27 January 1984, 1/1, ANCSHD.

76 "Report on Activities in Harare (01 – 04.04.84)," 10 April 1984, 161/3a, ANCL. "Report on Visit to Harare, Zimbabwe," 25 October 1984, 106/53, ANCL.

77 "Letter to George and Teddy signed Manto Tshabalala," 28 May 1984, 161/3a, ANCL.

78 "Report on the Mental Health Problems after a Tour of All ANC Centres in Angola and Lusaka," 1984, 29/4, ANCL. "Security Department Report: Prevailing Situation in Angola," 3 January

1984, 132/272, ANCL. "Recommendations of the MK Commission after Disturbances," February 1984, 132/272, ANCL. "Letter to the General Secretary Office signed [redacted]," 7 July 1984, 161/3a, ANCL.

79 Hippe and Pedersen, "Health Care in An Exile Community: Report on Health Planning in the ANC," 1987, 52, 31/8, ANCL.

80 "Work Report January to April 1985 at ANC – Solidarity Hospital, Mazimbu, 'Psychiatric Section,'" no date, Part II Additions, 42/107, ANCL.

81 "Letter to SG re Psychiatric patient [redacted] signed Stanley Mabizela," 26 March 1985, 128/240, ANCL.

82 "Letter to Slim (SOMAFCO) signed Henry Makgothi," 11 July 1985, 161/3b, ANCL.

83 "C.B.R. Programme," 1 August 1985, 38/113, ANCSD. "Community Based Rehabilitation Report, 1st August, 31st August," no date, 38/113, ANCSD.

84 "Raymond Mhlaba Rehabilitation Centre Community Based Monthly Report," 18 October 1985, 38/113, ANCSD.

85 "Meeting with Mazimbu Health Team," 7 July 1985, 161/3b, ANCL.

86 "Regional Health Report for the Year 1985," no date, 161/3b, ANCL.

87 "Quarterly report from Social Welfare Department for Directorate. Months: January, February, March, 1986," 26 June 1986, 131/257b, ANCL. "Six Monthly Report," May 1986, 131/275b, ANCL.

88 "ANC East Africa Regional Health Team: Mental Health Report," November 1986, 36/8, ANCT.

89 "Community Based Rehabilitation Team, Dakawa [Third Health Council Meeting]," no date [July–August 1986], 127/236, ANCL.

90 Hippe and Pedersen, "Health Care in An Exile Community," 1987, 28–9, 31/8, ANCL.

91 Interestingly, as she was finishing her term as social worker in Mazimbu, she welcomed the move to bring the Social Welfare Department under the wing of the Health Department. Ibid., 41. "Social Work Final Evaluation Report covering December, 1985–October 1987," September 1987, 65/39, ANCW.

92 Hippe and Pedersen, "Health Care in An Exile Community," 1987, 78, 31/8, ANCL.

93 Ibid., 91.

94 "Annual Regional Health Report East Africa from 1/1/86 to 27/3/87," no date, Part II Additions, 41/64, ANCL.

95 "Letter to Ralph Mgijima signed T.K. Maseko," 10 February 1987, Part II Additions, 9/28, ANCL.

96 "Social Work Final Evaluation Report covering December, 1985– October 1987," September 1987, 65/39, ANCW.

97 "Dakawa–Mazimbu Health Team Reports," November 1987, 14/19, ANCSD.

98 "Health Secretariat Meeting with the Emmasdale Clinic Committee on 1.11.88," 5 November 1988, Part II Additions, 42/104, ANCL.

99 "Psychiatric Services in the Region," 3 February 1989, Part II Additions, 6/7, ANCL.

100 "ANC Social Work Unit," 20 June 1990, 44/17, ANCW.

101 "Letter to Ralph Mgijima signed Freddy Reddy," 17 March 1990, Part II Addition, 6/8a, ANCL.

102 "Social Work Unit's Report on Lusaka," August 1990, Part II Additions, 37/18, ANCL.

103 "Paper on Material and other Assistance to the ANC in Support of Development Programmes for S. Africans in Exile," 22 June 1979, 3/30, Karis-Gerhart Papers. Also see, "Interview with Dr Freddy Reddy," 12, 9/7-1670, Hilda Bernstein Interviews.

104 "Letter to Whom it May Concern signed Dr Dlamini (Mbabane Government Hospital)," 28 April 1981, 111/89, ANCL.

105 See for instance, "Letter to the ANC signed Dr Lucieer," 6 October 1981, 96/5a, ANCL. Comrades were also frequently diagnosed with dagga-induced schizophrenia, and "the excessive use of alcohol or cannabis as casual factors to mental illness were attributed to the stressful exile [sic] and ineffective coping mechanisms." "Health Department Contribution on the Development of Dakawa November 17–19th, 1983," no date, 11/33, ANCSHD.

106 "Letter to the Secretary General signed Stanley Mabizela," 2 November 1981, 111/89, ANCL. "Letter to the Secretary General signed Florence Maleka," 11 June 1981.

107 WHO, *Health and Apartheid Part 1 & II*.

108 "Health and Apartheid in South Africa," November 1981, 51/67, ANCW.

109 Ibid.

110 "ANC Health Centre at Mazimbu, Morogoro, Tanzania," no date [1982], 160/1, ANCL.

111 "Kurasini Medical Centre Report on Proposed Extension and Conversion of Existing Buildings," 21 October 1982, 84/17, ANCL.

112 "Aide-memoire: Implementation of the recommendations and the plan of action of the Brazzaville Conference on Health and Apartheid," 17 May 1982, 112/91, ANCL.

113 See for instance, "Project Proposal to WHO for Extrabudgetary Funding – Mental Health and PHC Workshops," 1983, 11/34, ANCSD.

114 "Letter to 'Parties interested in the Mental Effects of the policy of Apartheid in South Africa' signed John Dommisse," September 1983, Part II Additions, 8/25, ANCL. "Letter to Arthur M. Sachler, MD signed John Dommisse," 3 July 1984, Part II Additions, 8/25, ANCL.

115 A study sponsored by the UN Centre Against Apartheid also called for the expulsion of South Africa: Jewkes, *The Case for South Africa's Expulsion*.

116 Burke, "Mental Health and Apartheid," 144–8. See also, "Unofficial W.P.A. Committee for the Expulsion of South Africa," June 1984, Part II Additions, 8/25, ANCL.

117 "Letter to Dr J. Dommisse signed Dr C.E.M. Viljoen/Secretary General," 19 June 1984, Part II Additions, 8/25, ANCL.

118 The World Federation for Mental Health is a nongovernment organisation that was established in 1948. The number of times that the federation meets per year is not clear. The federation's actions are included in this chapter because they show a gradual shift in opinion against apartheid policies and apartheid's effects on mental health in South Africa.

119 Dommisse, "The Psychological Effects," 61.

120 Dommisse reiterated these points in a second academic article published in 1987. Dommisse, "The State of Psychiatry," 749–61.

121 "Letter to Manto Tshabalala signed Tim Maseko," 9 June 1981, 112/90, ANCL.

122 "Interview with Dr Freddy Reddy," 19, 9/7-1670, Hilda Bernstein Interviews.

123 Fanon, *Black Skin, White Masks*, 100.

124 "Interview with Dr Freddy Reddy," 16, 9/7-1670, Hilda Bernstein Interviews.

125 "Health and Apartheid in South Africa," 10 November 1981, 51/67, ANCW.

126 Davis, *Cosmopolitans in Close Quarters*, 158.

127 "Unsigned letter to Andrew Masondo," 28 October 1981, 105/44, ANCL.

128 "Statement to the Truth and Reconciliation Commission," booklet, 19 August 1996, with appendices: Stuart, L. Skweyiya, and Motsuenyane Commission Reports, Report on Death of Thami Zulu, 19 August 1996, 3/99, Karis-Gerhart Papers.

129 Trewhela, *Inside Quatro*; Trewhela, "The Death of Albert Nzula," 27; Trewhela, "The ANC Prison Camps," 8–30; Trewhela, "A Namibian Horror."

130 Also see *Mutiny in the ANC, 1984* (Justice for Southern Africa/ Solidarity with Ex-SWAPO Detainees, 1996).

131 Ellis, *External Mission*, 179.

132 Macmillan, *The Lusaka Years*, 144, 249. Also see Ellis, "Mbokodo," 279–98; Ellis, "Politics and Crime," 622–36.

133 Macmillan, *The Lusaka Years*, 151.

134 The Stuart Commission, Skweyiya Commission, Motsueyane Commission, and the Jobodwana report were the focus of Ellis, "Mbokodo."

135 "Report: Commission of inquiry into Recent Developments in the People's Republic of Angola, March 14, 1984, Lusaka [Stuart Commission Report]," 33, 14 March 1984, 3/55, Karis-Gerhart Papers.

136 "Statement to the Truth and Reconciliation Commission," booklet, 19 August 1996, with appendices: Stuart, L. Skweyiya, and Motsuenyane Commission Reports, Report on Death of Thami Zulu, 19 August 1996, 3/99, Karis-Gerhart Papers.

137 Ibid., 12.

138 TRC, *Truth and Reconciliation Report*, 365.

139 Personal interview with Dr Vuyo Mpumlwana, 9 March 2016.

140 "Report of the Commission of the National Executive Committee appointed to investigate the allocation and utilization of the financial resources of the organization in regions of the Front Line States and Forward Areas, March 1984–July 1984," 31 July 1984, 3/56, Karis-Gerhart Papers.

141 "Letter to Alfred Nzo signed Manto Tshabalala," 12 December 1980, 111/89, ANCL.

142 Personal interview with Pia Mothander, 11 March 2016.

143 "Letter to the Secretary General Alfred Nzo signed Chief Representative Reddy Mazimbu," 3 December 1980, 95/5a, ANCL.

144 Personal interview with Pia Mothander, 11 March 2016.

145 "Memorandum on our Findings in the Muhimbili Psychiatric Unit," no date [1981], 112/90, ANCL.

146 "Letter to the Administrative Secretary in Lusaka signed the Chief Representative in Harare," 4 February 1984, Part II Additions, 9/28, ANCL.

147 "Medical Report," 22 February 1984, 160/1c, ANCL.

148 "The Report of the National Women's Executive Committee held in the Libala Offices of the Women's Secretariat from the 5th to the 8th April, 1984," no date, Part I Additions, 71/13, ANCL.

149 "Report on the Special Extended Meeting of the Secretary General's Office to Discuss the Pressing Problems of the Department of Health, 29th Nov–2 Dec 84, Lusaka," no date, 106/53, ANCL.

150 "Interview with Dr Freddy Reddy," 19, 9/7-1670, Hilda Bernstein Interviews.

151 Personal interview with Dr Vuyo Mpumlwana, 9 March 2016.

152 Dr Mpumlwana also discussed the fact that the ANC was not unique in its oppressive need for internal security. There are other accounts of human rights abuses within liberation movements. In particular, Dr Kalister Christine Manyame-Tazarurwa's book on the experiences of Zimbabwean women in the liberation struggle sheds light on this issue in the Zimbabwean context. Manyame-Tazarurwa, *Health Impact of Participation*.

153 "Meeting of the Regional Health Team with the National," 5, 15 August 1983, 8/20, ANCSHD. "Interview with Dr Freddy Reddy," 15–16, 9/7-1670, Hilda Bernstein Interviews.

154 "Interview with Dr Freddy Reddy," 15–16, 9/7-1670, Hilda Bernstein Interviews.

155 A view also shared in "Regional Health Meeting in Mazimbu," 31 December 1983, 33/72, ANCW.

156 "Letter to Alfred Nzo signed [redacted]," 24 September 1984, 128/240, ANCL.

157 "Report: Commission of inquiry into Recent Developments in the People's Republic of Angola, March 14, 1984, Lusaka [Stuart

Commission Report]," 3, 14 March 1984, 3/55, Karis-Gerhart Papers.

158 "Report on the Mental Health Problems after a Tour of All ANC Centres in Angola and Lusaka," 1984, 29/4, ANCL.

159 "Report: Commission of inquiry into Recent Developments in the People's Republic of Angola, March 14, 1984, Lusaka [Stuart Commission Report]," 6, 14 March 1984, 3/55, Karis-Gerhart Papers.

160 See for instance, "Health Department Contribution on the Development of Dakawa November 17–19th, 1983," no date, 11/33, ANCSHD.

161 Ibid.

162 "ANC Health Report to Directorate," May 1984, 9/31, ANCSD.

163 "Meeting of the Regional Health Team with the National," 5, 15 August 1983, 8/20, ANCSHD. "Interview with Dr Freddy Reddy," 1516, 9/7-1670, Hilda Bernstein Interviews.

164 "Report on the Mental Health Problems after a Tour of All ANC Centres in Angola and Lusaka," 1984, 29/4, ANCL.

Conclusion

1 "Paper by Chris Hani to the AIDS Workshop," May–June, 1990, Part II Additions, 64/25, ANCL.

2 "Draft Guidelines 930806 ANC Health Policy: Human Resources Development," 8 August 1983, 49/29b, LH.

3 Hammett, "Cuban Intervention," 63–81.

4 It should be noted that Tshabalala's health record does not state that alcoholism was the cause of her liver failure.

5 Shell and Qaga, "Trojan Horses," 24–7; Tsampiras, "Politics, Polemics, and Practice."

6 Klausen, *Abortion Under Apartheid*; Hodes, "HIV/AIDS in South African Documentary Film," 153–71; Hodes, "The Medical History of Abortion," 527–54; Mbali. "Mbeki's Denialism"; Mandisa Mbali, "A Long Illness."

7 "Medical committee ANC Secretary's Report," 2 July 1978, 37/29, ANCC.

Bibliography

Archival collections

African National Congress Archives (ANC),
University of Fort Hare, Alice:
    Canada series (ANCC)
    Finland Series (ANCF)
    Lusaka series (ANCL)
    Luthuli House (LH)
    Mozambique series (ANCM)
    Netherlands series (ANCNL)
    Oliver Tambo Papers (OTP)
    SOMAFCO Dakawa (ANCSD)
    SOMAFCO Health Department (ANCSHD)
    Swedish series (ANCS)
    Tanzania series (ANCT)
    Women's Section (ANCW)

University of the Western Cape, Mayibuye Centre, Cape Town:

Hilda Bernstein interviews
Interview with Dr Prenaiver Naicker, Harare
Interview with Dr Freddy Reddy (Norway, 1990)
Interview with Dr Gwendolyn Sello (Tanzania, 1989)

Historical Papers Research Archive, University of the Witwatersrand,
    Johannesburg
Federation of South African Women 1954–63
Karis-Gerhart Collection

Interviews

Borgå, Per. Interview by author. 2 October 2016; personal
  correspondence, March 2016–October 2016.
Mpumlwana, Vuyo. Interview by author. 9 March 2016.
Mothander, Pia. Interview by author. 11 March 2016.

Published Sources

Adepoju, Aderanti. "The Dimension of the Refugee Problem in Africa."
  African Affairs 81, no. 322 (1982): 21–35.
Ahlman, Jeffrey S. *Living with Nkrumahism: Nation, State, and Pan-
  Africanism in Ghana.* Urbana and Champaign: University of
  Illinois at Urbana-Champaign, 2011.
—. "Road to Ghana: Nkrumah, Southern Africa and the Eclipse of a
  Decolonizing Africa." *Kronos* 37, no. 1 (2011): 23–40.
Allman, Jean. "Nuclear Imperialism and the Pan-African Struggle
  for Peace and Freedom: Ghana, 1959–1962." *Souls* 10, no. 2 (2008):
  83–102.
Armstrong, Melissa. "Healthcare in Exile: ANC Health Policy and
  Health Care Provision in MK Camps, 1964 to 1989." *South African
  Historical Journal* 66, no. 2 (3 April 2014): 270–90.
—. "Militias, Maladies and Medicine: Towards a History of Health in
  Umkhonto weSizwe Camps." MSc Thesis, Oxford University, 2013.
Baldwin-Ragaven, Laurel, Leslie London, and Jeanelle De Gruchy. *An
  Ambulance of the Wrong Colour: Health Professionals, Human
  Rights and Ethics in South Africa.* Cape Town: University of Cape
  Town Press, 1999.
Barrell, Howard. *MK: The ANC's Armed Struggle.* London, UK: Penguin
  Books, 1990.
Baxter, Lawrence. "Doctors on Trial: Steve Biko, Medical Ethics, and the
  Courts." *South African Journal on Human Rights* 1 (1985): 137–51.
BBC Africa. "South Africa Local Elections: ANC Loses in Capital
  Pretoria." Accessed 6 August 2016. http://www.bbc.co.uk/
  indepthtoolkit/charts/SApolls?iframe=true&iframeUID=58363361d
  2fc0&initialWidth=592&childId=58363361d2fc0&parentUrl=http%3
  A%2F%2Fwww.bbc.com%2Fnews%2Fworld-africa-36997461.
Beinart, William. *The Political Economy of Pondoland.* Cambridge:
  Cambridge University Press, 1982.

Benatar, S.R. "Detention Without Trial, Hunger Strikes and Medical Ethics." *Law, Medicine & Health Care* 18 (1990): 140–5.

Bernstein, Hilda. *The Rift: The Exile Experience of South Africans.* London: Random House UK, 1994.

Bhasin, Tavishi, and Maia Carter Hallward. "Hamas as a Political Party: Democratization in the Palestinian Territories." *Terrorism and Political Violence* 25, no. 1 (2013): 75–93.

Bhebe, Ngwabi, and Gerald C. Mazarire. "'Paying the Ultimate Price': Zimbabwe and the Liberation of South Africa, 1980–1994." In *The Road to Democracy in South Africa*, vol. 5. Pretoria: UNISA Press, 2013.

Blanch, Hedelberto Lopez. "Cuba: The Little Giant Against Apartheid." In *The Road to Democracy in South Africa*, vol. 3. Pretoria: UNISA Press, 2008.

Bloom, Joshua, and Waldo E. Martin. *Black against Empire: The History and Politics of the Black Panther Party.* Oakland: University of California Press, 2013.

Bonner, Philip. *Kings, Commoners and Concessionaires: The Evolution of and Dissolution of the Nineteenth Century Swazi State.* Cambridge: Cambridge University Press, 1983.

Bonner, P., J. Sithole, B. Magubane, T. April, P. Delius, P. Gibbs, and J. Cherry. "The Turn to Armed Struggle." *The Road to Democracy in South Africa (1960–1970)*, vol. 1. Pretoria: UNISA Press, 2015.

Booth, Douglas. "Hitting Apartheid for Six? The Politics of the South African Sports Boycott." *Journal of Contemporary History* 38, no. 3 (2003): 477–93.

Bopela, Thula, and Daluxolo Luthuli. *Umkhonto We Sizwe: Fighting for a Divided People.* Johannesburg: Galago Publishing Co., 2005.

Bosgra, Sietse. "From Jan van Riebeeck to Solidarity with the Struggle: The Netherlands, South Africa and Apartheid." *The Road to Democracy in South Africa*, vol. 3. Pretoria: UNISA Press, 2006.

Bottoman, Wonga Welile. *The Making of an MK Cadre.* Pretoria; LiNc Publishers, 2010.

Bozzoli, Belinda, with Mmantho Nkotsoe. *Women of Phokeng: Consciousness, Life Strategy, and Migrancy in South Africa, 1900–1983.* Portsmouth, NH: Heinemann and London: James Currey Publishers, 1991.

Brown, Barbara B. "Facing the 'Black Peril': The Politics of Population Control in South Africa." *Journal of Southern African Studies* 13, no. 2 (1987): 256–73.

Bruce-Chwatt, L. J. "Chemoprophylaxis of Malaria in Africa: The Spent 'Magic Bullet.'" *British Medical Journal (Clinical Research Ed.)* 285, no. 6343 (11 September 1982): 674–6.

Bundy, Colin. "Cooking the Rice Outside the Pot? The ANC and SACP in exile–1960 to 1990." *Treading the Waters of History: Perspectives on the ANC.* Pretoria: Africa Institute of South Africa, 2014.

—. "National Liberation and International Solidarity: Anatomy of a Special Relationship." In *Southern African Liberation Struggles: New local, regional and global perspectives,* edited by Hilary Sapire and Chris Saunders, 212–28. Cape Town: University of Cape Town Press, 2013.

Burke, A.W. "Mental Health and Apartheid World Psychiatric Association Conference Report." *International Journal of Social Psychiatry* 31, no. 2 (1 June 1985): 144–8.

Burns, Catherine E. "Reproductive Labors: the Politics of Women's Health in South Africa, 1900–1960." PhD diss., Northwestern University, Illinois, 1995.

Butchart, Alexander. "The 'Bantu Clinic': A Genealogy of the African Patient as Object and Effect of South African Clinical Medicine, 1930–1990." *Culture, Medicine and Psychiatry* 21, no. 4 (1997): 405–47.

Butler, Larry, and Sarah Stockwell, eds. *The Wind of Change: Harold Macmillan and British Decolonization.* Basingstoke: Palgrave Macmillan, 2013.

Callinicos, Luli. "Oliver Tambo and the Dilemma of the Camp Mutinies in Angola in the Eighties." *South African Historical Journal* 64, no. 3 (2012): 587–621.

Cherry, Janet. *Spear of the Nation: Umkhonto weSizwe: South Africa's Liberation Army, 1960s–1990s.* Athens, OH: Ohio University Press, 2012.

Crane, Barbara B. "The Transnational Politics of Abortion." *Population and Development Review* 20 (1994): 241–62.

Cooper, Frederick. "Possibility and Constraint: African Independence in Historical Perspective." *The Journal of African History* 49, no. 2 (2008): 167–96.

Coovadia, Hoosen, Rachel Jewkes, Peter Barron, David Sanders, and Diane McIntyre. "The Health and Health System of South Africa:

Historical Roots of Current Public Health Challenges." *The Lancet* 374, no. 9692 (2009): 817–34.

Davis, Stephen. "The African National Congress, Its Radio, Its Allies and Exile." *Journal of Southern African Studies* 35, no. 2 (2009): 349–73.

—. *Cosmopolitans in Close Quarters: Everyday Life in the Ranks of Umkhonto We Sizwe (1961–present).* PhD diss., University of Florida, 2010.

—. "Training and Deployment at Novo Catengue and the Diaries of Jack Simons, 1977–1979." *Journal of Southern African Studies* 40, no. 6 (2014): 1325–42.

De Beer, Cedric. *The South African Disease: Apartheid Health and Health Services.* London: Africa World Press, 1986.

Delius, Peter. *The Land Belongs to Us: The Pedi Polity, the Boers, and the British in the Nineteenth-Century Transvaal.* Berkeley and Los Angeles: University of California Press, 1984.

Dlamini, Jacob. *Native Nostalgia.* Johannesburg: Jacana Media, 2009.

Dommisse, John. "The Psychological Effects of Apartheid Psychoanalysis Social, Moral and Political Influences." *International Journal of Social Psychiatry* 32, no. 2 (1 June 1986): 51–63.

—. "The State of Psychiatry in South Africa Today." *Social Science & Medicine (1982)* 24, no. 9 (1987): 749–61.

—. "World Medical Association and South Africa." *The Lancet* 334, no. 8674 (1989): 1280.

Dousemetzis, Harris. *The Man Who Killed Apartheid.* Johannesburg: Jacana Media, 2018.

Dufour, Pascale, Dominique Masson, and Dominique Caouette. *Solidarities Beyond Borders: Transnationalizing Women's Movements.* Vancouver: UBC Press, 2010.

Early, Bryan R. "'Larger than a Party, yet Smaller than a State': Locating Hezbollah's Place within Lebanon's State and Society." *World Affairs* 168, no. 3 (2006): 115–28.

Eklind, Christian, and Christopher Angenfelt. "From Bullets to Ballots – A Comparative Case Study of the Political Transition of ANC and Hamas." PhD diss., Lunds Universitet, 2015.

Ellis, Stephen. *External Mission: The ANC in Exile, 1960–1990.* London: Oxford University Press, 2013.

—. "The Genesis of the ANC's Armed Struggle in South Africa 1948–1961." *Journal of Southern African Studies* 37, no. 4 (2011): 657–76.

—. "Mbokodo: Security in ANC Camps, 1961–1990." *African Affairs* (1994): 279–98.

—. "Politics and Crime: Reviewing the ANC's Exile History." *South African Historical Journal* 64, no. 3 (2012): 622–36.

Ellis, Stephen, and Tsepho Sechaba. *Comrades against Apartheid: The ANC & the South African Communist Party in Exile*. Bloomington and Indianapolis: Indiana University Press, 1992.

Eriksen, Tore Linné. *Norway and National Liberation in Southern Africa*. Stockholm, Sweden: Nordic Africa Institute, 2000.

Everatt, David. "Alliance Politics of a Special Type: The Roots of the ANC/SACP Alliance, 1950–1954." *Journal of Southern African Studies* 18, no. 1 (1992): 19–39.

Fanon, Frantz. *Black Skin, White Masks*. New York: Grove Press, 2008.

Fieldhouse, Roger. *Anti-Apartheid: A History of the Movement in Britain: A Study in Pressure Group Politics*. London: Merlin Press, 2005.

Flint, Karen, and Julie Parle. "Healing and Harming: Medicine, Madness, Witchcraft and Tradition." In *Zulu Identities. Being Zulu, Past and Present*, edited by Benedict Carton, John Laband, and Jabulani Sithole, 312–21. Scottville: University of KwaZulu-Natal Press, 2008.

Foucault, Michel. *Madness and Civilization*. New York: Pantheon, 1965.

Gilder, Barry. *Songs and Secrets*. Johannesburg: Jacana Media, 2012.

Gleijeses, Piero. "Moscow's Proxy? Cuba and Africa 1975–1988." *Journal of Cold War Studies* 8, no. 2 (2006): 3–51.

"Google Maps." *Google Maps*. Accessed 22 March 2015. https://www.google.ca/maps/place/Morogoro,+Tanzania/@-6.8223375,37.6606178,3z/data=!4m2!3m1!1s0x185a5dc00cee7437:0xf0e8f2f705ae1dd1.

—. *Google Maps*. Accessed 3 March 2016. https://www.google.com/maps/d/edit?hl=en&mid=1-zmrhDp3cQQkoxy9t8_XpUokPec&ll=-15.710297566119701%2C22.05001859238223&z=6

—. *Google Maps*. Accessed 10 December 2016. https://www.google.com/maps/d/edit?hl=en&mid=1-zmrhDp3cQQkoxy9t8_XpUokPec&ll=-9.993670538972271%2C14.249504474426203&z=7

Gurney, Christabel. "The 1970s: Anti-Apartheid Movement's Difficult Decade." In *Southern African Liberation Struggles: New Local, Regional and Global Perspectives*, edited by Hilary Sapire and Chris Saunders, 229–50. Cape Town: University of Cape Town Press, 2013.

Hammett, Daniel. "Cuban Intervention in South African Health Care Service Provision." *Journal of Southern African Studies* 33, 1 (2007): 63–81.

Hassim, Shireen. *The ANC Women's League*. Athens, OH: Ohio University Press, 2015.

—. *Women's Organizations and Democracy in South Africa: Contesting Authority*. Madison: University of Wisconsin Press, 2006.

Hoad, Neville. "Thabo Mbeki's AIDS Blues: The Intellectual, the Archive, and the Pandemic." *Public Culture* 17, no. 1 (2005): 101–28.

Hodes, Rebecca. "HIV/AIDS in South African Documentary Film, c. 1990–2000." *Journal of Southern African Studies* 33, 1 (2007): 153–71.

—. "The Medical History of Abortion in South Africa, c. 1970–2000." *Journal of Southern African Studies* 39, 3 (2013): 527–42.

Houston, Gregory. "The Post-Rivonia ANC/SACP Underground." In *The Road to Democracy in South Africa: 1960–1970*, vol. 1. Pretoria: UNISA Press, 2004.

Houston, Gregory and Bernard Magubane. "The ANC Political Underground in the 1970s." In *The Road to Democracy in South Africa: 1970–1980*, vol. 2. Pretoria: UNISA Press, 2004.

—. "The ANC's Armed Struggle in the 1970s." *The Road to Democracy in South Africa: 1970–1980*, vol. 2. Pretoria: UNISA Press, 2004.

Houston, Gregory, Thami ka Plaatjie, and Thozama April. "Military Training and Camps of the Pan Africanist Congress of South Africa, 1961–1981." *Historia* 60, no. 2 (November 2015).

Information, Reed Business. *New Scientist*. Reed Business Information, 1977.

Jackson, Lynette A. "The Place of Psychiatry in Colonial and Early Postcolonial Zimbabwe." *International Journal of Mental Health* 28, no. 2 (1999): 38–71.

Jewkes, Rachel. *The Case for South Africa's Expulsion from International Psychiatry*. United Nations, 1984.

Jochelson, Karen. *The Colour of Disease: Syphilis and Racism in South Africa, 1880–1950*. Houndsmills, Basingstoke, Hampshire: Palgrave Macmillan, 2001.

Johnson, Erica. "Non-State Health Care Provision in Kazakhstan and

Uzbekistan: Is Politicisation a Model?" *Europe-Asia Studies* 66, no. 5 (28 May 2014): 735–58.

Jones, Charles Earl. *The Black Panther Party (Reconsidered)*. Baltimore: Black Classic Press, 1998.

Jones, Tiffany F. "Averting White Male (Ab)Normality: Psychiatric Representations and Treatment of 'Homosexuality' in 1960s South Africa." *Journal of Southern African Studies* 34, no. 2 (2008): 397–410.

—. *Dis-Ordered States: Views about Mental Disorder and the Management of the Mad in South Africa, 1939–1989*. PhD diss., Queen's University, 2004.

—. "Prospects of a Progressive Mental Health System in 1940's South Africa: Hereditarianism, Behaviourism and Radical Therapies." Paper given at the Workshop on South Africa in the 1940's: South African Research Centre. Queen's University, 2003.

—. *Psychiatry, Mental Institutions, and the Mad in Apartheid South Africa*. Routledge, 2012.

Joubert, Annekie. "History by Word of Mouth." In *Historical Memory in Africa: Dealing with the Past, Reaching for the Future in an Intercultural Context*, edited by Mamadou Diawara, Bernard Lategan, and Jörn Rüsen, 27–52. New York: Berghahn Books, 2010.

Ka Plaatjie, Thami. "The PAC's Internal Underground Activities.'" *The Road to Democracy in South Africa, 1970–1980*, vol. 2. Pretoria: UNISA Press, 2004.

—. "The PAC in exile." *The Road to Democracy in South Africa, 1970–1980*, vol. 2. Pretoria: UNISA Press, 2004.

Karis, Thomas, Gwendolen Margaret Carter, and Gail M. Gerhart. *From Protest to Challenge: Challenge and Violence, 1953–1964*. Stanford: Hoover Institution Press, 1972.

—. *From Protest to Challenge: Nadir and resurgence, 1964–1979*, vol. 5. Standford: Hoover Institution Press, 1972.

Keller, Richard. *Colonial Madness: Psychiatry in French North Africa*. Chicago: University of Chicago Press, 2007.

—. "Madness and Colonization: psychiatry in the British and French Empires, 1800–1962." *Journal of Social History* 35 (2001): 295–326.

Klausen, Susanne. *Abortion Under Apartheid: Nationalism, Sexuality, and Women's Reproductive Rights in South Africa*. Oxford and New York: Oxford University Press, 2015.

Laurenson, Helen, and Sally Swartz. "The Professionalization of Psychology within the Apartheid State 1948–1978." *History of Psychology* 14, no. 3 (2011): 249.

Lissoni, Arianna. "Transformations in the ANC External Mission and Umkhonto We Sizwe, C. 1960–1969." *Journal of Southern African Studies* 35, no. 2 (2009): 287–301.

Lissoni, Arianna, and Maria Suriano. "Married to the ANC: Tanzanian Women's Entanglement in South Africa's Liberation Struggle." *Journal of Southern African Studies* 40, no. 1 (2014): 129–50.

Lodge, Tom. *The ANC After Nkomati*. Johannesburg: South African Institute of Race Relations, 1985.

—. "State of Exile: The African National Congress of South Africa, 1976–86." *Third World Quarterly* 9, no. 1 (1987): 1–27.

Lonsdale, John. *South Africa in Question*. Portsmouth, NH: Heinemann, 1988.

Louw, Johann, and Sally Swartz. "An English Asylum in Africa: Space and Order in Valkenberg Asylum." *History of Psychology* 4, no. 1 (2001): 3.

Love, Janice. *The US Anti-Apartheid Movement: Local Activism in Global Politics*. Westport, CT: Praeger Pub Text, 1985.

Macmillan, Hugh. "After Morogoro: The Continuing Crisis in the African National Congress (of South Africa) in Zambia, 1969–1971." *Social Dynamics* 35, no. 2 (2009): 295–311.

—. "The 'Hani Memorandum'–introduced and Annotated." *Transformation: Critical Perspectives on Southern Africa* 69, no. 1 (2009): 106–29.

—. *The Lusaka Years: The ANC in Exile in Zambia, 1963 to 1994*. Johannesburg: Jacana Media, 2013.

—. "Morogoro and After: The Continuing Crisis in the African National Congress (of South Africa) in Zambia." In *Southern African Liberation Struggles: New local, regional and global perspectives*, edited by Hilary Sapire and Chris Saunders, 76–95. Cape Town: University of Cape Town Press, 2013.

Magubane, Bernard. "From Détente to the Rise of the Garrison State." *The Road to Democracy in South Africa, 1970–1980*, vol. 2. Pretoria: UNISA Press, 2006.

—. "Introduction to the 1970s: The Social and Political Context." *The Road to Democracy in South Africa, 1970–1980*, vol. 2. Pretoria: UNISA Press, 2006.

Magubane, Bernard, Philip Bonner, Jabulani Sithole, Peter Delius, Janet Cherry, Pat Gibbs, and Thozama April. "The Turn to Armed Struggle." *The Road to Democracy in South Africa, 1960–1970*, vol. 1. Pretoria: UNISA Press, 2004.

Mahone, Sloan. "The Psychology of Rebellion: Colonial Medical Responses to Dissent in British East Africa." *The Journal of African History* 47, no. 2 (2006): 241–58.

Mann, Gregory, and Baz Lecocq. "Between Empire, Umma, and the Muslim Third World: The French Union and African Pilgrims to Mecca, 1946–1958." *Comparative Studies of South Asia, Africa and the Middle East* 27, no. 2 (2007): 367–83.

Manyame-Tazarurwa, Kalister Christine. *Health Impact of Participation in the Liberation Struggle of Zimbabwe by Zanla Women Ex-Combatants in the Zanla Operational Areas.* Bloomington, IN: Author House, 2011.

Marks, Shula. "The Silent Scourge? Silicosis, Respiratory Disease and Gold-Mining in South Africa." *Journal of Ethnic and Migration Studies* 32, no. 04 (2006): 569–89.

Marks, Shula, and Neil Andersson. "Diseases of Apartheid." In *South Africa in Question*, edited by John Lonsdale, 172–99. London: Cambridge African Studies Centre with James Currey, 1985.

—. "Typhus and Social Control: South Africa, 1917–1950." In *Disease, Medicine and Empire: Perspectives on Western Medicine and the Experience of European Expansion*, edited by Roy Macleod and Milton Lewis, 257–83. London and New York: Routledge, 1988.

Mbali, Mandisa. "A Long Illness: Towards a History of NGO, Government and Medical Discourse around AIDS Policy-making in South Africa." Honours degree thesis, Durban, University of Kwa-Zulu/Natal, 2001.

—. "Mbeki's Denialism and the Ghosts of Apartheid and Colonialism for Post-Apartheid AIDS Policy-making." *Public Health Journal Club Seminar.* University of Natal–Durban, 2002.

McCulloch, Jock. *Asbestos: Its Human Cost.* St Lucia: University Queensland Press, 1986.

—. "Asbestos Mining in Southern Africa, 1893–2002." *International Journal of Occupational and Environmental Health* 9, no. 3 (2003): 230–5.

—. *Colonial Psychiatry and "the African Mind."* Cambridge. New York: Cambridge University Press, 1995.

—. "Women Mining Asbestos in South Africa, 1893–1980." *Journal of Southern African Studies* 29, no. 2 (1 June 2003): 413–32.

Mji, Diliza. "The World Medical Association in South Africa." *International Journal of Health Services* 15, no. 2 (April 1985): 351–3.

Monamodi, Isaac Seboko. *Medical Doctors under Segregation and Apartheid: A Sociological Analysis of Professionalization among Doctors in South Africa, 1900–1980*. PhD diss., Indiana University, 1996.

Morgenstierne, Christopher Munthe. *Denmark and National Liberation in Southern Africa: A Flexible Response*. Stockholm: Nordic Africa Institute, 2003.

Morrow, Sean. "Dakawa Development Centre: An African National Congress Settlement in Tanzania, 1982–1992." *African Affairs* 97, no. 389 (1998): 497–521.

Morrow, Sean, Brown Maaba, and Loyiso Pulumani. *Education in Exile: SOMAFCO, the African National Congress School in Tanzania, 1978 to 1992*. Cape Town: HSRC Press, 2004.

—. "Revolutionary Schooling? Studying the Solomon Mahlangu Freedom College, the African National Congress Liberation School in Tanzania, 1978 to 1992." *World Studies in Education* 3, no. 1 (2002): 23–37.

Murray, Bruce K. "Politics and Cricket: The D'Oliveira Affair of 1968." *Journal of Southern African Studies* 27, no. 4 (December 1, 2001): 667–84.

—. "The Sports Boycott and Cricket: The Cancellation of the 1970 South African Tour of England." *South African Historical Journal* 46, no. 1 (May 1, 2002): 219–49.

Mutiny in the ANC, 1984: As Told by Five of the Mutineers. London: Justice for Southern Africa/Solidarity with Ex-SWAPO Detainees, 1996.

Naidoo, Ricky. *The Fourth Dimension: The Untold Story of Military Health in South Africa*. Pretoria: South African Military Health Service, 2009.

Ndebele, Nhlanhla, and Noor Nieftagodien. "The Morogoro Conference: A Moment of Self-Reflection." *The Road to Democracy in South Africa, 1960-1970*, vol. 1. Pretoria: UNISA Press, 2004.

Ndlovu, Sifiso. "The ANC in Exile, 1960–1970." *The Road to Democracy in South Africa, 1960-1970*, vol. 1. Pretoria: UNISA Press, 2004.

—. "The ANC's Diplomacy and International Relations." *The Road to Democracy in South Africa, 1970–1980*, vol. 2. Pretoria: UNISA Press, 2006.

Nelson, Alondra. *Body and Soul: The Black Panther Party and the Fight against Medical Discrimination*. Minneapolis: University of Minnesota Press, 2011.

Nesbitt, Francis Njubi. *Race for Sanctions: African Americans against Apartheid, 1946–1994*. Bloomington and Indianapolis: Indiana University Press, 2004.

Nightingale, Elena O., Kari Hannibal, H. Jack Geiger, Lawrence Hartmann, Robert Lawrence, and Jeanne Spurlock. "Apartheid Medicine: Health and Human Rights in South Africa." *JAMA* 264, no. 16 (1990): 2097–102.

Nixon, Rob. "Apartheid on the Run: The South African Sports Boycott." *Transition*, no. 58 (1992): 68–88.

Nuwaha, Fred. "The Challenge of Chloroquine-Resistant Malaria in Sub-Saharan Africa." *Health Policy and Planning* 16, no. 1 (2001): 1–12.

Onslow, Sue. *Cold War in Southern Africa: White Power, Black Liberation*. Routledge, 2009.

Organisation of African Unity. "Lagos plan of action for the economic development of Africa, 1980–2000." OAU, 1980.

Packard, Randall M. "Industrialization, Rural Poverty, and Tuberculosis in South Africa, 1850–1950." *The Social Basis of Health and Healing in Africa*, no. 30 (1992): 104.

—. "The Invention of the 'Tropical Worker': Medical Research and the Quest for Central African Labor on the South African Gold Mines, 1903–36." *The Journal of African History* 34, no. 2 (1993): 271–92.

—. *The Making of a Tropical Disease—A Short History of Malaria*. Baltimore: Johns Hopkins University Press, 2007.

—. "Post-colonial Medicine." *Companion to medicine in the twentieth century* (2003): 97–112.

—. "Tuberculosis and the Development of Industrial Health Policies on the Witwatersrand, 1902–1932." *Journal of Southern African Studies* 13, no. 2 (1987): 187–209.

—. *White Plague, Black Labor: Tuberculosis and the Political Economy of Health and Disease in South Africa*, vol. 23. Berkeley and Los Angeles: University of California Press, 1989.

Panzer, Michael G. "Building a Revolutionary Constituency: Mozambican Refugees and the Development of the FRELIMO Proto-State, 1964–1968." *Social Dynamics* 39, no. 1 (1 March 2013): 5–23.

—. "Pragmatism and Liberation: FRELIMO and the Legitimacy of an African Independence Movement." *Portuguese Journal of Social Science* 14, no. 3 (2015): 323–42.

Parle, Julie. "Family Commitments, Economies of Emotions, and Negotiating Mental Illness in Late-Nineteenth to Mid-Twentieth-Century Natal, South Africa." *South African Historical Journal* (13 February 2014): 1–21.

—. *States of Mind: Searching for Mental Health in Natal and Zululand, 1868–1918*. Pietermaritzburg: University of Kwazulu Natal Press, 2007.

—. "Witchcraft or Madness? The Amandiki of Zululand, 1894–1914." *Journal of Southern African Studies* 29, no. 1 (2003): 105–32.

Peires, J.B. *The House of Phalo: A History of the Xhosa People in the Days of their Independence*. Johannesburg: Raven Press, 1981.

Potgieter, Eugéne. *Professional Nursing Education: 1860–1991*. Acad., 1992.

Robinson, Glenn E. "Hamas as Social Movement." In *Islamic Activism: A Social Movement Theory Approach*, edited by Quintan Wiktorowicz, 112–42. Bloomington: Indiana University Press, 2004.

Rubenstein, Leonard, and Leslie London. "The UDHR and the Limits of Medical Ethics: The Case of South Africa." *Health and Human Rights* (1998): 160–75.

Saebo, Marin. "A State of Exile: The ANC and Umkhonto we Sizwe in Angola, 1976–1989." Master's thesis, University of Natal, 2002.

Sandwell, Rachel. "'Love I Cannot Begin to Explain': The Politics of Reproduction in the ANC in Exile, 1976–1990." *Journal of Southern African Studies* 41, no. 1 (2015): 63–81.

Sapire, Hilary, and Chris Saunders. *Southern African Liberation Struggles: New Local, Regional and Global Perspectives*. Cape Town: University of Cape Town Press, 2012.

Sashidharan, S.P. "Psychiatrists and Detainees in South Africa." *The Lancet* 321, no. 8316 (1983): 128.

Saul, John. "Two Fronts of Anti-Apartheid Struggle: South Africa and Canada." *Transformation: Critical Perspectives on Southern Africa* 74, no. 1 (2010): 135–51.

Saunders, Chris. "Liberation Struggles in Southern Africa: New Perspectives." *South African Historical Journal* 62, no. 1 (2010).

Schmidt, Elizabeth. "Cold War in Guinea: The Rassemblement Démocratique Africain and the Struggle over Communism, 1950–1958." *Journal of African History* (2007): 95–121.

—. *Foreign Intervention in Africa: From the Cold War to the War on Terror*. Vol. 7. Cambridge: Cambridge University Press, 2013.

Searle, Charlotte. *Towards Excellence: The Centenary of State Registration for Nurses and Midwives in South Africa, 1891–1991*. Durban: Butterworths, 1991.

Seedat, Aziza. *Crippling a Nation: Health in Apartheid South Africa*. IDAF, 1984.

Sellström, Tor. *Liberation in Southern Africa: Regional and Swedish Voices: Interviews from Angola, Mozambique, Namibia, South Africa, Zimbabwe, the Frontline and Sweden*. Stockholm: Nordic Africa Institute, 2002.

—. "Some Factors behind Nordic Relations with Southern Africa." In *Regional Cooperation in Southern Africa: A Post-Apartheid Perspective*, edited by Bertil Oden and Haroub Othman, 13–46. The Scandinavian Institute of African Studies: Uppsala, 1989.

—. *Sweden and National Liberation in Southern Africa*. Vol. I, *Formation of a Popular Opinion (1950–1970)*. Stockholm: Nordiska Afrikainstitutet, 1999.

—. *Sweden and National Liberation in Southern Africa*. Vol. II, *Solidarity and Assistance, 1970–1994*. Stockholm: Nordic Africa Institute, 2002.

—. "Sweden and the Nordic Countries: Official Solidarity and Assistance from the West." In *The Road to Democracy in South Africa*, vol. 3. Pretoria: UNISA Press, 2006.

Shell, Robert, and Patricia Smonds Qaga. "Trojan Horses: HIV/AIDS and Military Bases in Southern Africa." In *Demographic Association of Southern Africa, Annual Workshop and Conference* (2002): 24–7.

Shubin, Vladimir Gennad'evich. *ANC: A View from Moscow*. Bellville: Mayibuye Books, 1999.

—. *The Hot "Cold War": The USSR in Southern Africa*. London: Pluto Press, 2008.

Shubin, Vladimir, and Marina Traikova. "There Is No Threat from the Eastern Bloc." *The Road to Democracy in South Africa*, vol. 3. Pretoria: UNISA Press, 2008.

Simpson, Thula, ed. *The ANC and the Liberation Struggle in South Africa: Essential Writings*. London: Routledge, 2018.

Simpson, Thula. "The ANC Underground in Swaziland, c. 1975–1982." In *Southern African Liberation Struggles: New local, regional and global perspectives*, edited by Hilary Sapire and Chris Saunders, 96–116. Cape Town: University of Cape Town Press, 2013.

—. *Umkhonto We Sizwe: The ANC's Armed Struggle*. Cape Town: Penguin Books, 2016.

Skinner, Rob. *The Foundations of Anti-Apartheid: Liberal Humanitarians and Transnational Activists in Britain and the United States, C. 1919–64*. Basingstoke: Palgrave Macmillan, 2010.

—. "The Moral Foundations of British Anti-Apartheid Activism, 1946–1960." *Journal of Southern African Studies* 35, no. 2 (2009): 399–416.

Soiri, Iina, and Pekka Peltola. *Finland and National Liberation in Southern Africa*. Stockholm: Nordic Africa Institute, 1999.

South African Democracy Education Trust. *The Road to Democracy – South Africans Telling Their Stories*. Johannesburg: Tsehai Publishers, 2008.

—. *The Road to Democracy in South Africa: 1970–1980*, vol. 2. Pretoria: UNISA Press, 2004.

South African History Online. "Dr Mantombazana 'Manto' Tshabalala-Msimang." Text, 4 June 2012. http://www.sahistory.org.za/people/dr-mantombazana-manto-tshabalala-msimang.

—. "Dr Nomava Eslinah Shangase." Text, 1 March 2012. http://www.sahistory.org.za/people/dr-nomava-eslinah-shangase.

Stapleton, Timothy J., and M. Maamoe. "An Overview of the African National Congress Archives at the University of Fort Hare." *History in Africa* 25 (1998): 413–22.

Stoler, Ann Laura. *Along the Archival Grain: Epistemic Anxieties and Colonial Common Sense*. Princeton NJ: Princeton University Press, 2010.

Stokke, Kristian. "Building the Tamil Eelam State: Emerging State Institutions and Forms of Governance in LTTE-Controlled Areas in Sri Lanka." *Third World Quarterly* 27, no. 6 (2006): 1021–40.

Susser, Mervyn, and Violet Padayachi Cherry. "Health and Health Care under Apartheid." *Journal of Public Health Policy* 3, no. 4 (1982): 455–75.

Suttner, Raymond. "The (Re-)Constitution of the South African Communist Party as an Underground Organisation." *Journal of Contemporary African Studies* 22, no. 1 (2004): 43–68.

Swanson, Maynard W. "The Sanitation Syndrome: Bubonic Plague and Urban Native Policy in the Cape Colony, 1900–1909." *Journal of African History* (1977): 387–410.

Swartz, Sally. "The Black Insane in the Cape, 1891–1920." *Journal of Southern African Studies* 21, no. 3 (1995): 399–415.

—. "Colonial Lunatic Asylum Archives: Challenges to Historiography." *Kronos* 34, no. 1 (2008): 285–302.

—. "IV. Lost Lives: Gender, History and Mental Illness in the Cape, 1891–1910." *Feminism & Psychology* 9, no. 2 (1999): 152–8.

—. "Shrinking: A Postmodern Perspective on Psychiatric Case Histories." *South African Journal of Psychology* 26, no. 3 (1996): 150–6.

Tarimo, E., and N. Reuben. "Tanzania's Solidarity with South Africa's Liberation." *The Road to Democracy in South Africa, African Solidarity,* vol. 5. Pretoria: UNISA Press, 2013.

Terretta, Meredith. "Cameroonian Nationalists Go Global: From Forest *Maquis* to a Pan-African Accra." *The Journal of African History* 51, no. 2 (2010): 189–212.

Thörn, Håkan. *Anti-Apartheid and the Emergence of a Global Civil Society.* Basingstoke: Palgrave Macmillan, 2006.

Tobias, Phillip V. "Apartheid and Medical Education: The Training of Black Doctors in South Africa." *Journal of the National Medical Association* 72, no. 4 (1980): 395.

Trewhela, Paul. "'A Namibian Horror: SWAPO's Prisons in Angola.'" *Searchlight South Africa* 4 (1990).

—. "The ANC Prison Camps: An Audit of Three Years, 1990–1993." *Searchlight South Africa* 3, no. 2 (1993): 8–30.

—. "The Death of Albert Nzula and the Silence of George Padmore." *Searchlight South Africa* 1, no. 1 (1988): 27.

—. *Inside Quatro: Uncovering the Exile History of the ANC and SWAPO.* Johannesburg: Jacana Media, 2009.

Truth and Reconciliation Commission. *Truth and Reconciliation Report,*

Volume 2, Chapter 4, "The Liberation Movements from 1960 to 1990." Accessed 14 November 2016. http://www.justice.gov.za/Trc/report/finalreport/Volume%202.pdf.

Tsampiras, Carla. "Politics, Polemics, and Practice: A History of Narratives about, and Responses To, AIDS in South Africa, 1980–1995." PhD diss., Rhodes University, Grahamstown, South Africa, 2012.

—. "Sex in a Time of Exile: An Examination of Sexual Health, AIDS, Gender, and the ANC, 1980–1990." *South African Historical Journal* 64, no. 3 (2012): 637–63.

UNHCR. "Report of the United Nations High Commissioner for Refugees (Covering the Period 1 April 1979 to 31 March 1980)." New York, 24 September 1980.

United Nations. "Yearbook of the United Nations 1981: Part 1 Section 2 Chapter 21 – Refugees." n.d.

—. "3201 (S-VI). Declaration on the Establishment of a New International Economic Order." 1 May 1974.

United Nations Centre against Apartheid, Mahler Halfdan, World Health Organization. "Health Implications of Apartheid in South Africa." Department of Political and Security Council Affairs, 1975. Accessed 20 February 2017. http://psimg.jstor.org/fsi/img/pdf/to/10.5555/al.sff.document.nuun1975_05_final.pdf.

Vansina, Jan. "Knowledge and Perceptions of the African Past." In *African Historiographies: What History for Which Africa*, edited by Bogumil Jewsiewicki and David Newbury, 28–41. Beverly Hills, CA: Sage, 1986.

—. *Oral Tradition: A Study in Historical Methodology.* New Brunswick, NJ: Transaction Publishers, 2006.

—. *Oral Tradition as History.* Madison: University of Wisconsin Press, 1985.

van der Heyde, Henri C., John Nolan, Valéry Combes, Irene Gramaglia, and Georges E. Grau. "A Unified Hypothesis for the Genesis of Cerebral Malaria: Sequestration, Inflammation and Hemostasis Leading to Microcirculatory Dysfunction." *Trends in Parasitology* 22, no. 11 (November, 2006): 503–8.

Vaughan, Megan. *Curing Their Ills: Colonial Power and African Illness.* Standford: Stanford University Press, 1991.

—. "Idioms of Madness: Zomba Lunatic Asylum, Nyasaland, in the colonial period." *Journal of Southern African Studies*, 9 (1983): 218–38.

Wernsdorfer, Walter, and David Payne. "The Dynamics of Drug Resistance in Plasmodium Falciparum." *Pharmacology & Therapeutics* 50, no. 1 (1991): 95–121.

Williams, Christian. "Exile History: An Ethnography of the SWAPO Camps and the Namibian Nation." PhD diss., University of Michigan, 2009.

—. "Living in Exile: Daily Life and International Relations at SWAPO's Kongwa Camp." *Kronos* 37, no. 1 (January 2011): 60–86.

—. "Practicing Pan-Africanism: International Relations at Kongwa Camp in 1960s Tanzania." Paper presented at 2013 Southern African Historical Society conference: *All for One, One for All? Leveraging National Interests with Regional Visions in Southern Africa*. Gaborone, Botswana.

Williams, Elizabeth. "Anti-Apartheid: The Black British Response." *South African Historical Journal* 64, no. 3 (2012): 685–706.

—. "Black British Solidarity With the Anti-apartheid Struggle: The West Indian Standing Conference and Black Action for the Liberation of Southern Africa." In *Southern African Liberation Struggles: New local, regional and global perspectives*, edited by Hilary Sapire and Chris Saunders, 251–73. Cape Town: University of Cape Town Press, 2013.

—. "'Until South Africa Is Free, We Shall Not Be Free!' Black British Solidarity with the Anti-Apartheid Struggle During the 1980s." PhD diss., Birkbeck: University of London, 2009.

Wellems, Thomas E., and Christopher V. Plowe. "Chloroquine-Resistant Malaria." *Journal of Infectious Diseases* 184, no. 6 (15 September 2001): 770–6.

White, Luise. *Speaking with Vampires: Rumor and History in Colonial Africa*. Berkeley and Los Angeles: University of California Press, 2000.

White, Luise, Stephan Miescher, and David William Cohen. *African Words, African Voices: Critical Practices in Oral History*. Bloomington: Indiana University Press, 2001.

Women's Global Network for Reproductive Rights. "History" (2014). Accessed 3 March 2017. http://wgnrr.org/who-we-are/history/.

World Bank, "Official Exchange Rate: (1979)." Accessed 2017. http://data.worldbank.org/indicator/PA.NUS.FCRF?end=1979&locations=TZ-DK-ZM-SE-GB-NL-MZ-US&name_desc=false&start=1979&view=bar.

—. "Official Exchange Rate: (1982)," Accessed 2017. http://data.worldbank.org/indicator/PA.NUS.FCRF?end=1982&locations=TZ-DK-ZM-SE-GB&name_desc=false&start=1982&view=bar.

—. "Official Exchange Rate: (1990)," Accessed 2017. http://data.worldbank.org/indicator/PA.NUS.FCRF?end=1991&locations=TZ-DK-ZM-SE-GB-NL&name_desc=false&start=1990&view=bar.

World Health Organization. *Health and Apartheid: Part 1. Report of an International Conference held at Brazzaville, People's Republic of the Congo, 16-20 November 1981; Part II. The Health Implications of Racial Discrimination and Social Inequality: An Analytical Report to the Conference. November, 1981.* Accessed 16 November 2016. http://apps.who.int/iris/bitstream/10665/37345/1/9241560797.pdf.

—. "Primary Health Care: Report of the International Conference on Primary Health Care." Alma-Ata, USSR, 1978/09/06-12. Accessed 19 February 2017. http://apps.who.int/iris/bitstream/10665/39228/1/9241800011.pdf.

—."WHO | Bridging the Gap in South Africa." Accessed 24 November 2016. http://www.who.int/bulletin/volumes/88/11/10-021110/en/.

—."WHO | Executive Summary." Accessed 8 January2017. http://www.who.int/whr/1998/media_centre/executive_summary6/en/.

Index

East Africa Regional Political Council (RPC), 129
education. *See* medical education
Education Department (ANC), 35, 141
Egypt, 5, 6, 25
Ellis, Stephen, 27, 190, 217n50
Emmasdale Clinic (Lusaka), 61–2, 181, 182, 229n61, 230n69
epilepsy, 264n9. *See also* mental health
Ethiopia, 25
exile, ANC in, 6–7, 25–7, 217n51. *See also* Department of Health
External Coordinating Committee (ANC), 221n106

family planning. *See* reproductive health
Family Planning Association (FPA), 113
Fanon, Frantz: *Black Skin, White Masks*, 188
Fansidar (antimalarial drug), 80, 81
Finnida, 65
Fiphaza, Ntabenkosi, 23
First, Ruth, 20
first aid courses, 25, 39–40, 133
First Moscow Medical State Institute, 18
Foucault, Michel: *Madness and Civilization*, 263n3
The Fourth Dimension (Naidoo), 213n2, 216n34, 235n113, 235n123, 250n7
Freedom Charter, 104
Frente de Libertação de

Moçambique (FRELIMO), 21–2, 28, 29–30, 97, 218n67
frontline states, 58, 87, 229n50

Gatsewe, Magdalene, 39
gender, 206
German Democratic Republic (GDR), 22, 26, 67
Ghana, 21
Goldberg, Denis, 6
Goldreich, Arthur, 6
government-in-waiting, 7, 109, 211n13. *See also* political legitimacy
Gqabi, A., 222n112
Guma, Lindelwa, 246n44

Hamas, 98
Hammett, Daniel, 204
Hani, Chris, 24–5, 203, 217n47
Hani Memorandum, 24, 217n47
Harare Psychiatric Unit (Zimbabwe), 166
Hashe, Zinto, 231n82
Hauli, J.G., 55, 59, 127, 169–70, 175, 266n41
Health and Apartheid conference (1981), 105–7, 168, 184–5, 246n37, 246n39
Health and Welfare Department (ANC), 25
Health Council (ANC), 42, 44, 89, 143, 221n111, 223n123
Health Department (ANC). *See* Department of Health
health secretariat: on abortions, 120; authority and interpersonal conflicts, 137, 141, 144, 149;

Solidarity Hospital; Mazimbu
(SOMAFCO) clinic
Mbali, Jackson, 23
Mbali, Mandisa, 205
Mbeki, Govan, 6
Mbeki, Thabo, 13, 213n2
Medical Association of South
Africa (MASA), 100–1, 108, 186
Medical Committee (ANC), 34–5,
202, 204. *See also* Department
of Health
medical education: in Angola, 68–
70; in Cuba, 204; opportunities
in exile, 17, 19; in Zambia, 57–8,
177, 228n47; in Zimbabwe, 64,
231n82
medical personnel: appeal for,
35; compensation, 41–2;
identification and recruitment,
17–20, 39–40, 44; infiltration
concerns with mental health
staff, 193–5, 266n41; Kongwa
camp, 23; Kurasini sickbay
issues, 127–9, 252n17, 252n26;
in Mazimbu, 51, 136, 145–6, 174,
257n76, 260n109
Medico International, 252n19
Medisch Komitee Angola (MKA),
51, 67, 132–6, 226n26, 250n1,
254n48
Mekgwe, Fish, 23
memoirs, exile, 212n17
mental health: about, 11, 155–8,
200–1, 206; addiction and,
174–6, 270n105; African Mental
Health Action Group, 64,
163, 165, 169, 185; in Angola,
177–8; apartheid and, 184–8;

colonialism and, 157–8; Dakawa
services, 62, 170, 172, 178–82;
depression and "combat
nostalgia," 168, 265n32; early
years, 159–60; epilepsy, 264n9;
Foucault on, 263n3; Health
and Apartheid conference, 168,
184–5; hereditary and parental
factors, 199–200; hypnosis
and acupuncture for, 173; from
idleness and boredom, 199;
infiltration concerns with new
staff, 193–5, 266n41; internal
security and, 156, 189–92, 197;
international interest in, 163;
Kurasini sickbay, 126–7, 169–70,
172, 174, 251n15; medical
education in, 177; perceived
ideal treatment, 176; perceived
reasons for mental illness,
183–5; plans for addressing,
170, 172; politicization of, 156,
185–7, 189; posttramautic stress
disorder (PTSD), 184; Reddy's
involvement, 168; referrals
to specialized hospitals, 167;
reports and surveys on, 167,
169–70; at SOMAFCO, 155, 168,
185; in South Africa, 160–3, *162*;
in students and youth, 187–8,
198–9; suicides, 159, 168, 190,
266n45; in Tanzania, 164–5, 169,
176–82; as tool to delegitimize,
192–3; traditional medicine
and, 173, 267n55; transitioning
patients back to South Africa,
182–3; treatment vs security
concerns, 195–7; WHO report

pregnancy, unplanned, 115–16, 198.
See also abortion; reproductive
health
primary healthcare delivery:
about, 11, 123–5, 153–4; conflicts,
effects on patients, 149–50;
definition of primary care,
46, 211n14; Kurasini sickbay
mismanagement, 126–32;
Mazimbu infrastructure
difficulties, 132–7; Mazimbu
staff and interpersonal
conflicts, 140–9; patient
MT's experience, 150–3,
262nn129–30; Tanzania, lack
of coordination, 125–6; WHO
"health for all" campaign, 101,
104–5, 122
"The Psychological Effects of
Apartheid" (1982 report), 169,
170, 176

Quenum, Comlan A.A., 86, 103–5,
168, 185, 245n32
quinine (antimalarial treatment),
76, 81, 238n147

Raadchelders, Lucia, 112
racism, institutional, 4, 114, 184, 188
Radebe, Mkhulu, 222n119
Radebe-Reed, Fiki, 33, 35, 109, 149
Randeree, Shaik Amhod Goolam, 35
Rantao, Simon (Tax Mosala), 23
Ratlabiane, Salele (Isaac Salele), 23,
228n44, 258n83
Raymond Mhlaba Rehabilitation
Centre (Dakawa), 178–82
Red Cross, 67, 163, 205

Reddy, Freddy: background
and exile, 19–20, 214n14;
first awareness of Health
Department, 35, 220n87;
interviews with Bernstein,
13; on mental health and
apartheid, 187–8; on mental
health and parental abuse, 200;
on mental health of youth, 194,
198–9; mental health work, 168,
173, 176, 178–80, 183, 195–7
"refugee mentality," concerns
about, 146, 224n10
Regional Committee for Africa
conference (WHO), 35
regional health teams (RHTs),
40–1. See also specific countries
reproductive health: about,
110–11, 120, 122; abortion
and unplanned pregnancy,
115–20, 198, 204, 249n74;
Depo-Provera, campaign
against, 111–12, 114, 247n59,
248n68; International Planned
Parenthood Federation (IPPF)
conference, 113; International
Tribunal and Meeting on
Reproductive Rights, 113–14,
248n64; policy development,
115
The Road to Democracy in South
Africa (publication), 13, 213n2,
243n2
Romania, 26, 67
Rwanda, 163

Saasa, Mmipe, 89
Saebo, Marin, 233n96

Soviet Union (USSR), 17–18, 22, 25–7
Soweto uprising (1976), 155
Special Programme of Technical Cooperation in Mental Health, 163
staff. *See* medical personnel
Stuart Commission, 177, 191, 198
students and youth: in ANC, 31, 219n71; mental health, 155, 168, 185, 187–8, 198–9
suicide, 159, 168, 190, 266n45
Swaziland, 32, 108, 163, 224n1, 246n37, 246n44
Sweden, 28–9, 30–1, 33, 68, 124, 218n62, 251n9
Swedish International Development Cooperation Agency (SIDA), 20, 29, 91, 163

Tambo, Oliver, 28, 31, 131, 160, 168
Tanzania: abortion, 115, 120; ANC, support for, 6, 11, 25, 51–2, 225n11; ANC asked to leave, 26–7, 217n50; bilateral relations, 46, 49–56, 93; civilian population in, 49; malaria, 78, 79–80, 85–90, 95, 225n20, 240n187, 241n191; maps, *xxi*, *48*; medical assistance from ANC nurses, 16–17, 214n4; mental health, 163–5, 169, 176–82; name, 211n11; "refugee mentality" concerns in, 146, 224n10; support for liberation movements, 21–2. *See also* Dakawa; Dar es Salaam; East Africa Regional Health Team;

Kongwa camp; Mazimbu
Technical Cooperation amongst the Developing Countries (TCDC), 7, 85
Thunyiswa, Kholeka, 17
Tikly, Mohammed, 115–16
traditional medicine, 102–3, 173, 267n55
Trewhela, Paul, 190; *Inside Quatro*, 190
Truth and Reconciliation Commission (TRC), 12, 156, 190–1
Tsampiras, Carla, 4, 205–6, 209n6
Tshabalala, Manto: on alcohol and drug abuse, 174–5; on ANC–Holland Solidarity Hospital construction, 134; in Angola, 68–9; anti-apartheid advocacy, 103–5, 245n32; background and exile, 17; at Committee of Experts on Primary Health Care in the Africa Region conference, 101; on communication issues, 41; on Dakawa healthcare, 52, 55; on Dommisse, 193; establishment of Health Department and, 33, 35, 37, 40; at Health and Apartheid conference, 105; health policy drafted by, 102; in health secretariat, 140, 222n119; interpersonal conflict, 37–8; at IPPF conference, 113; Kurasini sickbay and, 127, 129–31; liver failure, 205, 274n4; malaria and, 81–2, 84–6; Mazimbu health team, conflict with,

role, 140; patient MT and, 150–3; reproductive health policy development, 115; on women in army, 234n99

World Federation for Mental Health, 186, 271n118

World Health Organization (WHO): alcohol abuse and, 174; ANC observer status, 34, 101; anti-apartheid advocacy to, 103–5; apartheid investigation by, 99–100, 188; attempts to align with, 102–3; Biko murder and, 101; funding from, 6, 113, 127–8, 229n61; Health and Apartheid conference, 105–7, 168, 184–5, 246n37, 246n39; on healthcare in South Africa, 3; "health for all" campaign, 101, 104–5, 122; malaria and, 47, 76, 86; mental health, politicization of, and, 185–6; mental health model, 164–5; mental health partnerships in southern Africa, 156, 163–5, 168–70, 266n39; Regional Committee for Africa conference, 35; report on mental health in South Africa, 160–1, 163; on traditional medicine, 102–3

World Medical Association, 100–1, 187

World Psychiatric Association (WPA), 186–7

"Year of the Women" (1984), 111

Youth and Students' Section

(ANC), 24. *See also* students and youth

Yugoslavia, 26

Zambia: abortion, 115; ANC headquarters in, 6, 27, 56–7, 217n51; ANC population in, 57; bilateral relations, 46, 56–63, 93–4; health centres in, 58; housemanship training, 57–8, 228n47; map of medical points, *xxii*; mental health, 62, 163–5, 169–70, 181–2; transferring patients between Zimbabwe and, 63; two-tiered healthcare, 61; underutilization of ANC health facilities and overuse of Zambian facilities, 58–60, 229n51. *See also* Chainama Hills Psychiatric facility; Emmasdale Clinic; University Teaching Hospital

Zambia Regional Health Team (RHT), 40, 60, 92

Zimbabwe: ANC population, 231n81; bilateral relations, 46, 63–5, 94; as frontline state, 229n50; map of medical points, *xxii*; medical education in, 231n82; mental health, 163, 165–7, 177, 266n46; white settlers, 26

Zimbabwe African People's Union, 22

Zimbabwe Regional Health Team (RHT), 40

Zondy, Conny, 23

Zulu, Thami, 190